ENDING LIFE

ENDING LIFE

Ethics and the Way We Die

Margaret Pabst Battin

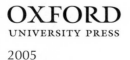

OXFORD
UNIVERSITY PRESS

2005

OXFORD
UNIVERSITY PRESS

Oxford University Press, Inc., publishes works that further
Oxford University's objective of excellence
in research, scholarship, and education.

Oxford   New York
Auckland   Cape Town   Dar es Salaam   Hong Kong   Karachi
Kuala Lumpur   Madrid   Melbourne   Mexico City   Nairobi
New Delhi   Shanghai   Taipei   Toronto

With offices in
Argentina   Austria   Brazil   Chile   Czech Republic   France   Greece
Guatemala   Hungary   Italy   Japan   Poland   Portugal   Singapore
South Korea   Switzerland   Thailand   Turkey   Ukraine   Vietnam

Copyright © 2005 by Margaret Pabst Battin

Published by Oxford University Press, Inc.
198 Madison Avenue, New York, New York 10016

www.oup.com

Oxford is a registered trademark of Oxford University Press

Library of Congress Cataloging-in-Publication Data
Battin, M. Pabst.
Ending life: ethics and the way we die / Margaret Pabst Battin.
   p. cm.
Includes bibliographical references and index.
ISBN-13 978-0-19-514026-2; 978-0-19-514027-9 (pbk.)
ISBN 0-19-514026-5; 0-19-514027-3 (pbk.)
1. Assisted suicide—Moral and ethical aspects.   2. Euthanasia—Moral and ethical aspects.
3. Death—Moral and ethical aspects.   I. Title.
R726 .B329 2005
179.7—dc22   2004049541

9 8 7 6 5 4 3 2
Printed in the United States of America
on acid-free paper

for Brooke Hopkins

Season of mists and mellow fruitfulness,
  Close bosom-friend of the maturing sun;
Conspiring with him how to load and bless
  With fruit the vines that round the thatch-eves run;
To bend with apples the moss'd cottage-trees,
  And fill all fruit with ripeness to the core . . .

—From John Keats, "To Autumn," 1819

CONTENTS

ENDING LIFE

Introduction

Ending Life: The Way We Do It, the Way We *Could* Do It

I want to talk in this collection about dying, about how we do it—and how we *could* do it, if we weren't so caught in conceptual confusion, misleading assumptions, bad argument, and political friction over this issue. How we die, and how we could die, is an issue under sustained debate in the United States and in much of the developed world. The currently visible controversies over voluntary euthanasia in the Netherlands and physician-assisted suicide in Oregon are, I believe, just iceberg-tips of a huge undercurrent of ongoing social ferment. Indeed, the social and political currents now in motion—some of which will be explored in this book—may well determine how we can and must die.

I have to confess that I've been thinking about this issue for twenty-five or thirty years. I go back and forth about it, and although I have a continuously articulated position in print I am still always plagued by the question of whether I should change my mind. You'll see some currents swirling forth, some eddying back, a process of continuing inquiry and reflection that moves like a river, sluggish here, rushing there, heading in one general direction but forever forming backwaters, meanders, waterfalls, and huge deep lakes along the way. How we do and how we could do our dying is still a live issue for me, a troubling one.

The Great Divide Concerning How We Die

To begin to see the theoretical poles that define the scope and central problematic of this issue, think first about Seneca, the Roman Stoic philosopher and statesman who lived from 4 BC to 65 AD, when Nero ordered him to commit suicide and he opened his veins. In Letter 70 of his *Moral Letters to Lucilius,* Seneca considers "the proper time to slip the cable." We make many mistakes, Seneca tells us here and in other texts, in thinking about death. Here are four: we assume (1) that death is bad, (2) that death later is better than death earlier, (3) that longer life is better than shorter life, and (4) that death is something that happens to us rather than something we control. All these assumptions seem completely obvious—to us. But here's what Seneca says:

> Living is not the good, but living well. The wise man therefore lives as long as he should, not as long as he can. He will observe where he is to live, with whom, how, and what he is to do. He will always think of life in terms of quality, not quantity. If he encounters many vexations which disturb his tranquillity, he will release himself. He will do this not only in an extreme exigency, but as soon as he begins to suspect Fortune he will look about him carefully to determine whether he ought to have done. He will consider it of no importance whether he causes his end or merely accepts it, whether late or early. He does not shrink as before some great deprivation, for not much can be lost from a trickle. Dying early or late is of no relevance, dying well or ill is. To die well is to escape the danger of living ill . . .
>
> Just as I choose a ship to sail in or a house to live in, so I choose a death for my passage from life. Moreover, whereas a prolonged life is not necessarily better, a prolonged death is necessarily worse. . . . A man's life should satisfy other people as well, his death only himself, and whatever sort he likes is best.[1]

Here's the core element of the Stoic view: that we—the wise man, in Stoic terms, or, translated into contemporary terms, each thinking, reflective one of us—that we are responsible for the timing and character of the deaths we die. We can't complain if death goes badly; it is up to us to seize the opportunity to ensure that it goes well. Sometimes this means suicide; sometimes this means dying quietly of old age in our own beds; sometimes this means a dramatic, public act like Cato's self-sacrifice in preference to slavery or Lucretia's suicide after she was raped.

There's an important theoretical point underneath Seneca's view—one it's taken me decades to understand. A self-embraced death, a suicide, Seneca argues, is not a premature end to a complete life. It isn't like a journey cut short, which is incomplete because you don't get there; rather, Seneca maintains, a life cut short can still be complete if it has been lived well—you do get there, so to speak; you've actually lived your whole life. The important thing, Seneca insists, is how well one lives, not how long. That means that the proper time to cut the cable could come at any point.

That's the Stoic view. But keep in mind all the considerations Seneca doesn't mention:

1. The impact of suicide on one's family—spouse, parents, children
2. The effect of suicide on one's fellows, coworkers, and those involved in joint work, projects, and other cooperative enterprises
3. The invidious role of depression and mental illness

4. The social framing of choices
5. The question of whether such an act, if many did it, would generate pressures on vulnerable persons, including the chronically ill, the elderly, people with disabilities, and others to do likewise, largely for reasons of social cost-saving
6. The question of whether there is some fundamental moral rule that prohibits killing oneself (Seneca certainly didn't think so)
7. The implications for an afterlife, if there is one

These are medieval, modern, and contemporary considerations. Seneca didn't address them, or at least he didn't pursue them much. But *we* have to. This is where the philosophical work begins, to try to sort out whether one form of concern takes priority over another, whether one's own sense of when it has become the proper time to slip the cable (which Seneca thinks you will almost instinctively know) is to be trumped by social and principled concerns, or the other way around.

Seneca and the other Stoic thinkers thought self-willed death, at the right time and for the right reasons, was a good thing—that way lay virtue. The Christian thinkers who followed them thought just the opposite: that issues about impact on society, on others, and especially fundamental religious/ethical law were central— one ought *never* act to deliberately end one's own life. That way lay sin. On the contrary, suffering, acceptance, the willing embrace of martyrdom—these were the ways in which the faithful should meet death: death should come at God's will, not man's. This is St. Thomas Aquinas's view of the morality of suicide, the issue that Seneca had also been addressing:

> . . . to kill oneself is altogether unlawful for three reasons. First, because every thing loves itself, it is thus proper for every thing to keep itself in being and resist decay as far as it can. Therefore, to kill oneself is contrary to natural inclination, and contrary to the charity according to which everyone ought to love himself. Hence self-killing is always a mortal sin, inasmuch as it stands against natural law and charity.
>
> Second, because every thing that is a part belongs to a whole, every man is part of a community, and as such is of the community. Therefore, he who kills himself injures the community . . .
>
> Third, because life is a gift divinely given to man, and subject to the power of Him "who kills and makes to live." Therefore, he who deprives himself of life sins against God . . . To God alone belongs the power over death and life . . .[2]

You don't have to be religious to have imbibed something of this view; it has become a fundamental part of Western culture, the notion that one ought not end one's own life. The other major monotheist religions have incorporated this view as well: Judaism had developed it (though with exceptions to avoid apostasy) by the time of the Talmudic period, and in Islam, the Prophet biography includes a categorical rejection of suicide, though it is currently under challenge in notions of *jihad*. In Western culture, of these three, it has been Christianity that has most resolutely rejected suicide.

Some later thinkers in the West, like Hume, sided with the Stoics; others, like Kant, argued for categorical prohibitions. Mme. de Staël, writing at the end of the

18th century, argued ardently for the liberty of suicide; she then changed her mind and, writing at the beginning of the 19th century, argued vehemently against suicide on essentially religious grounds. Nietzsche was for; Schopenhauer's view was guarded; Durkheim claimed it was an issue of social organization and not a moral issue at all. The rest, in a sense, is history—that descent from high theory to the knotty legacy of tension over right-to-die issues that is boiling up now in Oregon, in the Netherlands, in Switzerland, Canada, Germany, England, Belgium, Australia, Japan, everywhere in the developed world where death in the grasp of high-tech medicine is often seen as the unfortunate alternative.

Underlying this debate is what I think of as the Stoic/Christian divide about the individual's role in his or her own death: whether one's role should be as far as possible active, self-assertive, and responsible and may include ending one's own life—or, on the other hand, acceptant, obedient, and passive in the sense of being patient, where "allowing to die" is the most active step that should be taken. In the contemporary world we're still battling around the edges of this divide. When by a 51–49% majority and then again 60–40% Oregon legalizes physician-assisted suicide for people who are terminally ill; when Canada's Supreme Court rules 5–4 that physician-assisted suicide cannot be allowed for someone pleading for it in the final stages of ALS; when the Australian government reverses the Northern Territory's law permitting physician-assisted suicide and euthanasia in less than a year; when the Dutch Supreme Court rules that intolerable suffering can be mental as well as physical and thus an adequate basis for requesting euthanasia; when Britain's High Court and House of Lords reject a plea from a woman dying of ALS and the European Court of Human Rights in Strasbourg—where she travels in an ambulance—rules that her human rights are not being violated if she cannot be helped to die; when the U.S. Supreme Court rules 9–0 against a right to assistance in suicide but in effect leaves the matter up to the states; when the U.S. Attorney General moves to undercut Oregon's law with a reinterpretation of the Controlled Substances Act, the Ninth Circuit rules against this move, and the Attorney General files against just before he resigns, we should see these as just a few more skirmishes among the ongoing battles in this continuing conflict—part of the ongoing tension that results from the tectonic-plate collision of essentially Stoic and essentially Christian bodies of thought about a person's appropriate role in his or her own dying.

As members of contemporary culture, at least in the West, we almost all have deep-rooted allegiances to both, regardless of our surface affiliations and whether we're the slightest bit religious or not, and that's why this issue strikes such painful nerves. Not only does this tectonic-plate collision of deep-rooted bodies of thought affect our thinking about suicide, but it colors our attitudes toward all the other modern medical practices that come into play in treating (or not treating) the dying: do-not-resuscitate orders, withholding and withdrawing of life-prolonging treatment such as dialysis and respiratory support, the use of escalating levels of opioids, the withdrawal of artificial nutrition and hydration (especially in the practice known as terminal sedation), "letting die" in general, and many forms of "comfort care," as well as physician-assisted suicide and euthanasia. I've focused to a considerable extent on the various forms of assisted dying because that's where the issues are most vivid, but the Stoic/Christian divide underlies issues in all the ways we die—and *could* die.

In exploring these tensions in this collection of writings, I have at least five purposes in mind: to challenge assumptions about how we can and should die; to illuminate the structure of arguments for and against physician-assisted dying; to explore the morality of suicide (the deepest issue underlying the death-and-dying controversies that are visible in public debate); to speculate a bit about how the future might look and what we should be prepared for; and to look for possibilities of resolution in these ancient, yet new, debates. This collection is thoroughly diverse: it offers systematic essays, practical notes, historical explorations, policy analyses, cross-cultural comparisons, pieces with political implications, fiction, creative nonfiction, and essays on matters as varied as clinical suicide prevention, suicide bombing, serpent-handling, and the development of high-tech methods for non-drug-aided death. While this collection takes the argument over physician-assisted suicide as a central framework, many of these pieces are used here in a way that triangulates into this issue, so to speak, from comparatively unconventional vantage-points. Nearly everything in this collection has real relevance to the issues in physician-assisted suicide (though that may sometimes be difficult to see), but it also addresses the larger, tectonic-plate issue of the role a person may play in his or her own dying.

Most of these pieces have been written over the last dozen years, roughly since the publication of my earlier volume of essays *The Least Worst Death*—or, if you include "Roebeck" and "Terminal Procedure," one fiction, the other creative nonfiction, they stretch back almost thirty years. Some of the pieces, like "Euthanasia: The Way We Do It, the Way They Do It," have been continuously revised and updated, while others, like "Going Early, Going Late," "High-Risk Religion," and the creative pieces, remain deliberately unrevised, despite on the one hand huge advances in medicine or on the other considerable social change that has occurred since the original publication of those pieces. My general strategy has been to preserve insights where they remain relevant, and some of the earliest pieces I believe still offer insight in a way that more contemporary work no longer can. Still other pieces in this collection are quite new, written for this collection as it has taken shape—the piece puzzling over possible explanations for the same-day deaths of John Adams and Thomas Jefferson, for example. But despite its diversity in type and in time of composition, the pieces in this collection all nevertheless revolve around the central arguments in the death-and-dying debates.

On the Structure of the Argument over Physician-Assisted Dying

The death-and-dying debates, especially where they focus on physician-assisted dying—euthanasia and suicide—involve five central arguments—two pro, three con. These include two arguments for moral acceptance and/or legalization, the argument from autonomy or self-determination and the argument from the relief of pain and suffering, sometimes also called the argument from mercy. On the other side, the principal arguments against assisted dying include the argument from the intrinsic wrongness of killing, the argument concerning the integrity of the medical profession, and the argument about the potential for abuse, the so-called slippery-slope argument. The first of the pieces in this collection, "Euthanasia and Physician-Assisted Suicide," sketches an introduction to the overall issues of assisted dying; this exploration of the ethical framework is continued in "Is a Physician Ever Obligated to Help a Patient Die?"

The pieces in this volume, as well as those in *The Least Worst Death,* explore this overall argument, bit by bit. Some—indeed many—focus on or touch on issues of autonomy: for example, "Going Early, Going Late: The Rationality of Decisions about Physician-Assisted Suicide in AIDS," the case study "Scott Ames," the short novella "Robeck," the lengthy analysis of challenges to autonomy in religious contexts in "High-Risk Religion," and the future-oriented pieces "Genetic Information and Knowing When You Will Die," "Extra Long Life: Ethical Aspects of Increased Lifespan," and the closing piece, "Safe, Legal, Rare." Is autonomy central? How is it threatened? Should autonomy be recognized as central in public policy and law? Does the requirement of "informed consent" actually protect autonomy? Is autonomy even possible in the first place? Does religion enhance autonomy or get in the way? What are the implications in practice of recognizing autonomy at a theoretical level? The concept of autonomy has been on the ropes in philosophical discussion in recent years, but I still think it is crucial to the death-and-dying issues.

At the same time, some pieces focus on or touch on arguments about the other principal case in favor of assistance in dying—pain and suffering, both physical and psychological, what I sometimes like to call the argument from mercy or the argument from compassion. These include some of the same pieces, like "Scott Ames," and "Going Early, Going Late," as well as others, including "Is a Physician Ever Obligated to Help a Patient Die?" The futurist piece "Safe, Legal, Rare?" in particular considers whether adequate pain control would obviate any need for physician-assisted dying.

The principal claims on the "con" side of the argument over assisted dying are the claims that killing is intrinsically wrong, that allowing assistance in dying— especially *physician* assistance—would undermine the integrity of the medical profession, and that permitting the deliberate ending of life would pose risks of the so-called slippery slope and the possibility of abuse. This would involve both compromises to the integrity of physicians and direct economic and social pressures that oblige or force patients to choose assisted dying when they would not otherwise do so. A good many pieces here deal directly or indirectly with these issues. For example, "High-Risk Religion" deals with (among other things) expectations within a religiously defined community about risking death, while "Is a Physician Ever Obligated to Help a Patient Die?" deals with (among other things) whether the physician/patient relationship would be altered if assisted dying were allowed. "Euthanasia: The Way We Do It, The Way They Do It" articulates objections to various social policies about how we die, and in doing so argues that the one currently in force in the United States (except in Oregon) may not be the most suitable one, and indeed may be the most risky for patients in vulnerable groups.

Looking at both (or all) sides of the argument over assisted dying is something I've tried to be resolute about doing for years. This hasn't been a systematic effort, and most of these pieces aren't easily categorized under one or the other side of the argument. Rather, I've looked first at one part of the argument, then its opposite, then gone on to something else, then eddied back to the issues I find most deeply troubling and least amenable to resolution. Furthermore, since an interesting view must usually develop over time and rarely springs to life full-blown, many of the pieces in this and in my earlier book *The Least Worst Death* represent repeated and re-repeated attempts to face an issue—return trips often necessitated by something that has come to light in exploring another component of the picture. Despite this seemingly erratic pattern, this collection, together with the earlier one, is intended to examine the underlying philosophical components of the general argument about how we die and how we could die, especially focusing on assistance in dying.

Challenging Assumptions

Many of the pieces in this volume have a faintly Socratic cast, in that they involve challenging assumptions that are held ubiquitously but in a largely unquestioning way. These assumptions include at least four types.

Empirical Assumptions

Among the empirical assumptions challenged in this volume are many that play a substantial but unquestioned role in the discussion of end-of-life issues, such as the claim that there aren't big differences in the way that the advanced industrial nations with well-developed health care systems approach end-of-life issues, or that patients in vulnerable groups are the targets of extra pressure to die.

Values Assumptions

Some of the articles in this book focus on assumptions about values that are hidden, partly obscured, or evident but taken for granted in the public discussion. For example, all the proposals for legalization of physician-assisted suicide, including Oregon's Death with Dignity statute and ballot measures in Washington, California, Michigan, Maine, Hawaii, and elsewhere, have explicitly asserted that a physician is not obligated to provide a patient with assistance in suicide. I agree that this is an appropriate public policy, but in "Is a Physician Ever Obligated to Help a Patient Die?" I've tried to issue a warning for those who assume the answer is *no*.

It is widely assumed that physician-assisted suicide, if it is legalized, should remain rare, a last-resort option where pain and symptom control fail. Indeed, I've joined in arguing this way in other publications.[3] I think this too is appropriate as a matter of public policy—that it should be assumed that such cases are comparatively rare. Yet, examining the underlying values assumptions more closely from a philosophical point of view, I do not see the basis for such an assumption. That is the argument pursued in "Safe, Legal, Rare?"

It is widely assumed that religion and deeply held religious belief are "life-affirming" and stand opposed to any form of suicide or self-caused death. In "Primary Texts," "High-Risk Religion," and "The "Ethics of Self-Sacrifice," I try to show that religion is not nearly so simple.

Dichotomizing Assumptions about Practical Strategies

A widespread characteristic of thinking about end-of-life situations involves overly stark dichotomies—either/or dilemmas in which just two choices are offered. A number of the pieces included here challenge such assumptions in practical contexts: for example, "Scott Ames," which challenges the clinical choices proposed for dealing with a suicidal patient; multiple ways of interpreting the striking fact that John Adams and Thomas Jefferson both died on precisely the 50th anniversary of the signing of the Declaration of Independence; and recommendations for expanding the richness of social observation, in "Empirical Research in Bioethics: The Method of Oppositional Collaboration." These all combat dichotomizing assumptions about practical policies and reasoning with respect to dying.

Predictive Assumptions

The fourth kind of assumption at work in much of the discourse about end-of-life issues is a bit harder to detect, largely because such assumptions typically play a less conspicuous and less challenged (though just as important) role. These are predictive assumptions about the future. They are partly empirical, in the sense that they trade on projections from current empirical states of affairs; they are also partly value-laden, in that they very, very often reflect the ideological biases of whoever is making the prediction—or, rather, whoever is making the unchallenged, unquestioned predictive assumption that lies behind many sorts of claims about the future. Some of the articles in this volume—for example, "Genetic Information," "Extra Long Life," "Global Life Expectancies and International Justice: A Re-emergence of the Duty to Die?" the essay on NuTech, "New Life in the Assisted-Death Debate," and "Safe, Legal, Rare"—explore issues about the future; they seek to uncover, examine, and challenge both empirical and values assumptions that are typically made about the future in order to reflect on how a future might look different if such assumptions weren't in place.

Not all of these pieces are about physician-assisted dying or even dying in medical contexts. Some of them address what may seem to be unrelated topics—suicide bombing, laboratory research with dogs, and serpent-handling, for instance—but in fact they are all intended here to provide novel ways of looking at the central issues in the death-and-dying debates. For example, "The Ethics of Self-Sacrifice: What's Wrong with Suicide Bombing?" examines some of the basic arguments about the wrongness of killing, in this case self-killing for an understandable political purpose. "Terminal Procedure" takes a close-up look at killing in the interests of science. "High-Risk Religion," examining situations in which faithful adherence to a religious group's doctrines or practices may mean death, exposes some of the forms of social construction of choice that underlie fears of the slippery slope. "Robeck" moves beyond the question of self-willed death in terminal illness to pose the same question in the context of old age, where medical concerns are not at issue.

The Uses of Fiction and Creative Nonfiction

One of the serious risks of observation in bioethics—about how people live and how they go about dying—is that observation is easily theory-infected: this happens in accounts of suffering, autonomy, manipulation, pain, the mistreatment of vulnerable patients, and everywhere where we try to look at actual lives of people with whom bioethics is concerned. As "Oppositional Collaboration" points out, theory-infectedness is a real risk in bioethics and social observation generally: we see things that support the academic points we want to make, and overlook the rest.

It is, I think, an especially great risk in fiction, one reason I don't write fiction anymore. But I did many years ago—before there was a field of bioethics with its steady diet of puzzle cases and its ongoing flirtation with legal decisions and its romance with policymaking and, most important, its elaborate catechism of *autonomy/nonmaleficence/beneficence/justice.* Back in those years, the late 1960s and early 1970s, bioethics wasn't even a recognized field: journals like the *Hastings Center Report* had barely been established (first issue June 1971), Sam Gorovitz was just bringing together the group that edited the first bioethics text, *Moral Problems in Medicine* (not published until 1976), and graduate programs like that at Georgetown and Penn and Utah didn't offer specialization in bioethics. There weren't any big conventions and there weren't any TV interviews and there wasn't any "bioethics industry." But I was writing fiction then, and what would later come to be called "creative nonfiction," and I've included two of these pieces here. This is not just to support bioethics' comparatively new recognition of narrative as a respected form of investigation—including narrative in both nonfiction first-person accounts and in fictional constructions—but because I think it may preserve certain early intuitions about issues like autonomy, beneficence, paternalism, respect for persons, and ending life that are hard to capture in bioethics' academic discussions.

Whatever may be assumed in other quarters, fiction and its close cousin creative nonfiction are not irrelevant to theory. On the contrary, fiction and creative nonfiction may do a great deal to measure and assess theory and to force reflection on otherwise easy points. Indeed, it is tempting to see academic prose, creative nonfiction, and fiction as forming a kind of genre-continuum for exploring difficult social issues. For example, the academic essays presented in this collection are in general strongly autonomist, rooted in the view that a person should be free to live his or her life as he or she sees fit, provided, of course, that this does not cause substantial harm to others. But "Robeck" serves to complicate this view by showing that the issue of autonomy is not a simple matter at all—even if the principle should, as the essays in this volume argue or imply, remain unchanged. Similarly, while the essays in this volume also clearly assume that killing is in general wrong but argue that certain clearly voluntary cases of self-killing in terminal illness and perhaps old age are to be morally respected, "Terminal Procedure" serves to complicate these views by evoking a basic gut reaction about killing itself: it is hard to watch and hard to participate in, even when one's role is indirect and it happens, so to speak, off-stage.

Because these two pieces, one largely fictional, the other much closer to the genre of creative nonfiction, are "pre-theoretical" in the sense that I'd barely heard of bioethics at the time they were written and had little idea of bioethics' theoretical constructions, they offer a kind of view that is comparatively innocent of theory but reinforces and challenges later theoretical accounts. For example, the gut reaction on which "Terminal Procedure" trades (known in bioethics as the "yuck" factor) is often used as an argument in public policy discussion; the question this piece serves to raise is whether exploitation of the yuck factor is a legitimate move in rational argumentation or a bogus appeal to the emotions. I might venture a more careful answer to that question now, but I couldn't revise these pieces without the risk of theory-infection, so here they are, just as they were originally written.

"Terminal Procedure" was written around 1973, while I was taking a graduate class from the now-famous Daniel Dennett, when he was a young philosopher with an interesting theory on the way up—but although the account is influenced by Dennett's work, it is quite innocent of theory in bioethics. Since there wasn't any bioethics then, or at least I hadn't heard of it, I didn't have any developed views about autonomy, nonmaleficence, justice, all that. I just looked around and wrote about what I saw, what bothered and disturbed me. Desperate for space to work in while I was a graduate student—this was at the University of California at Irvine— I'd borrowed a desk in Michael Cole's neuropsychology lab. It was just an old, brown wooden desk over in the corner of the lab, where I thought I could get some work done. This happened a long time ago—the lab equipment seems antiquated now and the science being done outdated, long since incorporated in the basic understanding of the field, no longer new. There were people who worked in the lab where I was using that desk. A man I've named Boaz ran the lab, and there was a young dark-haired woman named Maia in the lab, nice people to work around, but there were 23 dogs with names like Mustard and Pablo and Francesca who would nuzzle around the base of my desk, let me scratch their heads, play with them when my attention drifted. This isn't fiction; this is the way it happened. Maia, the lab assistant who ran the experimental trials on these dogs, was absent from work the day of the events described in the piece, and I played her role. That's how I know something about killing, even if it was just dogs and even if it was indirect and even if it was done for an important scientific cause. I think it is crucial for bioethicists—like me—who talk and write about end-of-life topics like euthanasia and physician-assisted suicide and pulling the plug to keep in mind the unsettling, stomach-disturbing, conscience-trying unease that acquiescing in, or contributing indirectly to, or actively taking part in ending life can produce. This piece doesn't focus on the theoretical considerations bioethics offers about killing and letting die, life-termination and so on; it is about the way the "yuck" response can well up in one's throat, even though the ending of life is in the interests of science, even though the conditions are intended as humane, and even though in the end it involves dogs, not people. There is a lot in this volume of academic essays about how life ends and how we do and could make it end—all part of an extended exploration of the Stoic/Christian divide over the appropriate role of the individual in his or her own dying—but I've wanted you to know what killing has felt like to me.

Exploring the Future

Though considerations about the future properly begin with the historical selections like "Collecting the Primary Texts: Sources on the Ethics of Suicide" and "July 4, 1826," the essay wondering what could have happened to account for the fact that Adams and Jefferson died on the same significant day, it is the final group of selections that more directly explores the future. What will death and dying be like in our future? How will our underlying assumptions change? What technological advances will reshape this most basic fact of our lives? These pieces, especially "Genetic Information," "Extra Long Life," "Global Life Expectancies,", and "Scheduled Drugs versus NuTech" explore some of the ways our experience and practice with respect to our own deaths may change. These pieces are speculative, of course, in contrast to the several more empirically constrained pieces earlier in the volume, but it is the sort of speculation we cannot afford not to make if we are to consider not only how we do die but how we *could* be doing our dying. All the practices at issue in this volume are undergoing very rapid evolution—though it is sometimes difficult to foresee in what direction—and we cannot be content with analyses of them just as they are right now. Thus while this volume is partly analytic, in the usual mode of critical philosophers, it must also be partly visionary, in the mode of philosophers who use the analysis of predictive assumptions to speculate openly about the future.

Looking for Resolution

What about resolution? I've tried. I've been trying for many years; but I think the project of achieving resolution in the death-and-dying debates is overwhelmingly difficult. This is because, in part, the two huge tectonic plates of Stoic and Christian thinking are still in active collision in much of our thinking about these issues— the one a body of thought that insists that the individual be responsible for his or her own dying, the other a view that sees dying as something the individual must in the end accept. One view thinks of dying as something you do; the other sees it as something that happens to you. They're both partly right, of course; the trick is to capture these partial truths in a workable resolution.

There are hints and sketches everywhere in this volume of a potential resolution, but no official recipe. The last two selections offer differing approaches to the possibilities of resolution: "Oppositional Collaboration" says something about practical procedures in informal research that bear on how to seek resolution, while "Safe, Legal, Rare" says something about the content of resolution and—by going far beyond it—what it might look like. It's the closing paragraphs of the very first piece in this collection, the introduction to the death-and-dying debates "Euthanasia and Physician-Assisted Suicide," that first introduce the possibilities of resolution in proposing a notion of "advance personal policy making," and the final paragraphs of "Safe, Legal, Rare?" that sketch something of what this might look like in practice, but the full development of such a notion must remain for another day. Instead, in a sense, this volume itself serves as an exercise in advance personal policy making—you can tell what I'd want, what I wouldn't want, where I'd waffle, and what I'd resolutely seek. Yet I can hardly expect to impose these views on anyone else. In that sense, "advance personal policymaking" appropriately remains in the fullest sense an exercise for the reader.

Notes

1. Seneca, *Letters to Lucilius,* excerpts from Letter 70, in *The Stoic Philosophy of Seneca,* ed. and trans. Moses Hadas (New York: Norton, 1958).

2. Thomas Aquinas, *Summa Theologiae* 2a2ae, question 64, article 5, trans. Michael Rudick, unpublished text.

3. Timothy E. Quill and Margaret P. Battin, eds., *Physician-Assisted Dying: The Case for Palliative Care and Patient Choice* (Baltimore: The Johns Hopkins University Press, 2004).

DILEMMAS ABOUT DYING

1

Euthanasia and Physician-Assisted Suicide

Introduction

Something is amiss with the debate over euthanasia and physician-assisted suicide. When it emerged into public consciousness in the mid-1970s, the debate got off to a rousing start, as philosophers, doctors, theologians, public-policy theorists, journalists, social advocates, and private citizens became embroiled in the debate. On the one side were liberals, who thought physician-assisted suicide and perhaps voluntary active euthanasia were ethically acceptable and should be legal; on the other side were conservatives, who believed assisted dying was immoral and/or dangerous to legalize as a matter of public policy. Over the several decades in which this debate has been accelerating it has achieved a lively, florid richness, both as a philosophical dispute and as a broad, international public issue.

That is the good part. In this chapter I want to explore the richness of this debate by showing something of the terrain of the debate and the figures who have inhabited it, both the public figures and the academic ones partly behind the scenes. But I also want to explore the not-so-good part. I am particularly concerned with what has gone wrong in this debate—or, more precisely, what has not gone quite right just yet.

The Development of the Argument in the Assisted-Dying Debate

Although disputes over the moral status of suicide are found as far back as the First Intermediate Period of ancient Egypt, some two millennia BC, the debate about *physician-assisted* suicide and *physician-performed* euthanasia is new, occupying academic and public attention primarily in the late twentieth century and the early twenty-first. The emergence of this issue reflects a basic shift in the epidemiology of human mortality, a shift away from death due to parasitic and infectious disease (ubiquitous among humans in all parts of the globe prior to about 1850) to death in later life of degenerative disease (Olshansky and Ault 1987)—especially heart disease and cancer, which now together account for almost two-thirds of deaths in the developed countries. In earlier periods of human history, physicians could do little to stave off death; now, improvements in public sanitation, the development of immunization, the development of antibiotics, and the many technologies of modern medicine have combined to lengthen the human lifespan, particularly in the developed world. For much of human history, life expectancy hovered between 20 and 40; in the developed countries, at the beginning of the twenty-first century, it is nearing 80 and, unless infectious disease becomes more prevalent again, is expected to increase. The result is that, in the developed world, with its sophisticated health-care systems, the majority of the population in these countries dies at comparatively advanced ages of degenerative diseases with characteristically long down-hill courses, marked by a terminal phase of dying. On average, people die at older ages and in slower, far more predictable ways, and it is this new situation in the history of the world that gives rise to the assisted-dying issues to be explored here.

The debate over euthanasia and physician-assisted suicide pits arguments about autonomy and about relief of pain and suffering on the 'for' side, versus arguments about the intrinsic wrongness of killing, threats to the integrity of the medical profession, and potentially damaging social effects on the 'against' side.

Principal arguments *for* are:

- the argument from autonomy;
- the argument from relief of pain and suffering.

Principal arguments *against* are:

- the argument from the intrinsic wrongness of killing;
- the argument from the integrity of the profession;
- the argument from potential abuse: the slippery-slope argument.

It is to this overall schema that I will be referring in exploring the five component arguments to be examined below, which I will treat in the order indicated above, for reasons that will become evident later on. It is this overall schema that I will also have in mind in suggesting what seems to have gone wrong with the assisted-dying debate—or, rather, has not gone quite right just yet.

The focused debate over physician-assisted dying began in the wake of the

civil rights movements of the late 1960s and early 1970s, as many formerly disenfranchised or disregarded groups sought recognition of rights or a greater range
of rights than had previously been accorded them: blacks, women, people from
religious minorities, people with disabilities, and—gradually—medical patients, including patients with terminal illnesses. As in all these groups, the quest for greater
respect and a greater range of rights developed with increasing force. With the new
availability of antibiotics and technologies like intravenous lines, respirators, and
dialysis machines, medicine's capacity to extend the lives of dying patients had
begun to increase, but patients themselves were still regarded as 'patients'—comparatively passive subjects of medicine's ministrations. They were rarely understood
as agents of autonomous control, but rather as naive and frightened parties appropriately treated in paternalistic ways. In the 1960s, patients with fatal illnesses were
rarely (only about 10 percent of the time) told the truth about fatal prognoses.
Consent for experimentation was often ignored (as in the infamous Tuskegee syph-
ilis study), and consent for therapeutic treatment—fully informed and fully voluntary consent—comparatively rarely sought. Truth telling and autonomy were
hardly central values of medicine; doctors were expected to do what they thought
was best for patients, and—believing patients would be harmed if told they were
dying—routinely hid fatal diagnoses and urged patients to go on fighting as long
as they could.

Gradually, however, it came to be recognized that continuing all-out treatment
could be painful, dehumanizing, and pointless. Thanks in large part to Elizabeth
Kübler-Ross's influential book *On Death and Dying* (1969), by the mid-1970s it
was becoming socially possible to talk openly about death. Kübler-Ross had described a series of five stages through which the person who learns he or she is
terminally ill will pass in facing death (denial; anger; bargaining; depression; and
a final stage she called detachment but that became popularly known as acceptance); Kübler-Ross held that it was better for patients if the fact that they were
dying was openly acknowledged. The California Natural Death Act of 1976 marks
one of the earliest legal recognitions of this changing social perception, since it
enabled the patient who knew the truth to decline or discontinue treatment that
might otherwise prolong the process of dying; the law served to protect their physicians from prosecution for failure to treat. State by state, similar 'living-will'
legislation began to permit terminally ill patients to make advance choices about
withholding and withdrawing treatment, now that, with increasing frequency, they
were being told the truth that they were dying.

During this long process of transformation, several central figures emerged to
argue in favour of physician-assisted suicide. British journalist Derek Humphry,
widely recognized as the founder of the right-to-die movement, published *Jean's
Way* (1978), describing in heart-rending detail his assistance in the suicide of his
first wife, dying of cancer. By 1980, then in Los Angeles, Humphry founded the
Hemlock Society, a grassroots organization committed to the legalization of
physician-assisted suicide. The first philosophical voices in the new debate began
to be heard as well: philosophers like Tom Beauchamp, Ray Frey, Dan Brock,
David Mayo, and myself, in the United States, and those like John Harris and
Jonathan Glover in the United Kingdom, Carlos Prado in Canada, and Helga Kuhse

and Peter Singer in Australia all began to weigh in, largely supporting an autonomy-based view. Although they developed their views in somewhat different ways and responded quite differently to the various objections raised, they all subscribed to what might be called the argument from self-determination or autonomy. And, of course, they all faced the same objections from opponents.

The argument from autonomy is the first of the five components of the overall debate outlined above, one of the two principal arguments on the 'for' side. Because even this one component is too complex to examine fully here, I present it just as a schematic outline and will discuss only the more significant parts; it should be evident that its sequences of argument/objection/counter-objection could be extended in great detail through many more sub-arguments and counter-counter-objections.

Components of the Assisted-Dying Argument

The Argument from Autonomy (For)

Just as a person has the right to determine as much as possible the course of his or her own life, a person also has the right to determine as much as possible the course of his or her own dying. If a terminally ill person seeks assistance in suicide from a physician freely and rationally, the physician ought to be permitted to provide it.

- *Objection.* True autonomy is rarely possible, especially for someone who is dying. Not only are most choices socially formed, but in terminal illness depression and other psychiatric disturbances are likely to be a factor.
  - *Counter-objection.* Even if many choices are socially shaped, they must be respected as real choices.
  - *Counter-objection.* Rational suicide is possible, and it is possible for patients to make choices about dying without distortion by depression.
- *Objection.* One cannot impose on another an obligation to do what is morally wrong, even if one's own choice is made freely and rationally. Since suicide is wrong, the physician can have no obligation to assist in it.
  - *Counter-objection.* This merely assumes, but does not prove, that suicide in circumstances of terminal illness is morally wrong.
  - *Counter-objection.* The physician is not obligated to provide assistance in dying, but should be free to do so if he or she wishes.

Autonomy, involving both freedom from restriction (liberty) and the capacity to act intentionally (agency), is the central value to which this argument appeals, and respect for a person's autonomous choice the social principle it entails. In the context of end-of-life medical care, respecting autonomy for the dying patient not only means honouring as far as possible that person's choices concerning therapeutic and palliative care, including life-prolonging care if it is desired, but could also mean refraining from intervening to prevent that person's informed, voluntary, self-willed choice of suicide in preference to a slow, painful death, or even providing assistance in realizing that choice. Certainly, respect for autonomous choice had been understood (most fully by Kant) to involve respect for rational self-governance, and to be limited (as Mill had pointed out) by the harm principle: respect for a person's autonomous choice does not license just any old act—not crazed acts and not acts that harm others. But the principle does insist that free, considered, individual choice, where one is the architect of one's own life and the chooser of one's own deepest values, must be respected—including, at least as proponents interpret the principle, choices of physician-assisted suicide.

The early theorists were particularly concerned with what was called the issue of 'rational suicide'. The question was whether a person could rationally choose to die or whether such a choice was always a product of depression, a frequent concomitant of terminal illness that narrows one's view of the range of alternative futures, when the irrationality of the choice is compounded by the fact that the person making this choice can have no objectively confirmable belief about what might happen to him after suicide, at least assuming an agnostic view about whether there is or is not an afterlife. Certainly, such issues had been discussed as early as the time of Lucretius, but they took a new, more psychiatrically informed focus in the light of twentieth-century clinical theories of depression and other mental illness, as well as postmodernist claims that seemingly autonomous choices are actually socially formed. Could suicide be rational and rationally chosen? Could it be the product of a fully autonomous choice? Advocates of physician-assisted suicide said yes, taking this as a mainstay of their position.

The most direct, immediate response to the concept of 'rational suicide' was an objection to suicide itself on religious and ethical grounds, an objection most forcefully pursued by Catholic thinkers. This is the opening argument of the 'against' side in the schema above.

The Argument from the Intrinsic Wrongness of Killing (Against)

The taking of a human life is simply wrong (witness the commandment 'Thou shalt not kill'); since suicide is killing, suicide is also wrong.

- *Objection.* But killing is socially and legally accepted in self-defence, war, capital punishment, and other situations; if it can be accepted there it could be accepted where it is the voluntary, informed choice of the person who would be killed.
  - *Counter-objection.* In self-defence, war, and capital punishment, the person killed is guilty; in assisted suicide, the person killed is innocent.

Killing is understood as morally wrong in virtually all cultures and religious systems. Judaism, Christianity, Islam, Hinduism, Buddhism, Confucianism, and many other religious traditions prohibit killing; so do the moral and legal codes of virtually all social systems. Since suicide is a form of killing, this argument observes, suicide—and with it assisted suicide—is wrong ('sinful', 'taboo', 'reviled by God', and so on) as well. However, although this view is shared by all the major world traditions, it has been Roman Catholicism that has been most active in the political debate over physician-assisted suicide in Europe and the USA.

According to the teachings of Catholicism, suicide violates the biblical commandment 'Thou shalt not kill.' Self-killing can never be permitted, even in painful terminal illness, although if it is caused by depression or other psychopathology, it may be excused from ecclesiastical penalties like denial of funeral rites. It was Augustine in the early fifth century who first interpreted the commandment as a prohibition of suicide. Aquinas, in the thirteenth century, developed an extensive argument against suicide, arguing that because 'everything loves itself' and seeks to remain in being, suicide is unnatural; that suicide injures the community; and that suicide rejects God's gift of life. From Aquinas on, the position of the Catholic Church has been quite uniform: unless someone is driven by insanity and hence excused from blame, suicide is always wrong. (In practice, the Catholic Church has often assumed that suicide victims were emotionally disturbed or mentally ill, and on that ground has withheld blame and permitted church rites to be performed.) Catholic contributors to the contemporary debate over physician-assisted suicide in terminal illness, like Kevin Wildes (1993), John Finnis (1995), and John Noonan (1998), held this view; physician-assisted suicide, even if it could be 'rational', would still, in this view, be gravely wrong.

Proponents of physician-assisted suicide pointed out that, while killing is morally and legally regarded as wrong in general, in some exceptional circumstances—for instance, in war, self-defence, and (though now more controversially) capital punishment—it is accepted as morally permissible. Other religious traditions have different ranges of exceptions, though most accept killing in (legitimate) war and in self-defence. But, the objection goes, if killing could be morally acceptable in some or all of these circumstances like war, self-defence, and capital punishment, why not self-killing or self-directed killing in painful terminal illness, when the killing would be for good reason and any assistance offered in performing it occurs at the express request of the 'victim'?

A Catholic response, employed by a number of writers, seeks to distinguish between killing of the 'innocent' and killing of those who, guilty of aggressive or immoral actions, are not. Proponents of physician-assisted suicide point out that this gives a curious result: on this reasoning, 'innocent' patients who are terminally ill could not have physician-assisted suicide no matter how fervently they wanted it, but 'guilty' ones presumably could. Catholic thinkers appear to have found this response trivializing of the religious concept of innocence, and have made little response.

While the Catholic Church opposed directly caused dying even in painful terminal illness and had always held that suffering can be of redemptive value, the Church did not ignore the issue about pain. In 1958, Pope Pius XII issued his famous statement to anaesthesiologists 'The Prolongation of Life', in which he employed the traditional Principle of Double Effect to argue that, while death must never be intentionally caused, the physician may licitly use drugs for the control of pain even though foreseeing—though not intending—that this will cause an earlier death. The Pope was referring in particular to the use of opiates, especially morphine, which, it was widely understood, could depress respiration and so cause death. The principle of double effect rests on the observation that an act may have two ('double') or more effects, both an intended effect and a foreseen but unintended effect (as when a child is given castor oil: the intended effect is preservation of health; the foreseen but unintended effect is the bad taste of the medicine). Rigorously stated, the principle of double effect requires that four conditions be met: (1) the action must not be intrinsically wrong; (2) the agent must intend only the good effect, not the bad one; (3) the bad effect must not be the means of achieving the good effect; and (4) the good effect must be 'proportional' to the bad one—that is, outweigh it. The principle was used to argue that a dying patient could always be assured of an easy death, if given morphine with the intent to relieve his or her suffering, even if that were to mean that the death might occur earlier; this would still be to intend the good effect only—relieving the suffering— while the bad effect, death, was merely foreseen, not intended. Whether this was a tenable distinction was a subject of considerable dispute, but its role in the argument was clear: to deflect claims that death hastened with pain-killing drugs involved killing a human being.

Meanwhile, during the period in which this stage of the argument over assisted dying was being most forcefully argued, social expectations regarding terminal illness shifted from the earlier view that the dying patient ought to fight on as long as possible to the new view that forgoing treatment and discontinuing treatment were permissible, indeed acceptable and even normal. The 1976 case of Karen Ann Quinlan raised the issue of discontinuing the respirator for a permanently comatose patient; within a decade or so, discontinuation of respiratory support was to become routine. Over the years, not starting treatment, or, having once started, stopping treatment of all sorts became more common. While the earliest technologies to be regarded in this way were the conspicuous, highly invasive ones like dialyzers and respirators ('tubes and machines'), the practice gradually came to include withholding and withdrawing of all forms of life-sustaining treatment. Once it had become possible to recognize terminal illness as terminal, to discuss the approach of death with the patient, and to recognize that continuing treatment might prolong the process of dying but not stave off death altogether, it became increasingly possible to plan to 'negotiate' death. Respirators could be unplugged, dialysis discontinued, chemotherapy avoided, antibiotics and pressors simply not used. Most controversially, artificial nutrition and hydration could fail to be started, or discontinued once it was already in use.

Such practices were often referred to as 'letting die', not 'killing'. Though the principle of double effect that was held to draw an adequately bright line between them was inherited from Catholic thought, it was widely embraced in secular bioethics. Letting die seemed sharply distinguished from killing: to turn off the respirator was not to kill the patient, but simply to let the patient die of the underlying disease. The killing/letting-die distinction was supposed to draw an important line, to which virtually all conservatives in the debate subscribed; patients must never be deliberately, intentionally killed, but, if treatment were withheld or withdrawn, they could be allowed to die of natural causes—namely, the underlying disease.

However, early on in the debate, James Rachels had attacked this view in a short but highly influential paper that appeared in the *New England Journal of*

Medicine (1975). Imagine, he wrote in this now-famous paper, Smith and Jones, both of whom stand to inherit a sizeable fortune from their respective 6-year-old cousins, should the cousins die. One evening, while his cousin is taking his bath, Smith sneaks into the bathroom and drowns him. Meanwhile, Jones is also planning to drown his own cousin, who is also taking a bath, but, as Jones sneaks into the bathroom, the child hits his head and slips under the water. Jones does nothing to save him. Now both children are dead. Smith has killed his cousin; Jones has merely allowed his cousin to die. But both are seriously, equally wrong. Hence it cannot be, Rachels argued, that the distinction between killing and letting die is adequate to discriminate between ethically unacceptable and ethically acceptable cases, and indeed in some cases killing may be ethically more defensible than letting die.

Among such cases, proponents of legalization chorused, could be cases of painful terminal illness. In some such cases, they argued, the voluntary, deliberate termination of life involved in physician-assisted suicide or active voluntary euthanasia—even though they involve killing—could be ethically better than simply withdrawing treatment and thus consigning a pain-racked patient to a miserable end by letting the underlying disease cause death.

Opponents of assisted dying, religious and secular, have had little success in answering Rachels's point, especially as it has been developed more fully by later proponents, except to reaffirm the killing/letting-die distinction and to insist that pain can always be controlled (for a number of analyses, see Steinbock and Norcross 1994). They have turned instead to other points of opposition, particularly two closely related concerns about the consequences of legalization. The first of these, the argument concerning the integrity of the medical profession, is the second of the principal arguments against physician-assisted suicide; it has played a major role in the public opposition of physicians' groups like the AMA in opposing legalization.

The Argument from the Integrity of the Profession (Against)

Doctors should not kill; this is prohibited by the Hippocratic Oath. The physician is bound to save life, not take it.

- *Objection.* In its original version the Hippocratic Oath also prohibits doctors from performing surgery, providing abortifacients, and taking fees for teaching medicine. If the Oath can be modified to permit these practices, why not assistance in suicide, where the patient is dying anyway and seeks the physician's help?
    - *Counter-objection.* To permit physicians to kill patients would undermine the patient's trust in the physician.
        - *Counter-counter-objection.* Patients trust their physicians more when they know that their physicians will help them, not desert them as they die.

Doctors should not kill! thundered physicians like Willard Gaylin, Leon Kass, Edmund Pellegrino, and Mark Siegler (1988). For some opponents of assisted dying, this reflects a religiously based moral judgment about the intrinsic wrongness of killing; for others, it is the underlying axiom of medical practice to which the Hippocratic Oath alludes in stipulating that the physician shall give no deadly drug, not even when asked for it. For still others, it reflects concerns about the pressures under which physicians operate and the kinds of incentives to which they are subject. For example, Diane Meier, MD, a former proponent, changed her position to oppose legalization on the grounds that the conditions of medical practice in modern urban hospitals—immense time pressures, financial incentives against expensive treatment, little ongoing relationship with patients, and so on—could so severely compromise physician judgment in the matter of assisting a patient in dying that medical integrity would be sacrificed. For example, she noted, some 25 per cent of people in New York City have no health insurance. Many other physicians have made similar points, aware as they are of the circumstances in which they now practise. Although the argument concerning the integrity of the medical profession is closely related to the slippery-slope argument about the potential for abuse, since it intimates that doctors will become more callous in their treatment of patients, it is also an argument focused on the nature of trust. Patients will be unable to trust their physicians, the argument about integrity claims, since the nature of the physician's role will have changed to permit killing; this is to disrupt something essential to the bond that is established in the physician-patient relationship. Not only will it undermine trust, but it will change the physician as well, from healer to killer, from trusted helper to untrustworthy threat. On this argument, assisting in suicide or performing euthanasia will not only cause physicians personal anguish, as is sometimes observed in the Netherlands, but it will also lead to the corruption of their very nature as physicians.

Opponents, still stung by Rachel's dismantling of the theoretical distinction between killing and letting die, also began to emphasize more fully the second element of this counter-argument, an issue present in the debate from the start. This was the 'slippery-slope' claim that to allow even the few sympathetic cases of physician-assisted suicide or euthanasia where the patient fully autonomously chose it and would be spared great pain—these are the most compelling cases—would lead by gradual degrees down a slippery slope toward widespread abuse. Patients would be pressured by overwrought family members, callous physicians, or cost-conscious insurers into choosing an assisted death when they did not really want to die at all. They would be made to feel superfluous, burdensome, as if they *ought* to make such a request, or they might be forced into it by greedy heirs or circumstances deliberately made intolerable. This component of the overall argument, the third of the principal arguments against physician-assisted suicide, is a complex argument containing a variety of sub-arguments. It is the weightiest in the opposition's case—and, I believe, the one to be taken with greatest earnestness by all.

The Argument from Potential Abuse: The Slippery-Slope Argument (Against)

Permitting physicians to assist in suicide, even in sympathetic cases, may lead to situations in which patients are killed against their will.

- *Objection.* A basis for these predictions must be demonstrated before they can be used to suppress personal choices and individual rights.
  - *Counter-objection.* The bases for these predictions are increasing cost pressures, as well as greed, laziness, insensivity, prejudice, and other factors affecting physicians, family members, health-care institutions, and society.
    - *Counter-counter-objection.* It is possible, with careful design, to erect effective protections against abuse by doctors, families, institutions, or society.
  - *Counter-objection.* Vulnerable patients will be socially programmed to think of themselves as unworthy to remain alive, and the elderly, the chronically ill, the disabled, and others will be manœuvred into choosing to end their lives.
    - *Counter-counter-objection.* Only patients with documented terminal illnesses would be allowed this option.
      - *Counter-counter-counter-objection.* Restrictions of this sort cannot be enforced; pressures to die would spread beyond the terminally ill.
        - *Counter-counter-counter-counter-objection.* Where these practices are legal, there is no evidence of disparate impact on patients in vulnerable groups.

Slippery-slope arguments involve predictive empirical issues about possible future abuse. *If you let practice A happen now,* these arguments hold, *consequences B will occur, and they will be very, very bad.* To carry weight, there must be evidence to support such an argument; slope arguments take both causal and precedential forms in their efforts to provide such evidence, insisting either that practice A will cause consequence B, or that permitting practice A will set a precedent in the presence of which other causal forces will produce consequence B. Many versions of slope arguments in the end-of-life context point either to the suggestive character that some acts of assisted dying would have, thus causing more killing to occur, or to the way in which permitting some acts of assisted dying would loosen the barriers against killing and thus permit such forces as greed, impatience, prejudice, and so on to operate to produce killing on a wider scale.

The risks would be particularly great, many have argued, for those in vulnerable groups. For instance, Susan Wolf has sought to show that the impact of legalization would fall particularly heavily on women; Adrienne Asch has worried about the impact on people with disabilities; Leslie Francis has been concerned about the elderly. Still others have pointed to the likely impact of legalization on blacks and other racial minorities, on people with chronic illnesses, on people with mental illnesses, on people with developmental delays, and so on. To legalize assisted-dying practices at all would start the slide down this very treacherous slope, they have argued, particularly affecting vulnerable groups.

Patients need not even be members of vulnerable categories to be at risk of pressures from family, physicians, institutions, or social expectations in general. John Hardwig's well-known piece 'Is There a Duty to Die?' (1997) explored the way in which a person might come to think it appropriate to choose to end his life rather than constitute a 'burden' to his family. Were physician-assisted suicide a legal possibility, opponents argued, the pattern of reasoning Hardwig explores in his own case would also become expected of others in general. One would come to believe one had a 'duty to die.'

Virtually all opponents of assisted dying have employed some form of slippery-slope argument. For some, like Dan Callahan, Sissela Bok, and Yale Kamisar, the slippery-slope argument is a supplement to the view that intentionally causing death is morally wrong. For others, like Art Caplan, it is the central one: Caplan says that he would not object to physician aid-in-dying were it not for the risks of abuse. Much the same view characterized *When Death is Sought,* the report of the New York State Task Force on Life and the Law (1994), which took the risk of abuse as its primary reason for recommending against legalization of physician-assisted suicide. Similarly, the Canadian Supreme Court held in the 1993 case *Rodriguez v. British Columbia* that, although ALS patient Sue Rodriguez had good reason to want to end her life, the court could not permit her to do so because of the risks for others this would entail.

Even some proponents of physician-assisted suicide have been alert to the risks of the slippery slope. For instance, in an early paper titled 'Manipulated Suicide', I outlined the various mechanisms of potential abuse, including domestic abuse by families, professional abuse by physicians, and institutional abuse by health-care institutions, insurers, and government agencies, though I did not draw the conclusion that assisted dying ought therefore to be prohibited (Battin 1994: 195–204). Indeed, like many other proponents, I believe legalization and the openness it brings are the best protection against such abuse.

In the early days of the physician-assisted suicide debate, fuel was fed to the fire by data emerging from abroad: the Netherlands was beginning to recognize the legitimacy of voluntary active euthanasia and physician-assisted suicide. In a series of cases, euthanasia was increasingly legally tolerated, even though technically illegal, provided it met the guidelines for 'due care' established by the courts and the Royal Dutch Medical Association. The guidelines required that the patient's choice be voluntary and enduring; that the patient be undergoing or about to undergo intolerable suffering; that the patient have full information about his or her condition and prognosis; that all alternatives for relieving the suffering that are acceptable to the patient have been tried; that a second, independent physician be consulted; and that the physician report the action to the appropriate authorities. The physician who was faced with a conflict of duties between the obligation to prolong life and the obligation to relieve suffering would not be prosecuted for ending or helping end the patient's life under these guidelines, provided he or she acted with due care.

As news from the Netherlands began to reach the rest of the world, so did rumour. Opponents reacted to the developments in Holland with horror and also with distortion. Some, like Richard Fenigsen, a Dutch cardiologist, intimated that 20,000 people a year were being killed against their will; such grossly distorted claims were entertained or repeated by detractors around the world—for example, John Keown in England and a wide network of right-to-life writers in the USA.

The Dutch government issued a broad, systematic empirical study of end-of-life decisions known as the Remmelink Report in 1990, followed by two similar studies in 1995 and 2001 (see van der Maas 1996 and Onwuteaka-Philipsen 2003); these studies found that, in the period studied, somewhat over 3 percent of deaths were due to deliberately hastened death: voluntary active euthanasia, 2.5% of the total annual mortality of about 140,000, physician-assisted suicide, about 0.2%, and 'life-terminating treatment' where there was no current explicit request, about 0.7 percent (data from the 2001 study). In the 1990 study, there had been about 1,000 cases of euthanasia without current explicit consent; these notorious 'thousand cases' came to occupy a central role in the opponents' case against legalization in the USA and elsewhere, despite the fact that these cases nearly all involved people who had made antecedent enquiries or who were no longer competent and could no longer make requests (Pijnenborg et al. 1993). Proponents' pleas to look at the actual data emanating from the Netherlands, which does not exhibit a pattern of abuse and shows no victimization of vulnerable groups, have largely fallen on deaf ears.

Slippery-slope arguments are often extremely effective in swaying public opinion, and have been central to the opposition's case. Proponents, however, have argued that there is no adequate evidence to support the case against legalization of physician-assisted suicide and euthanasia, and what little evidence there is—especially that from the Netherlands—seems to cut the other way. The second report of the Remmelink Commission, covering all forms of assisted death in the Netherlands between 1990 and 1995, found that the rates of euthanasia and assisted suicide had not changed substantially since the first report five years earlier, and concluded that, 'in our view, these data do not support the idea that physicians in the Netherlands are moving down a slippery slope' (van der Maas et al. 1996: 1705). To the opposition's rebuttal that these studies covered only a decade and that the real danger lay in the future, proponents replied that the conclusions of slippery-slope arguments about social change can never be confirmed in advance of the future they predict. But neither can they be disconfirmed, at least in the broad social contexts in which they are usually used, and they have tremendous—though often unwarranted—persuasive power. Furthermore, slippery-slope arguments tend to be one-sided: used in the contexts of social debate, such arguments are almost always employed to present evidence favouring one side of a picture but not evidence favouring the other, and hence do not invite comparisons of value or probability assessment among various predicted outcomes. By their very nature, slippery-slope arguments tend to be unreliable—though, of course, this does not entail that the bad consequences predicted could not materialize.

The difficulties of slippery-slope arguments are well known to social commentators. Particularly troubling is the issue of the appropriate weight to be given to slope arguments versus other considerations. Suppose slippery-slope evidence did suggest that some patients would be abused—how should this weigh against the freedoms of other patients to make specific end-of-life choices? Slippery-slope arguments hold that practice *A* should be prevented in order to prevent undesirable outcome *B,* but in their usual forms do not assess arguments about the moral consequences of suppressing *A,* nor the relative likelihood that *B* and *A* will occur.

Meanwhile, heightened awareness of the conditions of dying invited renewed focus on the second central argument made by proponents for the ethical acceptability and legalization of assisted dying, which for some time had formed the core of its intuitive appeal. No patient should have to endure pointless terminal suffering, proponents of assisted dying argued, and, if pain cannot be controlled, then the patient should be able to avoid such suffering by means of an earlier, easier death. With this we return to the second principal component of the argument in favour of physician-assisted suicide, the argument that pain and suffering ought to be relieved where possible, sometimes also called the argument from mercy.

The Argument from Relief of Pain and Suffering (For)

No person should have to endure pointless terminal suffering. If the physician is unable to relieve the patient's suffering in other ways acceptable to the patient and the only way to avoid such suffering is by death, then as a matter of mercy death may be brought about.

- *Objection.* Thanks to techniques of pain management developed by Hospice and others, it is possible to treat virtually all pain and to relieve virtually all suffering.
  - *Counter-objection.* 'Virtually all' is not 'all'; if some pain or suffering cannot be treated, there will still sometimes be a need to avoid them by directly caused death.
    - *Counter-counter-objection.* Complete sedation can be used where pain cannot be controlled.
      - *Counter-counter-counter-objection.* Complete sedation means complete obtundation, and, because the patient can no longer communicate or perceive, is equivalent to causing death. If these are permitted, why not more direct methods of bringing about death?
- *Objection.* Even if it involves pain and suffering, the dying process can be valuable as a positive, transformative experience of new intimacy and spiritual growth.
  - *Counter-objection.* There can be no guarantee of a positive, transformative experience.

Allowing patients to try to avoid pain and suffering, proponents argued, would in some cases mean allowing physician-assisted suicide and, a few also argued, allowing euthanasia as well, at least euthanasia in its root sense, *eu-thanatos,* Greek for 'good death.' (Although in the USA and other countries the term 'euthanasia' was often understood in its post-Nazi sense as referring to politically motivated genocidal killing, in contrast, 'euthanasia' has been understood in the Netherlands in the Greek sense of 'good death.') The Netherlands provided a relevant example: in the Netherlands, euthanasia and physician-assisted suicide were coming to be legally tolerated for a person facing intolerable suffering (though not necessarily terminally ill), where that suffering could not be relieved by any methods acceptable to the patient (a patient with amyotrophic lateral sclerosis (ALS), or Lou Gehrig's

disease, could not be forced onto a respirator, for example): the avoidance of suffering was what was central. What counted as intolerable suffering was to be defined by the patient; there were no objective criteria for this.

As the increasing acceptance of assisted dying in the Netherlands was coming
to light, so also was a greater range of empirical data in the USA and elsewhere
about what actually was happening to dying patients. The conditions of dying in
America were bad: inadequately treated pain was rampant, choices were ignored,
patients were consigned to 'living deaths' hooked to tubes and machines, and medical science in its relentless drive for progress ignored the human well-being of
dying patients in favour of prolonging merely biological life. As the SUPPORT
study of 1995 found, half of conscious patients in a sample of tertiary-care hospitals
were reported by family members to have suffered moderate to severe pain (though
this may have involved other symptoms as well) at least 50 per cent of the time
during their last three days of life (SUPPORT Principal Investigators 1995). The
conditions of dying in America, as in many countries with advanced, highly technologically developed health-care systems, were often inhumane. Small wonder that
some patients might want to avoid them by an earlier, easier death.

In the public mind, however, the issue of physician-assisted suicide had come
to be associated with the name of Jack Kevorkian, MD, a retired anesthesiologist
who, more perhaps than any other person, kept the issue before the press. Kevorkian
was a crusader for legalization of physician-assisted suicide: again and again, he
assisted the suicides of people suffering from conditions ranging from Alzheimer
disease to ALS. He responded to patients' claims of untreatable, intolerable suffering; like the Dutch, he did not require that the patient be terminally ill. Over a
period of years, Kevorkian provided assistance in the suicides of well over 100
people; he was tried repeatedly, but it was not until he performed euthanasia by
injecting a lethal drug (rather than assisted in suicide by providing means of death
that the patient could operate him or herself) on nationwide television in 1998 that
he was convicted of second-degree murder and imprisoned. Kevorkian served in
the minds of many as the spectre of what could go wrong with physician-assisted
suicide, though he was a hero to others.

If Kevorkian was seen by some as the bad doctor, there was a good doctor on
the scene too, Timothy Quill, MD. Quill provided his leukaemia patient Diane with
a prescription for a lethal drug, which she took some months later, and he then
described his role in her death in the *New England Journal of Medicine* (Quill
1991). The ensuing legal events became one of the central episodes in the history
of the development of the assisted-dying argument: a New York State grand jury
simply refused to indict him. Articulate in expressing his conviction that a bad
death should be treated as a 'medical emergency'—that is, that it is urgent that the
physician act to help the patient avoid terminal suffering and pain—Quill also holds
the view that a physician's assistance in suicide should be a 'last resort,' that final
measure to turn to when all other ways of avoiding suffering have failed. Quill has
become one of the central, though more moderate, figures among proponents.

The argument from mercy, that pain and suffering are to be relieved, is understood to support the claim that good medicine involves helping a patient avoid
pain and suffering in dying, and that it is within the physician's role as reliever of

suffering to help a patient achieve an easier death. This concern is also central in the view of a number of other physicians. Marcia Angell, MD, associate editor and then editor of the *New England Journal of Medicine,* Christine Cassel, MD, and Howard Brody, MD, are among the more moderate voices on the scene, subscribing to Quill's view that physician-assisted suicide should be viewed as a 'last resort,' something to turn to only in the most difficult cases. Even if rare, such proponents argue, physician-assisted dying nevertheless needs legal protection. Still others believe it may be a reasonable, normal way of bringing life to an end.

But pain can be controlled, objects a chorus of physicians on the other side, opposing any form of assisted dying. Cicely Saunders, MD, one of the earliest and most revered figures in the controversy, has not merely claimed that pain can be controlled but has pioneered effective ways of doing so: she developed the Hospice technique, especially effective with cancer pain, of administering pain medication before the onset of pain symptoms, making it possible to break the cycle of recurrent breakthrough pain. Saunders is a true pioneer, having done perhaps more than any other to change the actual circumstances of dying in modern, highly technologically developed societies—the grim circumstances that provoked the original movement concerning voluntary euthanasia and assisted suicide. Palliative care, now a recognized medical speciality, focuses first on the recognition, treatment, and prevention of pain: its practitioners advocate better attention to pain management in terminally ill patients, more reliable assessment of pain, the use of escalating, ladder-type schedules of pain management, antecedent interception of pain before it begins (the technique pioneered by Hospice), and more thorough training of physicians and restructuring of provider incentives to provide better pain management. Palliative care also involves attention to the question of what to do in those cases in which pain cannot be adequately managed: here, it advocates the use of pain control even in contexts in which it is foreseen, though not intended, that a shorter life may result; and, in very extreme cases, it accepts the use of terminal sedation: sedating the terminally ill patient into unconsciousness, and then withholding or withdrawing artificial nutrition and hydration that would be required to keep an unconscious patient alive.

The first Hospice in the USA was opened in 1974, and since that time work in palliative care has been carried on by a wide range of pain specialists, including palliative-care and Hospice physicians like Kathleen Foley, MD, and Joanne Lynn, MD, both known for their work on pain, pain assessment, and social issues related to pain. Like many others who are opposed to the legalization of physician-assisted suicide and any form of euthanasia, these pain-specialist physicians see the solution to the public debate in improved methods of pain control, symptom control, and increased resources for pain research, as well as more thorough instruction for medical students and physicians in pain-control techniques, destruction of myths about addiction, and other forms of progress in palliative care. Better pain control means less call for assisted suicide, they say.

Pain control techniques do not always work, retort proponents of aid-in-dying. There are still some situations in which perfect pain control is not possible, and in any case there is an immense gap between theoretical capacities for pain control and the actual situations of dying. Not all patients receive the kind of expert palliative care that is theoretically possible, and in some cases even the theory is inadequate. Timothy Quill's urging that a bad death be regarded as a medical emergency is not an idle abstraction: there really are cases in which pain and suffering are intolerable.

To this charge, opponents of physician-assisted suicide—for example, philosopher Bernard Gert and physician Ira Byock—recommend the practice known as terminal sedation. Terminal sedation, they insist, allows the patient whose pain is intolerable to find relief, but still preserves the delicate line between killing and letting die. Terminal sedation has been the last-resort darling of many opponents in the debate.

Proponents of physician-assisted suicide—philosophers Gerald Dworkin and R. G. Frey come to mind—issue a double rejoinder. First, terminal sedation hardly preserves the line between killing and letting die: by sedating a patient and then failing to provide nutrition or hydration, the physician is foreseeably and deliberately ending his life; there is no safe line here. They claim that 'those who oppose medically assisted dying themselves favor policies that cannot be morally distinguished from the policies we favour and they oppose' (Dworkin et al. 1998:3). Dworkin and Frey's move here exposes the confusion of the opposition in trying to draw a line between allowing to die (which the opposition accepts) and causing to die (which it says it rejects); terminal sedation is functionally equivalent to killing the patient—that is, causing the end of his life. David Orentlicher puts the point more boldly: to accept terminal sedation, as the US Supreme Court did in its joint decision (1997) in *Washington v. Glucksberg* and *Vacco v. Quill,* is to 'embrace euthanasia.'

Secondly, perhaps more importantly, the unsatisfactoriness of recourse to terminal sedation shows that the avoidance of pain is not all there is to the debate. For some, maybe most, patients who seek assistance in dying, pain is not the issue as much as its control. This view—in many ways, a return to the autonomist view with which the debate started—is to some degree borne out by the data from the Netherlands covering the period 1985–2001 and from Oregon, where physician-assisted suicide has been legal since 1997. In the Netherlands, according to the Remmelink studies, pain is a factor in the choices of patients who receive euthanasia or assisted suicide in less than half the cases; it is the sole factor in just a tiny fraction. In the period during which assisted suicide has been legal in Oregon—from 1997 through 2003 there were 171 cases (Oregon Dept. of Human Services, 2004)—there is no evidence that there were any cases for pain alone. Patients fear future pain and want to avoid future hard deaths; but for most of them, it is retaining control, remaining capable of being the architects of their own lives, that is central. Even if all pain could be controlled—as terminal sedation will do, though in a way that proponents find unacceptable—this would not resolve the issue. Rather, the issue has to do with respecting terminally ill patients' own choices about how they want to die, rather than—as proponents would put it—forcing them to accept their physicians' or health-care institutions' models of appropriate terminal care.

In a sense, the debate at the moment stands right here. It is a stand-off between, on the one side, opponents who rely on the claim that pain can be controlled and that improvements in pain-control capacities are what is needed, and, on the other side, proponents who insist that the real issue is not only pain but autonomy, self-determination, and personal control.

The Skewed Nature of the Debate

Most of these arguments on both sides of the debate, including the five principal arguments sketched so far, merit exploration in much greater detail. This has been a schematic review, intended to provide a road map for fuller exploration. But the components of the argument examined so far must also all be seen as part of a larger, overall argument, a larger argument whose structure has itself become problematic. This is an issue about how the debates are conducted and what turf, so to speak, they occupy.

Take, as a specimen of the difficulty, the book *Euthanasia and Physician-Assisted Suicide: For and Against* (Dworkin et al. 1998), which, while admirable in many respects, illustrates the central problem at the core of the assisted dying debate. The authors of this short volume are three well-known philosophers mentioned earlier, Gerald Dworkin, R. G. Frey, and Sissela Bok. It is an excellent book, and its distinguished authors argue with considerable clarity, rigour, and sensitivity about many of the deepest issues in the euthanasia debates. This book has everything central to the debate: discussions of the difference between killing and letting die, the distinction between foreseeing and intending, the tenuous relationship between allowing and causing. It discusses the principle of double effect, the risks of the slippery-slope, the delicate matter of the integrity of the medical profession. Indeed, this small book is an excellent model of the entire debate.

But its structure tells us much about the debate as a whole. On the first page of the first chapter of this little book, Dworkin—arguing on the 'for' side of the issue, attacks the opposition, represented in this case by Kass, Siegler, and the view of other opponent physicians that 'doctors should not kill.' Only a few pages later, at the beginning of the second short chapter, Frey, likewise arguing the 'for' side of the debate, also begins by attacking the opposition: he shows how the opposition's position concerning pain control and terminal sedation fails to be coherent, and why, as we have seen earlier, the normative asymmetry often alleged between them does not hold. However, Sissela Bok, defending the 'against' view in the second part of the book, does something different: while she reviews some of the sorts of arguments Dworkin and Frey make, she largely addresses concerns about the social effects of acceptance or legalization of physician-aided dying.

All three authors are making moves entirely characteristic of the current debate, including all the moves we have already discussed here. What both Dworkin and Frey do, on the 'for' side, is to move straight to the attack against their opponents. Their argument is an adroit *reductio* in which contradictions in the opponents' position are exposed, pointing out that, although opponents of physician-assisted suicide say they do not accept physician-assisted suicide or euthanasia, they in fact accept practices like terminal sedation that are functionally equivalent to these. But, in running this clever, sophisticated argument, Dworkin and Frey, on the 'for' side, make a problematic move of their own. What they do is *assume* the principles on which their side of the argument is based, principles of autonomy and freedom from suffering, without explicitly or directly defending these principles.

We might assume that this defence would be easy to mount. The principle of autonomy, or self-determination, or liberty, is a familiar, fundamental principle in ethical theory, and might seem to need little direct defence. So too, it might be argued, is the principle that pain and suffering ought to be relieved where possible, perhaps a straightforward utilitarian claim. But neither Dworkin nor Frey, both philosophers of considerable distinction and skill, defends these issues directly, though here is where the really interesting philosophical work might occur.

Meanwhile, Bok, defending the 'against' position, exploits its strongest point: the slippery-slope argument sketched above that the legalization or acceptance of euthanasia or physician-assisted suicide would lead to pressures on vulnerable patients, that people would be edged or forced into dying when that was not their choice. While Bok considers other arguments, this is her central claim. Bok's concerns are important, crucial ones. But they are the only ones she considers decisive: thus one cannot join the discussion with her about anything else except this issue. Thus, both in their 'attack' against the opposition's position and in their direct discussion of the points Bok will raise, Dworkin and Frey are as it were lured into fighting the rest of the battle on what is essentially Bok's turf, the slippery-slope set of concerns about social effects. They score points against elements of her positions; but she gains the home-court advantage. Consequently, although defeated in the initial manœuvre and outclassed in the technical argumentation over the issues of causation and intention, Bok in a sense wins the day, even though the arguments she uses about the slippery slope are not fully persuasive. Her achievement lies in the fact that she is able to cast the slippery-slope issue as the *central* one, the one on which, it is assumed, views about legalization will stand or fall. Both sides end up allowing the slippery-slope issues of abuse to take the main court, and, implicitly, to be the issue on which practical policy measures like legalization turn. Dworkin and Frey argue that the slippery-slope argument does not succeed; Bok argues that it does; but all seem to agree that, if it did succeed, it would prove decisive in issues of policy. While this one small book—and it is a text intended for classroom use at that, in a series designed as 'For and Against'—is only a small part of the immense literature on euthanasia and physician-assisted suicide, it is uncannily representative of the skewed nature of the debate. This skewed argument is the not-so-good part of the debate I have wanted to explore.

There are two distinct problems with this relocation of the debate over euthanasia and physician-assisted suicide on slippery-slope turf. For one thing, as we have seen, slippery-slope arguments involve predictive empirical issues about possible future abuse, and the evidence for such claims cannot be firm; however, slippery-slope arguments cannot be disconfirmed either, at least not in the weak sense that undesirable consequences *B* could always follow *A*, whether or not they were actually caused by *A* or caused by some other force in the presence of *A* as a precedent. Slippery-slope arguments are always around; they rarely dissipate until long after the social change in question has already taken place. However, because of their power to persuade, especially in a broad, public context, slippery-slope arguments tend to block out other major concerns that should be regarded as central too, or perhaps as still more central. Thus, on both counts, the structure and location of the debate skew the answer.

There is an additional problem with the for-and-against structure of the euthanasia debate, also mirrored in the Dworkin, Frey, and Bok book. This structure of adversarial debate is used effectively in many areas of human discourse, including philosophy and in particular bioethics. A *for-and-against* argumentative format is not just a universally good idea; rather, a *for-and-against* format may or may not be appropriate to a particular topic, depending on, among other things, the degree of infancy or maturity of the debate. A new social and ethical issue, just breaking open into explicit debate when it may have been festering unrecognized beneath the surface of public consciousness for years, needs the kind of philosophical exploration that *for-and-against* analysis yields: the elements of the debate need to be isolated, identified, catalogued, and critiqued. But after a debate begins to mature, it becomes time to pursue attempts at resolution: here, the search should be for common elements, points of agreement, ways of reaching both practical and theoretical consensus about the issue at hand. There have been many, many *for-and-against* works on the issue of physician-aided dying, including treatises, popular articles, edited collections, and assemblages of amicus briefs to the US Supreme Court. The Dworkin, Frey, and Bok volume, like much of my own work, properly counts among these. Certainly, the debate has evolved considerably over time, so that proponents are less likely to argue for absolute-autonomy views that patients should be free to do whatever they want and are more likely to support guidelines and safeguards for the practice of physician-assisted suicide, while opponents are less likely to argue that patients have an obligation to try to continue to live at whatever cost and more likely to accept death-hastening strategies like disconnecting ventilators or undergoing terminal sedation. But there are comparatively few works that attempt to seek genuine consensus, though I believe the debate has now matured enough to demand them. New, evolved structures of reflective consideration, not just debate, will suit the issue better; it is time for all of us to move on.

The Possibility of Concession and Compromise

Two things must happen in the debate over physician-aided dying if it is to avoid calcification and extended political friction, as has been the case, for example, with the abortion debate. It has one advantage over the abortion debate that makes resolution seem more plausible; in the assisted-dying debate, unlike the abortion debate, there is no third party analogous to the fetus whose ontological status and vulnerability to harms are under dispute. However, in many other ways the assisted-dying debate has many of the trappings of the abortion debate: noisy rhetoric, hostile sides entrenched over an issue constructed as 'choice' versus 'killing,' and (though this remains more pronounced for the abortion debate) the development of a political 'litmus test' over the issue.

Nevertheless, there are some things that would make the assisted-dying debate far more open to resolution. First, the debate needs to enlarge the range within which it is conducted. This involves expanding the scope of the issue or issues that are seen as central beyond slippery-slope concerns to the positive case that is offered for accepting and legalizing euthanasia and/or physician-assisted suicide. There are basic philosophical issues here about autonomy and self-determination, freedom and control, about the moral issues in suicide: these need direct scrutiny.

As I have said, one might think these would be easy to defend. After all, the central notions of liberty—of self-determination and autonomy, about freedom to choose how to live one's life—are said to be central to the liberal traditions of Western culture. Here, popular discussion in the physician-assisted suicide debate may have an edge over academic dispute: chatlines, letters to the editor, popular books, and other vehicles of public discussion are full of ringing appeals to freedom, self-determination, and 'get-government-off-my-back' conceptions of individual liberty in matters of dying. But the philosophers are strangely reluctant to take these issues on, knowing, of course, how complex they can be. What is the appropriate scope of individual autonomy, anyway? This is an issue under debate throughout the entire history of philosophy, but still ready for fresh re-examination in the light of the new circumstances of dying.

Indeed, the discussion of autonomy in the context of death and dying might even help illuminate the issue of autonomy in general. If there are certain kinds of actions, like enslavement or murder, that one ought not to undertake, is bringing about one's own death one of them? How is such action to be described, in any case: as 'suicide', or 'self-deliverance', or 'aid-in-dying', or 'hastened death', or in any of the various euphemisms and derogatory labels employed in the public debates? Does an individual have a basic right to (try to) avoid pain and suffering, and, if so, is this perhaps the obverse of the right to pursue happiness, or is it rooted in some deeper, more basic interest? If, as Buchanan and Brock (1989) have argued, competence in decision making is task specific (one may be competent to decide whom to have watch the delivery of one's baby but not competent to decide what anaesthetic to use, or competent to refuse treatment but not competent to balance one's cheque book), the question remains whether competence to decide on a course of medical action that will result in one's death (like physician-assisted suicide while in severe, terminal pain) requires a high standard of competence (as is often assumed), or a low one, so that a terminally ill patient who is suffering severely and wants to die need not meet demanding standards of competence. It is not that these issues are unknown in the academic debates over physician-aided dying but that they have not been cast as *central;* it is the slippery-slope argument that has been largely cast as central, when it may well be secondary to these more fundamental conceptual issues. This is not to say that the slippery-slope argument is not important; it is, enormously so. But it is not the only important thing about this issue. Of course, to restructure the debate so that these more fundamental issues become central does not entail that the debate will be resolved in favour of the 'pro' side, but means only that the debate must focus more directly on the deeper issues at hand.

A centrist, consensus position beyond this for-and-against polarization may already seem to be emerging, particularly in practical medical contexts. The palliative-care movement in particular, as we have already seen, claims to offer a solution to the end-of-life dilemmas over pain and suffering that seem to have given rise to the issues of euthanasia and physician-assisted suicide in the first place: better pain control will mean less call for physician-assisted suicide, and, until such time as the science of pain control has been perfected, measures like terminal sedation can always be employed in cases of intractable terminal pain.

But while there is some progress here—indeed real growth—towards a more mature phase of the debate, I do not think its direction will be straight ahead. In almost every way the new attention being given to palliative care is an excellent development. But the construction of the position dedicated to palliative care as a *centrist* position is not, I think, fully warranted. It may seem to be so, since it elides the distinction between killing and letting die and thus may appear to dissolve it. But palliative care does not provide a compromise between the 'pro' and 'con' positions, at least not an adequate compromise, and it is not really centrist. While it permits more extensive pain control, and while it permits actions that are functionally equivalent to euthanasia and physician-assisted suicide, it still does not permit active euthanasia or physician-assisted suicide in the senses that many advocates have in mind. Palliative care answers just one of the underlying concerns of the 'pro' side, relief from pain and suffering; it does not address the other basic principle, autonomy, very well at all, particularly since such ostensible compromises as terminal sedation have the effect of placing the patient in a position of absolute loss of control while undergoing the sedation process. After all, many thinkers support the legalization of physician-assisted suicide and/or voluntary active euthanasia because they support the desire that some terminally ill patients express for control over the timing, character, and circumstances of their deaths— not so much because they fear pain, but because they want to be the architects of the ends of their lives. The palliative-care movement certainly represents progress towards a partial consensus, but it does not yet represent full resolution of the issues between the 'for' and 'against' sides of the debate.

A more mature phase of the intellectual discussion may also seem to be beginning. Some works advance the discussion towards resolution by reserving judgement on the theoretical and policy issues while exploring the realities of concrete application, whether the practices in question are legalized or remain underground. For example, the report of the American Psychological Association's task force on physician-assisted suicide includes an extended discussion of the multiple roles psychologists can play in end-of-life decisions as well as the practical considerations and challenges they face in becoming more active in the end-of-life arena. (American Psychological Association Working Group on Assisted Suicide 2000). The US Supreme Court's 1997 joint decision in *Washington v. Glucksberg* and *Vacco v. Quill* may also seem to be a comparatively mature, consensus-seeking decision, since it did not actually side with either the 'pro' or the 'con' factions in the debate (although, because the decision held that there is no constitutional right to physician-assisted suicide, it is sometimes seen as defeat for the 'pro' side); rather, it side-stepped the moral issue by turning the matter over to the individual states.

However, many discussions that claim to or are perceived to seek consensus are not fully successful: they still want resolution on one side or the other of the same continuing battle. For example, Linda Emanuel's 'Facing Requests for Physician-Assisted Suicide' (1998*a*) advises physicians how to deal with patients who seek assistance in suicide, and thus to some extent allows recognition of the issue, but, after a lengthy series of steps designed to deflect the patient into other forms of care, tells physicians to reject the request if it persists at the end: this is not compromise or resolution; this is to side with the 'against' faction, even after a seemingly sensitive discussion. More negatively, the Supreme Court's decision can be read not as paving the way for resolution, but as evasion of the issue. Meanwhile, also apparently unwilling to cooperate in the search for resolution, some writers on the 'pro' side continue to call for legalization without much attention to slippery-slope issues at all. It is difficult to find a writer with a foot firmly planted on each side of the fence, or, better still, for whom there is no longer any fence at all. I do not yet see the kind of genial, comprehensive summation of the issue that is sensitive to the concerns of both sides, one that manages synthesis without ignoring or trivializing the principal concerns on both sides, one that could be called a real resolution of the issues, one that could elicit consensus and agreement at both policy and practical levels.

On the contrary, many authors seem to assume the problem will just go away, if pain control can be sufficiently improved and medicine's enthusiasm for prolonging life beyond a reasonable point can be restrained. Others see a political pattern of worsening escalation as conservative politicians consider federal measures that would preclude the use of scheduled drugs for the purpose of ending life, leading Hemlock, Ergo!, Last Rights Publications, the Voluntary Euthanasia Research Foundation, and other right-to-die groups in the USA and abroad to develop new technologies for bringing about death that do not rely on prescription drugs at all. (I have discussed both these points at greater length elsewhere; see Chapters 15 and 17, this volume.) These 'NuTech' methods under development by the more resolute proponents include devices like hypoxic masks and tents, plastic bags (the 'Exit Bag'), helium inhalation devices, scuba-based 'Debreathers,' and other technologies for producing an easy death; they can be operated by family members or friends or by the patient him or herself. These NuTech measures have the effect of taking the matter of assisted suicide out of the hands of physicians altogether: the deed can be done within the intimate circle of patient, family, or friends, and the medical establishment is no longer involved. Like the Pain Relief Promotion Act and its successors developed by opponents of physician-assisted suicide, NuTech ups the stakes on the proponent side as well: the matter is now beyond medicine's control.

Perhaps real resolution is not possible and consensus a silly dream. But perhaps resolution and consensus are possible; it is the moment at which the current discussion ought to begin in earnest to try to seek them, and in the final section I want to sketch how I think this resolution might proceed. After all, these are not trivial social issues, and the circumstances in which these dilemmas arise—where, as a result of the epidemiological transition in the causes of mortality, death at the conclusion of long, terminal illness awaits an ever-increasing proportion of the population in the developed world—are what the future increasingly brings.

Can the Dispute over Physician-Assisted Suicide Be Resolved?

In my optimistic moments, I do think it is possible to reach resolution in this debate in a way that will satisfy most of the concerns of most parties to the debate. Consider the principal tension: autonomy, on the one hand, versus the risks of the slippery slope, on the other. Relief of pain, I think, along with concerns about the integrity of the medical profession and the moral status of killing, are comparatively secondary, since pain control is not really an *issue* but a matter of practical inadequacy (virtually all parties agree that pain control and access to it ought to be improved); since the intrinsic-wrongness-of-killing argument falls to its counterexamples of war and self-defence without adequate rebuttal, and since concerns about the integrity of the medical profession are so closely related to slippery-slope concerns. At root, what remains is a tension between what the patient really wants, at the deepest, most reflective level, and what limitations may be placed on his or her choices to protect the interests of other parties or society as a whole.

These are real tensions, not to be minimized; they explain why the slippery-slope issues have such prominence. But the tension can be reduced by reinspecting the temporal location of decision making about dying. Typically, medicine has been structured so that decisions about aspects of terminal care are delayed as long as possible, often until a crisis occurs and a decision must be made immediately. By this time, the patient is in distress, the family is in distress, and many peripheral aspects of the decision are swept aside. Advance directives play some role, but they have many deficiencies: they may have been executed in casual, inadequately informed circumstances, they may be too specific, too general, or not fully clear; and in any case they are often ignored. But, in typical decision-making situations, things need to be done right away: doctors are busy, schedules are tight; the readings on the monitors are already slipping. Decision making in crisis is different in character from reflective decision making well in advance, and part of what gives rise to the current tension over end-of-life decision making is the fact that institutional structures and conventional medical practice favour urgent, last-minute decision making rather than reflective anticipation. It is an institutional pattern, not necessarily a human one.

But the decisions at hand are decisions about issues basic to end-of-life care—about whether it may be acceptable to forgo or discontinue treatment in order to let death occur; about whether one should always try to obliterate pain completely, even at the cost of obliterating consciousness, or regard some pain as acceptable; about whether forgoing nutrition and hydration is a welcome strategy or a repugnant charade; and about whether active aid-in-dying is morally permissible or morally wrong. Patients—that is, people—often form their ideas about these things long in advance, indeed long before the start of an illness that might lead to practical questions about dying, and what they develop is a kind of personal philosophy about these issues—a more general, reflective view, often idiosyncratically their own, a view broad and deep enough to govern specific practical questions.

If decision making takes place earlier, in the more leisured space of life when real reflection is possible, it is far less likely to be decision making that is warped by intense institutional or familial pressures. Of course, patients cannot decide the precise details of their care far in advance, since it is not clear what illnesses and what circumstances will arise. And, of course, some patients change their minds over time, sometimes in response to specific life experiences. Just the same, patients can certainly indicate the kinds of things they would seek and they would avoid— their personal view, a view they develop and refine over time. To convey this personal philosophy is, we might say, to articulate a 'personal end-of-life policy'— it is to express what sorts of things one would favour and what one would not. This is not quite the same thing as executing an advance directive—that is, executing a restrictive, stipulative document with legal force and thus incurring many of the difficulties of combining formal advance directives with physician aid-in-dying (Francis 1993); it is rather a matter of making one's basic values and preferences a matter of record in one's medical history and in one's family's or friends' ongoing lore, revising it if it evolves, as the basis for all further discussion. Factors that contribute to one's 'personal policy' may include one's religious convictions or the absence of them, one's sense of the meaning of life, one's personal style as a risk-taker or risk-minimizer, and so on, but are hardly reducible to these. Advance reflective decision making—or, better, *advance personal policy making,* as it might be called, both satisfies the principle of autonomy but protects against the slippery slope, the two deepest core concerns in the debate. Some people will want the kind of terminal care that emphasizes palliation and uses only a limited range of means; others will want direct, open assistance in the self-termination of their own lives; still others will want many options in between. Advance directives in the conventional sense capture only a part of this, and they are characteristically executed much further along in a terminal process; they govern specific medical procedures once a terminal course has begun. *Advance personal policy making* is grander, if you will; it involves the antecedent, lifelong, philosophically reflective exploration and articulation of one's deeper commitments about living and dying, alert to shifts it may undergo but sensitive to the most basic elements of one's convictions. Advance directives, limited and specific as they characteristically are, might be seen as the tip of the personal-choice iceberg, so to speak—the telltale symptom of an underlying personal philosophy that could be expressed as a personal policy, but hardly the whole thing.

A second component is also necessary for full resolution. Briefly sketched, it involves the notion of a social 'default' disposition for troubling cases concerning death and dying. A default specifies what happens if no contrary instructions are specified instead: it is what you get if you do not choose something else. A full consensus might articulate a default policy about treatment of the dying, and this would be the standard, 'normal' way to resolve dilemmas about the prolongation of life, the control of pain, and so on, in the modern, industrialized world, where life characteristically ends after a prolonged period of deterioration or terminal illness. But the very notion of 'default' presupposes that there are other options as well, and a default arrangement is morally tolerable *only* provided it offers a fuller range of choice. (If there are no other options, it can hardly be said to be a 'default'.) Thus I can imagine an approach that concedes to conservatives some unease about the slippery slope and allows the establishment of a default (such a default might, for example, permit withholding and withdrawing treatment as well as the use of 'double-effect' opiates in controlling pain) but that does not establish terminal sedation or physician-aided dying as a norm; it would have to ensure that options remain open for alternative ways of approaching death. These alternatives would have to include both more conservative and more liberal options: seeking more extensive treatment even where it is viewed as futile, seeking terminal sedation, seeking physician-assisted suicide, and (perhaps) seeking voluntary active euthanasia. That there be other options besides the default, both more conservative and more liberal, is a non-negotiable demand.

This is not yet to explore this conjecture in full detail, but it is the kind of direction in which I think the discussion of euthanasia and physician-assisted suicide should now go, in both the public and the academic areas. The benefits of polarized, *for-and-against* discussion have now been largely gained in ongoing argument about assisted dying; it is time to turn to exploring the possibilities for resolution. *Advance personal policy making* together with public policy that recognizes a *default-with-other-options* may be only one of these, though I think it is a promising combination for both theory and practice. Certainly, there may be other fruitful avenues for exploration, but it is high time to turn to the consideration of such possibilities. After all, the majority of people in developed countries will die the kinds of deaths from diseases with long terminal courses in which these issues arise, and it is crucial to find ways of resolving the debates. If these debates continue to fuel public polarization and political controversy, it could make all our deaths worse; it resolution can be found, that would be a gain for us all.

Note

From Hugh LaFollette, ed., *Oxford Handbook of Practical Ethics.* Oxford: University Press, 2003, pp. 673–704. By permission of Oxford University Press.

Reference

American Psychological Association Working Group on Assisted Suicide and End of Life Decisions (2000). *Report to the Board of Directors.* Washington: American Psychological Association; http://www.apa.org/pi/aseolf.html.

Angell, Marcia (1997). Editorial: 'The Supreme Court and Physician-Assisted Suicide—the Ultimate Right'. *New England Journal of Medicine,* 336: 50–3.

Arras, John D. (1997). 'Physician-Assisted Suicide: A Tragic View.' *Journal of Contemporary Health Law and Policy,* 13: 361–89.

Asch, Adrienne (1998). 'Distracted by Disability.' *Cambridge Quarterly of Health Care Ethics,* 7/1: 77–87.

Baron, C. H., Bergstresser, C., Brock, D. W., Cole, G. F., Dorfman, N. S., Johnson, J. A. et al. (1996). 'A Model State Act to Authorize and Regulate Physician-Assisted Suicide.' *Harvard Journal of Legislation,* 33: 1–34.

Battin, Margaret P. (1982). *Ethical Issues in Suicide.* Englewood Cliffs, NJ: Prentice Hall; rev. ed. 1985; trade-titled *The Death Debate* (1996).

—— (1994). *The Least Worst Death: Essays in Bioethics on the End of Life.* Oxford: Oxford University Press.

———— (1998). 'Physician-Assisted Suicide: Safe, Legal, Rare?' in Battin et al. (1998), 63–72.

———— (2000). 'On the Structure of the Euthanasia Debate: A Review of Dworkin, Frey, and Bok, *Euthanasia and Physician-Assisted Suicide. For and Against,*' in Review Symposium on Euthanasia and Physician-Assisted Suicide. *Journal of Health Politics, Policy, and Law,* 25/2: 415–30.

———— (2001). 'New Life in the Assisted-Death Debate in the US: Scheduled Drugs vs. NuTech,' in A. Klijn, F. Mortier, M. Trappenburg, and M. Otlowski (eds.), *Regulating Physician-Negotiated Death* (special issue of *Recht der Werkelijkheid, Dutch/Flemish Journal of Law & Society*). s-Gravenhage: Elsevier, 49–63.

Battin, Margaret P., Rhodes, Rosamond, and Silvers, Anita (1998). *Physician-Assisted Suicide: Expanding the Debate.* New York: Routledge.

Beauchamp, Tom L. (ed.) (1996). *Intending Death: The Ethics of Assisted Suicide and Euthanasia.* Upper Saddle River, NJ: Prentice Hall.

Beauchamp, Tom L., and Perlin, Seymour (1978) (eds.), *Ethical Issues in Death and Dying.* Englewood Cliffs, NJ: Prentice Hall.

Brock, Dan W. (1993). *Life and Death: Philosophical Essays in Biomedical Ethics.* Cambridge: Cambridge University Press.

Brody, Howard (1992). 'Assisted Death—a Compassionate Response to a Medical Failure.' *New England Journal of Medicine,* 327: 1384–8.

Buchanan, Allen E., and Brock, Dan W. (1989). *Deciding for Others: The Ethics of Surrogate Decision Making.* Cambridge: Cambridge University Press.

Byock, Ira (1997*a*). 'Physician-Assisted Suicide is not an Acceptable Practice,' in R.F. Weir (ed.), *Physician-Assisted Suicide.* Bloomington, IN: University of Indiana Press, 107–35.

———— (1997*b*). *Dying Well: The Prospect for Growth at the End of Life.* New York: Riverhead Books.

Callahan, Daniel (1992). 'When Self-Determination Runs Amok.' *Hastings Center Report,* 22: 52–5.

———— (1993). *The Troubled Dream of Life: Living with Mortality.* New York: Simon & Schuster.

———— (1997). 'Self-Extinction: The Morality of the Helping Hand,' in Robert F. Weir (ed.), *Physician-Assisted Suicide.* Bloomington, IN: University of Indiana Press, 69–85.

Campbell, Courtney S. (1992). 'Sovereignty, Stewardship, and the Self: Religious Perspectives on Euthanasia,' in R.I. Misbin (ed.), *Euthanasia: The Good of the Patient, the Good of Society.* Frederick, MD: University Publishing Group, 165–82.

Caplan, Arthur L., Snyder, Lois and Faber-Langedoen, K. (2000). 'The Role of Guidelines in the Practice of Physician-Assisted Suicide.' University of Pennsylvania Center for Bioethics Assisted Suicide Consensus Panel. *Annals of Internal Medicine,* 132: 476–81.

Cassel, Christine K., and Meier, Diane E. (1990). 'Morals and Moralism in the Debate over Euthanasia and Assisted Suicide.' *New England Journal of Medicine,* 323: 750–2.

Cassell, Eric J. (1991). *The Nature of Suffering and the Goals of Medicine.* New York: Oxford University Press.

Conwell, Yates, and Caine, Eric (1991). 'Rational Suicide and the Right to Die—Reality and Myth.' *New England Journal of Medicine,* 325/15: 1100–3.

Dresser, Rebecca, and Whitehouse, Peter J. (1994). 'The Incompetent Patient on the Slippery Slope.' *Hastings Center Report,* 24/4: 6–12.

Dworkin, Gerald, Frey, R. G., and Bok, Sissela (1998). *Euthanasia and Physician-Assisted Suicide: For and Against.* Cambridge: Cambridge University Press.

Dworkin, Ronald (1993). *Life's Dominion—an Argument about Abortion and Euthanasia.* London: HarperCollins.

Dworkin, Ronald, Nagel, Thomas, Nozick, Robert, Rawls, John, Scanlon, Thomas, and Thomson, Judith Jarvis (1997). 'Assisted Suicide: The Philosophers' Brief.' *New York Review of Books* (27 Mar.), 41–7; also in Battin et al. (1998), app. C.

Emanuel, Ezekiel J., and Battin, Margaret P. (1998). 'What are the Potential Cost Savings from Legalizing Physician-Assisted Suicide?' *New England Journal of Medicine,* 339/ 3: 167–72.

Emanuel, Ezekiel J., Fairclough, D. L., Daniels, E. R., and Clarridge, B. R. (1996). 'Euthanasia and Physician-Assisted Suicide: Attitudes and Experiences of Oncology Patients, Oncologists, and the Public.' *Lancet,* 347: 1805–10.

Emanuel, Linda L. (1998*a*). 'Facing Requests for Physician-Assisted Suicide: Toward a Practical and Principled Clinical Skill Set.' *Journal of the American Medical Association,* 280/7: 643–47.

—— (ed.) (1998*b*). *Regulating How We Die: The Ethical, Medical, and Legal Issues Surrounding Physician-Assisted Suicide.* Cambridge, MA: Harvard University Press.

Feldman, Fred (1992). *Confrontations with the Reaper: A Philosophical Study of the Nature and Value of Death.* New York: Oxford University Press.

Fenigsen, Richard (1989). 'The Case against Dutch Euthanasia.' *Hastings Center Report,* 19: suppl. 22–30.

Field, M. J., and Cassel, Christine (1997) (eds.), *Approaching Death: Improving Care at the End of Life.* Washington: National Academy of Science Press.

Finnis, John (1995). 'A Philosophical Case against Euthanasia' and other essays in Keown (1995*b*), 23–36, 46–56, 62–72.

Foley, Kathleen M. (1991). 'The Relationship of Pain and Symptom Management to Patient Requests for Physician-Assisted Suicide.' *Journal of Pain and Symptom Management,* 6: 289–97.

—— (1997). 'Competent Care for the Dying Instead of Physician-Assisted Suicide.' *New England Journal of Medicine,* 336/1: 54–8.

Foley, Kathleen M., and Hendin, Herbert (1999). 'The Oregon Report. Don't Ask Don't Tell.' *Hastings Center Report,* 29: 37–42.

Foot, Philippa (1984). 'Killing and Letting Die,' in Jay L. Garfield and Patricia Hennessey (eds.). *Abortion and Legal Perspectives.* Amherst, MA: University of Massachusetts Press, 177–85.

Francis, Leslie Pickering (1993). 'Advance Directives for Voluntary Euthanasia: A Volatile Combination?' *Journal of Medicine and Philosophy,* 18/3: 297–322.

Gaylin, Willard, Kass, Leon R., Pellegrino, Edmund D., and Siegler, Mark M. (1988). 'Doctors Must Not Kill.' *Journal of the American Medical Association,* 259: 2139–40.

Gert, Bernard, Bernat, James L., and Mogielnicki, R. Peter (1994). 'Distinguishing between Patients' Refusals and Requests'. *Hastings Center Report,* 24/4: 13–15.

Glover, Jonathan (1977). *Causing Death and Saving Lives.* Harmondsworth: Penguin.

Gomez, Carlos F. (1991). *Regulating Death: Euthanasia and the Case of the Netherlands.* New York: Free Press.

Gorovitz, Samuel (1992). *Drawing the Line: Life, Death, and Ethical Choices in an American Hospital.* New York: Oxford University Press.

Hardwig, John (1997). 'Is There a Duty to Die?' *Hastings Center Report,* 27/2: 34–42.

Harris, John (1975). 'The Survival Lottery'. *Philosophy,* 50/191: 81–7.

—— (1985). *The Value of Life.* London: Routledge & Kegan Paul.

Hedberg, Katrina, Hopkins, David and Southwick, Karen (2002). 'Legalized Physician-

Assisted Suicide in Oregon, 2001'. *New England Journal of Medicine,* 346/6: 450–2, also citing data and references for previous years.

Hendin, Herbert (1996). *Seduced by Death: Doctors, Patients, and the Dutch Cure.* New York: W.W. Norton.

Humphry, Derek (1984–6). *Let Me Die Before I Wake.* Eugene, OR: Hemlock Society.

——— (1992). *Final Exit: The Practicalities of Self-Deliverance and Assisted Suicide for the Dying.* New York: Dell.

Humphry, Derek, and Clement, Mary (1998). *Freedom to Die: People, Politics, and the Right-to-Die Movement.* New York: St. Martin's Press.

Humphry, Derek, with Wickett, Ann (1978). *Jean's Way.* London and New York: Quartet Books.

Kamisar, Yale (1958). 'Some Non-Religious Views Against Proposed "Mercy Killing" Legislation.' *Minnesota Law Review,* 42: 966–1004.

Kamm, Frances M. (1993). *Morality, Mortality.* New York: Oxford University Press.

Kass, Leon (1993). 'Is There a Right to Die?' *Hastings Center Report* (Jan.–Feb.), 34–43.

Keown, John (1995a). 'Euthanasia in the Netherlands: Sliding Down the Slippery Slope?' *Notre Dame Journal of Law, Ethics, and Public Policy,* 9/2: 407–48.

——— (1995b). *Euthanasia Examined: Ethical, Clinical, and Legal Perspectives.* Cambridge: Cambridge University Press.

Kluge, Eike-Henner (1975). *The Practice of Death.* New Haven: Yale University Press.

Kübler-Ross, Elizabeth (1969). *On Death and Dying.* New York: Macmillan.

Kuhse, Helga (1987). *The Sanctity-of-Life Doctrine in Medicine: A Critique.* New York: Oxford University Press.

Kuhse, Helga, and Singer, Peter (1994). *Individuals, Humans, Persons: Questions of Life and Death.* Sankt Augustin: Academia Verlag.

Lynn, Joanne (1986) (ed.). *By No Extraordinary Means: The Choice to Forgo Life-Sustaining Food and Water.* Bloomington, IN: Indiana University Press.

——— (1992). 'Should Doctors Hasten Death?' *Dartmouth Medicine,* 17/2: 34–41.

Mayo, David J. (1983). 'Contemporary Philosophical Literature on Suicide: A Review'. *Suicide and Life-Threatening Behavior,* 13/4: 313–45.

Mayo, David J., and Wikler, Daniel (1979). 'Euthanasia and the Transition from Life to Death'. in M. Robinson and J. Pritchard (eds.), *Medical Responsibility: Paternalism, Informed Consent, and Euthanasia.* Clinton, NJ: Humana Press, 720–35.

Meier, Diane E. (1992). 'Physician-Assisted Dying: Theory and Reality'. *Journal of Clinical Ethics,* 3/1: 35–7.

Miller F. G., Quill, T. E., Brody, H., Fletcher, J. C., Gostin, L. O., Meier, D. E. (1994). 'Regulating Physician-Assisted Death'. *New England Journal of Medicine,* 331: 119–23.

Misbin, Robert I. (1992). *Euthanasia: The Good of the Patient, The Good of Society.* Frederick, MD: University Publishing Group.

Momeyer, Richard W. (1988). *Confronting Death.* Bloomington, IN: Indiana University Press.

New York State Task Force on Life and the Law (1994). *When Death Is Sought: Assisted Suicide and Euthanasia in the Medial Context.* Albany, NY: New York State Task Force on Life and the Law.

Noonan, John T. (1998). 'Dealing with Death'. *Notre Dame Journal of Law, Ethics, and Public Policy,* 112/2: 387–400.

Nuland, Sherwin B. (1994). *How We Die: Reflections on Life's Final Chapter.* New York: Knopf.

Olshansky, S. Jay, and Ault, A. Brian (1987). 'The Fourth Stage of the Epidemiologic

Transition: The Age of Delayed Degenerative Disease', in Timothy M. Smeeding et al. (eds.), *Should Medical Care Be Rationed By Age?* Totowa, NJ: Rowman & Littlefield, 11–43.

Olshansky, S. J., Rogers, R. G., Carnes, B. A., and Smith, L. (2000). 'Emerging Infectious Diseases: The Fifth Stage of the Epidemiologic Transition?' *World Health Statistics Quarterly,* 51/2–4: 207–17.

Onwuteaka-Philipsen, Bregje D., et al., 'Euthanasia and other end-of-life decisions in the Netherlands in 1990, 1995, and 2001.' *Lancet* 263, (2003): 395–399.

Oregon Department of Human Services, *Sixth Annual Report on Oregon's Death with Dignity Act,* March 10, 2004, www.dhs.state.or.us/publichealth/chs/pas/ar-index/cfm.

Orentlicher, David (1997). 'The Supreme Court and Physician-Assisted Suicide: Rejecting Assisted Suicide but Embracing Euthanasia'. *New England Journal of Medicine,* 337: 1236–9.

Pijnenborg, Loes, van der Maas, Paul J., van Delden, Johannes J. M., and Looman, Caspar W. N. (1993). 'Life Terminating Acts without Explicit Request of Patient'. *Lancet,* 341: 1196–9.

Pius XII (1958). 'The Prolongation of Life' (address to a congress of anaesthesiologists), in *The Pope Speaks,* 4/4: 393–8.

Prado, C. G. (1998). *The Last Choice: Preemptive Suicide in Advanced Age.* 2nd edn. Westport, CT: Praeger.

Quill, Timothy E. (1991). 'Death and Dignity—a Case of Individualized Decision Making'. *New England Journal of Medicine,* 324/10: 691–4.

——— (1996). *A Midwife through the Dying Process: Stories of Healing and Hard Choices at the End of Life.* Baltimore: Johns Hopkins University Press.

Quill, Timothy E., Cassel, Christine, and Meier, Diane E. (1992). 'Care of the Hopelessly Ill—Proposed Clinical Criteria for Physician Assisted Suicide'. *New England Journal of Medicine,* 327/19: 1380–4.

Quill, Timothy E., Dresser, Rebecca, and Brock, Dan W. (1997). 'The Rule of Double Effect—a Critique of its Role in End-of-Life Decision Making'. *New England Journal of Medicine,* 337: 1768–71.

Rachels, James (1975). 'Active and Passive Euthanasia'. *New England Journal of Medicine,* 292: 78–80. (Follow-up articles in Steinbock and Norcross 1994.)

——— (1986). *The End of Life: Euthanasia and Morality.* New York: Oxford University Press.

Rodriguez v. British Columbia 519, 3 SCR (1993).

Rosenberg, Jay F. (1982). *Thinking Clearly About Death.* Englewood Cliffs, NJ: Prentice Hall.

Saunders, Cicely (1976). 'Living with Dying'. *Values and Ethics in Health Care,* 1: 227–42.

Singer, Peter (1987). 'Uncertain Voyage,' in Philip Pettit (ed.), *Metaphysics and Morality.* New York: Blackwell, 154–72.

Society for Health and Human Values (1995). *Physician-Assisted Suicide: Toward a Comprehensive Understanding.* Report of the Task Force on Physician-Assisted Suicide of the Society for Health and Human Values. *Academic Medicine,* 70: 583–90.

Steinbock, Bonnie, and Norcross, Alastair (1994) (eds.), *Killing and Letting Die.* 2nd edn. New York: Fordham University Press.

SUPPORT Principal Investigators (1995). 'A Controlled Trial to Improve Care for Seriously Ill Hospitalized Patients: The Study to Understand Prognoses and Preferences for Outcomes and Risks of Treatments (SUPPORT).' *Journal of the American Medical Association,* 274/20: 1951–98.

Tolle, Susan W., and Snyder, Lois (1996). 'Physician-Assisted Suicide Revisited: Comfort and Care at the End of Life,' in Lois Snyder (ed.), *Ethical Choices: Case Studies for Medical Practice*. Philadelphia: American College of Physicians, 17–23.

Vacco v. Quill, 521 US 793 (1997).

van der Maas, Paul J., van Delden, Johannes J. M., and Pijnenborg, Loes (1992). *Euthanasia and other Medical Decisions Concerning the End of Life: An Investigation Performed upon Request of the Commission of Inquiry into the Medical Practice Concerning Euthanasia* [known as the Remmelink Report], published in full in English as a special issue of *Health Policy,* 22/1–2.

van der Maas, Paul J. et al. (1996). 'Euthanasia, Physician-Assisted Suicide and Other Medical Practices Involving the End of Life in the Netherlands, 1990–1995' [known as the second Remmelink Report]. *New England Journal of Medicine,* 335/22: 1699–705.

van der Wal, Gerrit et al. (1996). 'Evaluation of the Notification Procedure for Physician-Assisted Death in the Netherlands.' *New England Journal of Medicine,* 335/22: 1706–11.

Wanzer, Sidney H., Federman, D. D., Adelstein, S. J., Cassel, C. K., Cassem, E. H., Cranford, R. D. et al. (1989). 'The Physician's Responsibility toward Hopelessly Ill Patients: A Second Look.' *New England Journal of Medicine,* 320: 844–8.

Washington v. Glucksberg, 521 US 702 (1997).

Weir, Robert F. (ed.) (1997). *Physician-Assisted Suicide*. Bloomington, IN: Indiana University Press.

Wildes, Kevin W. (1993). 'Conscience, Referral, and Physician-Assisted Suicide.' *Journal of Medicine and Philosophy,* 18/3: 323–8.

Wolf, Susan (1996). 'Physician-Assisted Suicide in the Context of Managed Care.' *Duquesne Law Review,* 34: 455–79.

2

Euthanasia

The Way We Do It, the Way They Do It

Because we tend to be rather myopic in our discussions of death and dying, especially about the issues of active euthanasia and assisted suicide, it is valuable to place the question of how we go about dying in an international context. We do not always see that our own cultural norms may be quite different from those of other nations and that our background assumptions and actual practices differ dramatically—even when the countries in question are all developed industrial nations with similar cultural ancestries, religious traditions, and economic circumstances. I want to explore the three rather different approaches to end-of-life dilemmas prevalent in the United States, the Netherlands, and Germany—developments mirrored in Australia, Belgium, Switzerland, and elsewhere in the developed world—and consider how a society might think about which model of approach to dying is most appropriate for it.

Three Basic Models of Dying

The Netherlands, Germany, and the United States are all advanced industrial democracies. They all have sophisticated medical establishments and life expectancies over 75 years; their populations are all characterized by an increasing proportion of older persons. They are all in what has been called the fourth stage of the epidemiologic transition[1]—that stage of societal development in which it is no longer the case that the majority of the population dies of acute parasitic or infectious diseases, often with rapid, unpredictable onsets and sharp fatality curves (as was true in earlier and less developed societies); rather, in modern industrial societies, the majority of a population—estimated in Europe at about 66–71%—dies of degenerative diseases, especially delayed-degenerative diseases that are characterized by late, slow onset and extended decline.[2] This is the case throughout the developed world. Accidents and suicide claim some, as do infectious diseases like AIDS, pneumonia, and influenza, but most people in highly industrialized countries die from heart disease (by no means always suddenly fatal); cancer; atherosclerosis; chronic obstructive pulmonary disease; diabetes, liver, kidney, or other organ disease; or degenerative neurological disorders. In the developed world, we die not so much from attack by outside diseases but from gradual disintegration. Thus, all three of these modern industrial countries—the United States, the Netherlands, and Germany—are alike in facing a common problem: how to deal with the characteristic new ways in which we die.

Dealing with Dying in the United States

In the United States, we have come to recognize that the maximal extension of life-prolonging treatment in these late-life degenerative conditions is often inappropriate. Although we could keep the machines and tubes—the respirators, intravenous lines, feeding tubes—hooked up for extended periods, we recognize that this is inhumane, pointless, and financially impossible. Instead, as a society we have developed a number of mechanisms for dealing with these hopeless situations, all of which involve withholding or withdrawing various forms of treatment.

Some mechanisms for withholding or withdrawing treatments are exercised by the patient who is confronted by such a situation or who anticipates it. These include refusal of treatment, the patient-executed do-not-resuscitate (DNR) order, the living will, and the durable power of attorney. Others are mechanisms for decision by second parties about a patient who is no longer competent or never was competent, reflected in a long series of court cases from *Quinlan, Saikewicz, Spring, Eichner, Barber, Bartling, Conroy, Brophy,* and the trio *Farrell, Peter,* and *Jobes* to *Cruzan.* These cases delineate the precise circumstances under which it is appropriate to withhold or withdraw various forms of therapy, including respiratory support, chemotherapy, dialysis, antibiotics in intercurrent infections, and artificial nutrition and hydration. Thus, during the past quarter-century, roughly since *Quinlan* (1976), the United States has developed an impressive body of case law and state statutes that protects, permits, and facilitates the characteristic American strategy of dealing with end-of-life situations. These cases provide a framework for withholding or withdrawing treatment when physicians and family members believe there is no medical or moral point in going on. This has sometimes been termed *passive euthanasia;* more often it is simply called *allowing to die.*

Indeed, "allowing to die" has become ubiquitous in the United States. For example, a 1988 study found that of the 85% of deaths in the United States that occurred in health-care institutions, including hospitals, nursing homes, and other facilities, about 70% involved electively withholding some form of life-sustaining treatment.[3] A 1989 study found that 85–90% of critical care professionals said they were withholding or withdrawing life-sustaining treatments from patients who were "deemed to have irreversible disease and are terminally ill."[4] A 1997 study of limits to life-sustaining care found that between 1987–88 and 1992–93, recommendations to withhold or withdraw life support prior to death increased from 51% to 90% in the intensive-care units studied.[5] Rates of withholding therapy such as ventilator support, surgery, and dialysis were found in yet another study to be substantial, and to increase with age.[6] A 1994/95 study of 167 intensive-care units—all the ICUs associated with U.S. training programs in critical care medicine or pulmonary and critical care medicine—found that in 75% of deaths, some form of care was withheld or withdrawn.[7] It has been estimated that 1.3 million American deaths a year follow decisions to withhold life support;[8] this is a majority of the just over 2 million American deaths per year.

In recent years, the legitimate use of withholding and withdrawing treatment has increasingly been understood to include practices likely or certain to result in death. The administration of escalating doses of morphine in a dying patient, which, it has been claimed, will depress respiration and so hasten death, is accepted under the (Catholic) principle of double effect, provided the medication is intended to relieve pain and merely foreseen but not intended to result in death; this practice is not considered killing or active hastening of death. The use of "terminal sedation," in which a patient dying in pain is sedated into unconsciousness while artificial nutrition and hydration are withheld, is also recognized as medically and legally acceptable; it too is understood as a form of "allowing to die," not active killing. With the single exception of Oregon, where physician-assisted suicide became legal in 1997,[9] withholding and withdrawing treatment and related forms of allowing to die are the only legally recognized ways we in the United States go about dealing with dying. A number of recent studies have shown that many physicians—in all states studied—do receive requests for assistance in suicide or active euthanasia and that a substantial number of these physicians have complied with one or more such requests; however, this more direct assistance in dying takes place entirely out of sight of the law. Except in Oregon, *allowing to die,* but not *causing to die,* has been the only legally protected alternative to maximal treatment legally recognized in the United States; it remains America's—and American medicine's—official posture in the face of death.

Dealing with Dying in the Netherlands

In the Netherlands, although the practice of withholding and withdrawing treatment is similar to that in the United States, voluntary active euthanasia and physician assistance in suicide are also available responses to end-of-life situations.[10] Active euthanasia, understood as the termination of the life of the patient at the patient's explicit and persistent request, is the more frequent form of directly assisted dying, and most discussion in the Netherlands has concerned it rather than assistance in suicide, though the conceptual difference is not regarded as great: many cases of what the Dutch term *euthanasia* involve initial self-administration of the lethal dose by the patient but procurement of death by the physician, and many cases of what is termed *physician-assisted suicide* involve completion of the lethal process by the physician if a self-administered drug does not prove fully effective. Although until

2002 they were still technically illegal under statutory law—and even with legalization remain an "exception" to those provisions of the Dutch Penal Code that prohibit killing on request and intentional assistance in suicide—active euthanasia and assistance in suicide have long been widely regarded as legal, or rather *gedoogd,* legally "tolerated," and have in fact been deemed justified (not only non-punishable) by the courts when performed by a physician if certain conditions were met. Voluntary active euthanasia (in the law, called "life-ending on request") and physician-assisted suicide are now fully legal by statute under these guidelines. Dutch law protects the physician who performs euthanasia or provides assistance in suicide from prosecution for homicide if these guidelines, known as the conditions of "due care," are met.

Over the years, the guidelines have been stated in various ways. They contain six central provisions:

1. That the patient's request be voluntary and well-considered
2. That the patient be undergoing or about to undergo intolerable suffering, that is, suffering that is lasting and unbearable
3. That all alternatives acceptable to the patient for relieving the suffering have been tried, and that in the patient's view there is no other reasonable solution
4. That the patient have full information about his or her situation and prospects
5. That the physician consult with a second physician who has examined the patient and whose judgment can be expected to be independent
6. That in performing euthanasia or assisting in suicide, the physician act with due care

Of these criteria, it is the first that is held to be central: euthanasia may be performed only at the *voluntary* request of the patient. This criterion is also understood to require that the patient's request be a stable, enduring, reflective one—not the product of a transitory impulse. Every attempt is to be made to rule out depression, psychopathology, pressures from family members, unrealistic fears, and other factors compromising voluntariness, though depression is not in itself understood to necessarily preclude such choice. Euthanasia may be performed *only* by a physician, not by a nurse, family member, or other party.

In 1991, a comprehensive, nationwide study requested by the Dutch government, popularly known as the Remmelink Commission report, provided the first objective data about the incidence of euthanasia and physician-assisted suicide.[11] This study also provided information about other medical decisions at the end of life, particularly withholding or withdrawal of treatment and the use of life-shortening doses of opioids for the control of pain, as well as direct termination. The Remmelink report was supplemented by a study focusing particularly carefully on the characteristics of patients and the nature of their euthanasia requests.[12] Five years later, the researchers from these two studies jointly conducted a major new nationwide study replicating much of the previous Remmelink inquiry, providing empirical data both about current practice in the Netherlands and change over a five-year period.[13] A third replication of the nationwide study was published in 2003.[14]

About 140,000 people die in the Netherlands every year, and of these deaths, about 30% are sudden and unexpected, while the majority are predictable and foreseen, usually the result of degenerative illness comparatively late in life. Of the total deaths in the Netherlands, according to the 2001 data, about 20.2% involve decisions to withhold or withdraw treatment in situations where continuing treatment would probably have prolonged life; another 20.1% involve the "double effect" use of opioids to relieve pain but in dosages probably sufficient to shorten life. Only a small fraction of people who die do so by euthanasia—about 2.4%—and an even smaller fraction, 0.2%, do so by physician-assisted suicide. Of patients who do receive euthanasia or physician-assisted suicide, about 80 percent have cancer, while 3% have cardiovascular disease and 4% neurological disease, primarily ALS.

However, the 1990 Remmelink report had also revealed that another 0.8% of patients who died did so as the result of life-terminating procedures not technically called euthanasia, without explicit, current request. These cases, known as "the 1000 cases," unleashed highly exaggerated claims that patients were being killed against their wills. In fact, in about half of these cases, euthanasia had been previously discussed with the patient or the patient had expressed in a previous phase of the disease a wish for euthanasia if his or her suffering became unbearable ("Doctor, please don't let me suffer too long"); and in the other half, the patient was no longer competent and was near death, clearly suffering grievously although verbal contact had become impossible.[15] In 91% of these cases without explicit, current request, life was shortened by less than a week, and in 33% by less than a day.

Over the next decade, as revealed in the 1995 and 2003 nationwide studies, the proportion of cases of euthanasia rose slightly (associated, the authors conjectured, with the aging of the population and an increase in the proportion of deaths due to cancer, that condition in which euthanasia is most frequent); the proportion of cases of assisted suicide had remained about the same. The proportion of cases of life termination without current explicit request declined slightly to 0.7%, down from the notorious 1,000 to about 900. In 1990, a total of 2.9% of all deaths had involved euthanasia and related practices; by 2001 this total was about 3.7%.[16] In the early days of openly tolerated euthanasia, comparatively few cases were reported as required to the Public Prosecutor; there has been a dramatic gain since reporting procedures have been revised to require reporting to a review committee rather than to the police, and about 54% are now reported. However, there are no major differences between reported and unreported cases in terms of the patient's characteristics, clinical conditions, or reasons for the action.[17] Euthanasia is performed in about 1:25 of deaths that occur at home, about 1:75 of hospital deaths, and about 1:800 of nursing home deaths. The Netherlands has now established regional review committees for such cases and has initiated hospice-style pain management programs complete with 24-hour phone-in consultation services for physicians confronted by euthanasia requests.

Although euthanasia is thus not frequent, a small fraction of the total annual mortality, it is nevertheless a conspicuous option in terminal illness, well known to both physicians and the general public. There has been very widespread public discussion of the issues that arise with respect to euthanasia during the last quarter-century, and surveys of public opinion show that public support for a liberal euthanasia policy has been growing: from 40% in 1966 to 81% in 1988, then to about 90% by 2000. Doctors, too, support the practice, and although there has been a vocal opposition group, it has remained in the clear minority. Some 57% of Dutch physicians say that they have performed euthanasia or provided assistance in suicide, and an additional 30% say that although they have not actually done so, they can conceive of situations in which they would be prepared to do so. Ten percent say they would never perform it but would refer the patient to another physician. The proportion of physicians who say they not only would not do so themselves but would not refer a patient who requested it to a physician who would dropped from 4% in 1990 to 3% in 1995 to 1% in 2001. Thus, although many physicians who have performed euthanasia say that they would be most reluctant to do so again and that "only in the face of unbearable suffering and with no alternatives would they be prepared to take such action,"[18] all three nationwide studies have shown that the majority of Dutch physicians accept the practice. Surveying the changes over the 5-year period between 1990 and 1995, the authors of the nationwide study also commented that the data do not support claims of a slippery slope.[19] Work now in progress shows no such pattern either.[20]

In general, pain alone is not the basis for deciding upon euthanasia, since pain can, in most cases, be effectively treated. Only a third of Dutch physicians think that adequate pain control and terminal care make euthanasia redundant, and that number has been dropping. Rather, the "intolerable suffering" mentioned in the second criterion is understood to mean suffering that is intolerable in the patient's (rather than the physician's) view, and can include a fear of or unwillingness to endure *entluistering,* that gradual effacement and loss of personal identity that characterizes the end-stages of many terminal illnesses. In very exceptional circumstances, the Supreme Court ruled in the *Chabot* case of 1994, physician-assisted suicide may be justified for a patient with nonsomatic, psychiatric illness like intractable depression, but such cases are extremely rare and require heightened scrutiny.

In a year, about 35,000 patients seek reassurance from their physicians that they will be granted euthanasia if their suffering becomes severe; there are about 9,700 explicit requests, and about two-thirds of these are turned down, usually on the grounds that there is some other way of treating the patient's suffering. In 14% of cases in 1990, the denial was based on the presence of depression or psychiatric illness.

In the Netherlands, many hospitals now have protocols for the performance of euthanasia; these serve to ensure that the legal guidelines have been met. However, euthanasia is often practiced in the patient's home, typically by the general practitioner who is the patient's long-term family physician. Euthanasia is usually performed after aggressive hospital treatment has failed to arrest the patient's terminal illness; the patient has come home to die, and the family physician is prepared to ease this passing. Whether practiced at home or in the hospital, it is believed that euthanasia usually takes place in the presence of the family members, perhaps the visiting nurse, and often the patient's pastor or priest. Many doctors say that performing euthanasia is never easy but that it is something they believe a doctor ought to do for his or her patient when the patient genuinely wants it and nothing else can help.

Thus, in the Netherlands a patient who is facing the end of life has an option not openly practiced in the United States, except Oregon: to ask the physician to bring his or her life to an end. Although not everyone in the Netherlands does so—indeed, over 96% of people who die in a given year do not do so in this way—it is a choice legally recognized and widely understood.

Facing Death in Germany

In part because of its very painful history of Nazism, German medical culture has insisted that doctors should have no role in directly causing death. As in the other countries with advanced medical systems, withholding and withdrawing of care is widely used to avoid the unwanted or inappropriate prolongation of life when the patient is already dying, but there has been vigorous and nearly universal opposition in German public discourse to the notion of active euthanasia, at least in the horrific, politically motivated sense associated with Nazism. In the last few years, some Germans have begun to approve of euthanasia in the Dutch sense, based on the Greek root, *eu-thanatos,* or "good death," a voluntary choice by the patient for an easier death, but many Germans still associate euthanasia with the politically motivated exterminations by the Nazis and view the Dutch as stepping out on a dangerously slippery slope.

However, although under German law killing on request (including voluntary euthanasia) is illegal, German law has not prohibited assistance in suicide since the time of Frederick the Great (1742), provided the person is *tatherrschaftsfähig,* capable of exercising control over his or her actions, and also acting out of *freiverantwortliche Wille,* freely responsible choice. Doctors are prohibited from assistance in suicide not by law but by the policies and code of ethics of the Bundesärztekammer, the German medical association.[21] Furthermore, any person, physician or otherwise, has a duty to rescue a person who is unconscious. Thus, medical assistance in suicide is limited, but it is possible for a family member or friend to assist in a person's suicide, for instance by providing a lethal drug, as long as the person is competent and acting freely and the assister does not remain with the person after unconsciousness sets in.

Taking advantage of this situation, a private organization, the Deutsche Gesellschaft für Humanes Sterben (DGHS), or German Society for Dying in Dignity, has developed; it provides support to its very extensive membership in many end-of-life matters, including choosing suicide as an alternative to terminal illness. Of course, not all Germans are members of this organization, and many are not sympathetic with its aims, yet the notion of self-directed ending of one's own life in terminal illness is widely understood as an option. Although since 1993 the DGHS has not itself supplied such information for legal reasons, it tells its members how to obtain the booklet "Departing Drugs," published in Scotland, and other information about ending life, if they request it, provided they have been a member for one year and have not received medical or psychotherapeutic treatment for depression or other psychiatric illness during the last three years. The information includes a list of prescription drugs, together with the specific dosages necessary for producing a certain, painless death. The DGHS does not itself sell or supply lethal drugs;[22] rather, it recommends that the member approach a physician for a prescription for the drug desired, asking, for example, for a barbiturate to help with sleep. If necessary, the DGHS has been willing to arrange for someone to obtain drugs from neighboring countries, including France, Italy, Spain, Portugal, and Greece, where they may be available without prescription. It also makes available the so-called Exit Bag, a plastic bag used with specific techniques for death by asphyxiation. The DGHS provides and trains family members in what it calls *Sterbebegleitung* (accompaniment in dying), which may take the form of simple presence with a person who is dying but may also involve direct assistance to a person who is committing suicide, up until unconsciousness sets in. The *Sterbebegleiter* is typically a layperson, not someone medically trained, and physicians play no role in assisting in these cases of suicide. Direct active *Sterbehilfe*—active euthanasia—is illegal under German law. But active indirect *Sterbehilfe,* understood as assistance in suicide, is not illegal, and the DGHS provides counseling in how a "death with dignity" may be achieved in this way.

To preclude suspicion by providing evidence of the person's intentions, the DGHS also provides a form—printed on a single sheet of distinctive purple paper—to be signed once when joining the organization, documenting that the person has reflected thoroughly on the possibility of "free death" *(Freitod)* or suicide in terminal illness as a way of releasing oneself from severe suffering, and expressing the intention to determine the time and character of one's own death. The person then signs this "free death directive" or "suicide decision declaration" *(Freitodverfügung)* again at the time of the suicide, leaving it beside the body as evidence that the act is not impetuous or coerced. The form also requests that, if the person is discovered before the suicide is complete, no rescue measures be undertaken. Because assisting suicide is not illegal in Germany (provided the person is competent and in control of his or her own will, and thus not already unconscious), there has been no legal risk for family members, the *Sterbebegleiter,* or others in reporting information about the methods and effectiveness of suicide attempts, and, at least in the past, the DGHS has encouraged its network of regional bureaus, located in major cities throughout the country, to facilitate feedback. On this basis it has regularly updated and revised the drug information provided. There has been no legal risk in remaining with the patient to assist him or her at the bedside—that is, at least until recent legal threats.

Open, legal assistance in suicide has been supported by a feature of the German language that makes it possible to conceptualize it in a comparatively benign way. While English, French, Spanish, and many other languages have just a single primary word for suicide, German has four: *Selbstmord, Selbsttötung, Suizid,* and *Freitod,* of which the latter has comparatively positive, even somewhat heroic connotations.[23] Thus German speakers can think about the deliberate termination of their lives in a linguistic way not easily available to speakers of other languages. The negatively rooted term *Selbstmord* ("self-murder") can be avoided; the comparatively neutral terms *Selbsttötung* ("self-killing") and *Suizid* ("suicide") can be used, and the positively rooted term *Freitod* ("free death") can be reinforced. The DGHS has frequently used *Freitod* rather than German's other, more negative terms to describe the practice with which it provides assistance.

No reliable figures are available about the number of suicides with which the DGHS has assisted, and, as in the Netherlands and Oregon, the actual frequency of directly assisted death is probably small: most Germans who die as a result of medical decision making, like most Dutch and most Americans, die as treatment is withheld or withdrawn or as opiates are administered in doses that foreseeably but not intentionally shorten life—that is, by being "allowed to die." Yet it is fair to say, both because of the legal differences and the different conceptual horizons of German-speakers, that the option of self-produced death outside the medical system is more clearly open in Germany than it has been in the Netherlands or the United States.

In recent years, the DGHS has decreased its emphasis on suicide, now thinking of it as a "last resort" when pain control is inadequate—and turned much of its attention to the development of other measures for protecting the rights of the terminally ill, measures already available in many other countries. It distributes newly legalized advance directives, including living wills and durable powers of attorney, as well as organ-donation documents. It provides information about pain control, palliative care, and Hospice. It offers information about suicide prevention. Yet, despite various legal threats, it remains steadfast in defense of the terminally ill patient's right to self-determination, including the right to suicide, and continues to be supportive of patients who make this choice.

To be sure, assisted suicide is not the only option open to terminally ill patients in Germany, and the choice may be infrequent. Reported suicide rates in Germany are only moderately higher than in the Netherlands or the United States, though there is reason to think that terminal-illness suicides in all countries are often reported as deaths from the underlying disease. Although there is political pressure from right-to-die organizations to change the law to permit voluntary active euthanasia in the way understood in the Netherlands, Germany is also seeing increasing emphasis on help in dying, like that offered by Hospice, that does not involve direct termination. Whatever the pressures, the DGHS is a conspicuous, widely known organization, and many Germans appear to be aware that assisted suicide is available and not illegal even if they do not use its services.

Objections to the Three Models of Dying

In response to the dilemmas raised by the new circumstances of death, in which the majority of people in the advanced industrial nations die after an extended period of terminal deterioration, different countries develop different practices. The United States, with the sole exception of Oregon, legally permits only withholding and withdrawal of treatment, "double effect" uses of high doses of opiates, and terminal sedation, all conceived of as "allowing to die." The Netherlands permits these but also permits voluntary active euthanasia and physician-assisted suicide. Germany rejects physician-performed euthanasia but, at least until recent legal threats, permits assisted suicide not assisted by a physician. These three serve as the principal types or models of response to end-of-life dilemmas in the developed world. To be sure, all of these practices are currently undergoing evolution, and in some ways they are becoming more alike: Germany is paying new attention to the rights of patients to execute advance directives and thus to have treatment withheld or withdrawn, and public surveys reveal considerable support for euthanasia in the Dutch sense, voluntary active aid-in-dying under careful controls. In the Netherlands, a 1995 policy statement of the Royal Dutch Medical Association expressed a careful preference for physician-assisted suicide over euthanasia, urging that physicians encourage patients who request euthanasia to administer the lethal dose themselves as a further protection for voluntary choice. And, in the United States, the Supreme Court's 1997 ruling that there is no constitutional right to physician-assisted suicide has been understood to countenance the emergence of a "laboratory of the states" in which individual states, following the example of Oregon, may in the future move to legalize physician-assisted suicide, though as of this writing no such further measures have yet succeeded. An attempt by U.S. Attorney General John Ashcroft to reinterpret the Controlled Substances Act to prohibit the use of scheduled drugs for the purpose of causing death and thus undercut Oregon's statute was rejected at the appellate level in 2004, though his further appeal may take the issue to the U.S. Supreme Court. Nevertheless, among these three countries that serve as the principal models of approaches to dying, there remain substantial differences, and while there are ethical and practical advantages to each approach, each approach also raises serious moral objections.

Objections to the German Practice

German law does not prohibit assisting suicide, but postwar German culture and the German physicians' code of ethics discourages physicians from taking an active role in causing death. This gives rise to distinctive moral problems. For one thing, if the physician is not permitted to assist in his or her patient's suicide, there may be little professional help or review provided for the patient's choice about suicide. If patients make such choices essentially outside the medical establishment, medical professionals may not be a position to detect or treat impaired judgment on the part of the patient, especially judgment impaired by depression. Similarly, if the patient must commit suicide assisted only by persons outside the medical profession, there are risks that the patient's diagnosis and prognosis will be inadequately confirmed, that the means chosen for suicide will be unreliable or inappropriately used, that the means used for suicide will fall into the hands of other persons, and that the patient will fail to recognize or be able to resist intrafamilial pressures and manipulation. While it now makes efforts to counter most of these objections, even the DGHS itself has been accused in the past of promoting rather than simply supporting choices of suicide. Finally, as the DGHS now emphasizes, assistance in suicide can be a freely chosen option only in a legal context that also protects the many other choices a patient may make—declining treatment, executing advance directives, seeking Hospice care—about how his or her life shall end.

Objections to the Dutch Practice

The Dutch practice of physician-performed active voluntary euthanasia and physician-assisted suicide also raises a number of ethical issues, many of which have been discussed vigorously both in the Dutch press and in commentary on the Dutch practices from abroad. For one thing, it is sometimes said that the availability of physician-assisted dying creates a disincentive for providing good terminal care. There is no evidence that this is the case; on the contrary, Peter Admiraal, the anesthesiologist who has been perhaps the Netherlands' most vocal defender of voluntary active euthanasia, insists that pain should rarely or never be the occasion for euthanasia, as pain (in contrast to suffering) is comparatively easily treated.[24] In fact, pain is the primary reason for the request in only about 5% of cases. Instead, it is a refusal to endure the final stages of deterioration, both mental and physical, that primarily motivates the majority of requests.

It is also sometimes said that active euthanasia violates the Hippocratic oath. The original Greek version of the oath does prohibit the physician from giving a deadly drug, even when asked for it; but the original version also prohibits the physician from performing surgery and from taking fees for teaching medicine, neither of which prohibitions has survived into contemporary medical practice. At issue is whether deliberately causing the death of one's patient—killing one's patient, some claim—can ever be part of the physician's role. "Doctors must not kill," opponents insist,[25] but Dutch physicians often say that they see performing euthanasia—where it is genuinely requested by the patient and nothing else can be done to relieve the patient's condition—as part of their duty to the patient, not as a violation of it. As the 1995 nationwide report commented, "a large majority of Dutch physicians consider euthanasia an exceptional but accepted part of medical practice."[26] Some Dutch do worry, however, that too many requests for euthanasia or assistance in suicide are refused—only about ⅓ of explicit requests are actually honored. One well-known Dutch commentator points to another, seemingly contrary concern: that some requests are made too early in a terminal course, even shortly after diagnosis, when with good palliative care the patient could live a substantial amount of time longer.[27] However, these are concerns about how euthanasia and physician-assisted suicide are practiced, not about whether they should be legal at all.

The Dutch are also often said to be a risk of starting down the slippery slope, that is, that the practice of voluntary active euthanasia for patients who meet the criteria will erode into practicing less-than-voluntary euthanasia on patients whose problems are not irremediable and perhaps by gradual degrees will develop into terminating the lives of people who are elderly, chronically ill, handicapped, mentally retarded, or otherwise regarded as undesirable. This risk is often expressed in vivid claims of widespread fear and wholesale slaughter—claims based on misinterpretation of the 1,000 cases of life-ending treatment without explicit, current request, claims that are often repeated in the right-to-life press in both the Netherlands and the United States. Work now in progress on the impact of legalized physician-assisted dying in the Netherlands and Oregon shows that these claims are simply not true: except for patients with AIDS, the rates of assisted dying show no evidence of disparate impact on ten groups of potentially vulnerable patients: the elderly, women, the uninsured (not applicable in the Netherlands, where all are insured), people with low educational status, the poor, racial minorities (except Asians in Oregon; data not available in the Netherlands), people with physical disabilities or chronic illness, mature minors, and people with psychiatric illness.[28] However, it is true that in recent years the Dutch have begun to agonize over the problems of the incompetent patient, the mentally ill patient, the newborn with serious deficits, and other patients who cannot make voluntary choices, though these are largely understood as issues about withholding or withdrawing treatment, not about direct termination.[29]

What is not often understood is that this new and acutely painful area of reflection for the Dutch—withholding and withdrawing treatment from incompetent patients—has already led in the United States to the emergence of a vast, highly developed body of law: namely, the long series of cases beginning with *Quinlan* and culminating in *Cruzan*. Americans have been discussing these issues for a long time and have developed a broad set of practices that are regarded as routine in withholding and withdrawing treatment from persons who are no longer or never were competent. The Dutch see Americans as much further out on the slippery slope than they are because Americans have already become accustomed to second-party choices that result in death for other people. Issues involving second-party choices are painful to the Dutch in a way they are not to Americans precisely because *voluntariness* is so central in the Dutch understanding of choices about dying. Concomitantly, the Dutch see the Americans' squeamishness about first-party choices—voluntary euthanasia, assisted suicide—as evidence that we are not genuinely committed to recognizing voluntary choice after all. For this reason, many Dutch commentators believe that the Americans are at a much greater risk of sliding down the slippery slope into involuntary killing than they are.

Objections to the American Practice

The German, Dutch, and American practices all occur within similar conditions—in industrialized nations with highly developed medical systems where a majority of the population die of illnesses exhibiting characteristically extended downhill courses—but the issues raised by the American response to this situation—relying on withholding and withdrawal of treatment—may be even more disturbing than those of the Dutch or the Germans. We Americans often assume that our approach is "safer" because, except in Oregon, it involves only letting someone die, not killing them; but it, too, raises very troubling questions.

The first of these issues is a function of the fact that withdrawing and especially withholding treatment are typically less conspicuous, less pronounced, less evident kinds of actions than direct killing, even though they can equally well lead to death. Decisions about nontreatment have an invisibility that decisions about directly causing death do not have, even though they may have the same result; hence there is a much wider range of occasions in which such decisions can be made. One can decline to treat a patient in many different ways, at many different times—by not providing oxygen, by not instituting dialysis, by not correcting electrolyte imbalances, and so on—all of which will cause the patient's death. Open medical killing also brings about death but is much more overt and conspicuous. Consequently, letting die offers many fewer protections. In contrast to the standard slippery-slope argument, which sees killing as riskier than letting die, the more realistic slippery-slope argument warns that because our culture relies primarily on decisions about nontreatment and practices like terminal sedation construed as "allowing to die," grave decisions about living or dying are not as open to scrutiny as they are under more direct life-terminating practices, hence are more open to abuse. Indeed, in the view of one influential commentator, the Supreme Court's 1997 decision in effect legalized active euthanasia, voluntary and nonvoluntary, in the form of terminal sedation, even as it rejected physician-assisted suicide.[30]

Second, reliance on withholding and withdrawal of treatment invites rationing in an extremely strong way, in part because of the comparative invisibility of these decisions. When a health-care provider does not offer a specific sort of care, it is not always possible to discern the motivation; the line between believing that it would not provide benefit to the patient and that it would not provide benefit worth the investment of resources in the patient can be very thin. This is a particular problem where health-care financing is decentralized, profit-oriented, and nonuniversal, as in the United States, and where rationing decisions without benefit of principle are not always available for easy review.

Third, relying on withholding and withdrawal of treatment can often be cruel. Even with Hospice or with skilled palliative care, it requires that the patient who is dying from one of the diseases that exhibits a characteristic extended, downhill course (as the majority of patients in the developed world all do) must, in effect, wait to die until the absence of a certain treatment will cause death. For instance, the cancer patient who forgoes chemotherapy or surgery does not simply die from this choice; he or she continues to endure the downhill course of the cancer until the tumor finally destroys some crucial bodily function or organ. The patient with ALS who decides in advance to decline respiratory support does not die at the time this choice is made but continues to endure increasing paralysis until breathing is impaired and suffocation occurs. Of course, attempts are made to try to ameliorate these situations by administering pain medication or symptom control at the time treatment is withheld—for instance, by using opiates and paralytics as a respirator is withdrawn—but these are all ways of disguising the fact that we are letting the disease kill the patient rather than directly bringing about death. But the ways diseases kill people can be far more cruel than the ways physicians kill patients when performing euthanasia or assisting in suicide.

End-of-Life Practices in Other Countries

In most of the developed world dying looks much the same. As in the United States, the Netherlands, and Germany, the other industrialized nations also have sophisticated medical establishments, enjoy extended life expectancies, and find themselves in the fourth stage of the epidemiological transition, in which the majority of their populations die of diseases with extended downhill courses. Dying takes place in much the same way in all these countries, though the exact frequency of withholding and withdrawing treatment, of double-effect use of opiates, and euthanasia and physician-assisted suicide varies among them. Indeed, new data is rapidly coming to light.

In Australia, a replication of the Remmelink Commission study originally performed in the Netherlands found that of deaths in Australia that involved a medical end-of-life decision, 28.6% involved withholding or withdrawing treatment; 30.9% involved the use of opiates under the principle of double effect, and 1.8% involved voluntary active euthanasia (including 0.1% physician-assisted suicide), though neither are legal.[31] But the study also found—this is the figure that produced considerable surprise—that some 3.5% of deaths involved termination of the patient's life without the patient's concurrent explicit request. This figure is five times as high as that in the Netherlands. In slightly more than a third of these cases (38%), there was some discussion with the patient, though not an explicit request for death to be hastened, and in virtually all of the rest, the doctor did not consider the patient competent or capable of making such a decision. In 0.5% of all deaths involving medical end-of-life decisions, doctors did not discuss the choice of hastening of death with the patient because they thought it was "clearly the best one for the patient" or that "discussion would have done more harm than good."[32]

A 2003 study of six European countries—Belgium, Denmark, Italy, the Netherlands, Sweden, and Switzerland—found that in all countries studied, about a third of deaths are sudden and unexpected; among the other two-thirds, the frequency of death following end-of-life decisions ranged from 23% in Italy to 51% in Switzerland. "Double-effect" deaths and direct termination without explicit current request were found everywhere. However, patients and relatives were more likely to be involved in decisionmaking where assistance in dying is legal and the frequency comparatively high—Switzerland and the Netherlands—and while rates of voluntary euthanasia were highest in the Netherlands, rates of euthanasia without current, explicit consent were higher in all five other countries. Rates of physician-assisted suicide were highest in Switzerland (0.36% of all deaths); 92% of such deaths involved the participation of a right-to-die organization.[33]

End-of-life practices in these and other developed countries tend to follow one of the three models explored here. For example, Canada's practices are much like those of the United States, in that it relies on withholding and withdrawing treatment and other forms of allowing to die, but, in the 1993 case, *Rodriquez v. British Columbia,* the Supreme Court of Canada narrowly rejected physician-assisted suicide. Australia's Northern Territory briefly legalized assisted dying in 1997, but the law was overturned after just four cases. The United Kingdom, the birthplace of the Hospice movement, stresses palliative care but also rejects physician-assisted suicide and active euthanasia. After the British courts rejected the poignant request of ALS patient Diane Pretty to be allowed to receive assistance in dying from her husband, she then traveled to Strasbourg to the European Court of Human Rights; early in 2002 it ruled that her human rights were not being violated and refused her request; she died not long thereafter. Late in 2001, Belgium legalized active euthanasia but not physician-assisted suicide; despite the latter, Belgium's law is patterned fairly closely after the Dutch law.

Switzerland has been particularly active in right-to-die issues. Like that of Germany, Switzerland's law does not criminalize assisted suicide, but unlike Germany, Switzerland does not impose a duty to rescue that makes medical assistance in suicide difficult. Rather, assisted suicide is not illegal if done without self-interest. Switzerland now has at least four right-to-die organizations, including Exit Deutsche Schweiz, Exit International, and Dignitas—in part analogues of Oregon's Compassion in Dying and the "Caring Friends" program of the Hemlock Society (now End-of-Life Choices)—and Germany's DGHS, that provide information, counseling, instruction, and personal guidance, as well as other support to terminally ill patients who choose suicide—or, as it is usually called in German-speaking Switzerland, where this is most common, *Freitod.* However, the Swiss groups are also able to provide such patients with an accompaniment team that consults with the patient to make sure that the choice of suicide is voluntary, secures a prescription from a physician for the lethal medication, and will deliver it to the person at a preappointed time. They also maintain "safe houses" where a person can go to die. These organizations encourage family members to be present when the patient takes the drug, if he or she still wants to use it, and Dignitas operates a safe house for patients traveling from abroad for this purpose. In general, the Swiss organizations provide extensive help to the patient who chooses this way of dying, though in keeping with Swiss law, they all insist that the patient take the drug himself or herself, either orally or (in an alternative permitted since 1997), through an intravenous line or feeding tube.[34] In Switzerland, as in Germany, assisted suicide is legal, but euthanasia is not. In 2002, about 500 people, approximately 0.4% of the 60,000 people in German-speaking Switzerland who died, died by assisted suicide.[35] Terminally ill Germans, Britons, and others now often travel to Switzerland to end their lives.

In contrast, practices in less developed countries look very, very different. In these countries, especially the least developed, background circumstances are different: life spans are significantly shorter, health-care systems are only primitively equipped and grossly underfunded, and many societies have not passed through to the fourth stage of the epidemiologic transition: in these countries, people die earlier, they are more likely to die of infectious and parasitic disease, including AIDS, and degenerative disease is more likely to be interrupted early by death from pneumonia, sepsis, malnutrition, and other factors in what would otherwise have been a long downhill course. Dying in the poorer countries continues to be different from dying in the richer countries, and the underlying ethical problem in the richer countries—what practices concerning the end of life to adopt when the majority of a population dies of late-life degenerative diseases with long downhill courses—is far less applicable in the less developed parts of the world.

The Problem: A Choice of Cultures

In the developed world, we see three sorts of models in the three countries just examined in detail. While much of medical practice in them is similar, they do offer three quite different basic options in approaching death. All three of these options generate moral problems; none of them, nor any others we might devise, is free of moral difficulty. The question, then, is this: for a given society, which practices about dying are, morally and practically speaking, best?

It is not possible to answer this question in a less-than-ideal world without attention to the specific characteristics and deficiencies of the society in question. In asking which of these practices is best, we must ask which is best *for us.* That we currently employ one set of these options rather than others does not prove that it is best for us; the question is whether practices developed in other cultures or those not yet widespread in any culture would be better for our own culture than that which has so far developed here. Thus, it is necessary to consider the differences between our own society and these other societies in the developed world that have real bearing on which model of approach to dying we ought to adopt. This question can be asked by residents of any country or culture: which model of dying is best *for us?* I have been addressing this question from the point of view of an American, but the question could be asked by any member of any culture, anywhere.

First, notice that different cultures exhibit different degrees of closeness between physicians and patients—different patterns of contact and involvement. The German physician is sometimes said to be more distant and more authoritarian than the American physician; on the other hand, the Dutch physician is often said to be closer to his or her patients than either the American or the German physician. In the Netherlands, basic primary care is provided by the *huisarts,* the general practitioner or family physician, who typically lives in the neighborhood, makes house calls frequently, and maintains an office in his or her own home. This physician usually also provides care for the other members of the patient's family and will remain the family's physician throughout his or her practice. Thus, the patient for whom euthanasia becomes an issue—say, the terminal cancer patient who has been hospitalized in the past but who has returned home to die—will be cared for by the trusted family physician on a regular basis. Indeed, for a patient in severe distress, the physician, supported by the visiting nurse, may make house calls as often as once a day, twice a day, or even more frequently (after all, the physician's office is right in the neighborhood) and is in continuous contact with the family. In contrast, the traditional American institution of the family doctor who makes house calls has largely become a thing of the past, and although some patients who die at home have access to hospice services and receive house calls from their long-term physician, many have no such long-term care and receive most of it from staff at a clinic or from house staff rotating through the services of a hospital. Most Americans die in institutions, including hospitals and nursing homes; in the Netherlands, in contrast, the majority of people die at home. The degree of continuing contact that the patient can have with a familiar, trusted physician and the degree of institutionalization clearly influence the nature of the patient's dying and also play a role in whether physician-performed active euthanasia, assisted suicide, and/ or withholding and withdrawing treatment is appropriate.

Second, the United States has a much more volatile legal climate than either the Netherlands or Germany; its medical system is highly litigious, much more so than that of any other country in the world. Fears of malpractice actions or criminal prosecution color much of what physicians do in managing the dying of their patients. Americans also tend to develop public policy through court decisions and to assume that the existence of a policy puts an end to any moral issue. A delicate legal and moral balance over the issue of euthanasia, as has been the case in the Netherlands throughout the time it was understood as *gedoogd,* tolerated but not fully legal, would hardly be possible here.

Third, we in the United States have a very different financial climate in which to do our dying. Both the Netherlands and Germany, as well as virtually every other industrialized nation, have systems of national health insurance or national health care. Thus the patient is not directly responsible for the costs of treatment, and consequently the patient's choices about terminal care and/or euthanasia need not take personal financial considerations into account. Even for the patient who does have health insurance in the United States, many kinds of services are not covered, whereas the national health care or health insurance programs of many other countries provide multiple relevant services, including at-home physician care, home nursing care, home respite care, care in a nursing home or other long-term facility, dietician care, rehabilitation care, physical therapy, psychological counseling, and so on. The patient in the United States needs to attend to the financial aspects of dying in a way that patients in many other countries do not, and in this country both the patient's choices and the recommendations of the physician are very often shaped by financial considerations.

There are many other differences between the United States on the one hand and the Netherlands and Germany, with their different options for dying, on the other, including differences in degrees of paternalism in the medical establishment, in racism, sexism, and ageism in the general culture, and in awareness of a problematic historical past, especially Nazism. All of these cultural, institutional, social, and legal differences influence the appropriateness or inappropriateness of practices such as active euthanasia and assisted suicide. For instance, the Netherlands' tradition of close physician-patient contact, its comparative absence of malpractice-motivated medicine, and its provision of comprehensive health insurance, together with its comparative lack of racism and ageism and its experience in resistance to Nazism, suggest that this culture is able to permit the practice of voluntary active euthanasia, performed by physicians, as well as physician-assisted suicide, without risking abuse. On the other hand, it is sometimes said that Germany still does not trust its physicians, remembering the example of Nazi experimentation, and, given a comparatively authoritarian medical climate in which the contact between physician and patient is quite distanced, the population could not be comfortable with the practice of physician-performed active euthanasia or physician-assisted suicide. There, only a wholly patient-controlled response to terminal situations, as in non-physician-assisted suicide, is a reasonable and prudent practice.

But what about the United States? This is a country where (1) sustained contact with a personal physician has been decreasing, (2) the risk of malpractice action is perceived as substantial, (3) much medical care is not insured, (4) many medical decisions are financial decisions as well, (5) racism remains high, with racial and ethnic minorities tending to receive lower quality health care,[36] and (6) the public has not experienced direct contact with Nazism or similar totalitarian movements. Thus, the United States is in many respects an untrustworthy candidate for practicing active euthanasia. Given the pressures on individuals in an often atomized society, encouraging solo suicide, assisted if at all only by nonprofessionals, might well be open to considerable abuse too.

However, there are several additional differences between the United States and both the Netherlands and Germany that may seem peculiarly relevant here. First, American culture is more confrontational than many others, including Dutch culture. While the Netherlands prides itself rightly on a long tradition of rational discussion of public issues and on toleration of others' views and practices, the United States (and to some degree also Germany) tends to develop highly partisan, moralizing oppositional groups, especially over social issues like abortion. In general, this is a disadvantage, but in the case of euthanasia it may serve to alert the public to issues and possibilities it might not otherwise consider, especially the risks of abuse. Here the role of religious groups may be particularly strong, since in discouraging or prohibiting suicide and euthanasia (as many, though by no means all, religious groups do), they may invite their members to reinspect the reasons for such choices and encourage families, physicians, and health-care institutions to provide adequate, humane alternatives.

Second, though this may at first seem to be not only a peculiar but a trivial difference, it is Americans who are particularly given to self-analysis. This tendency not only is evident in the United States' high rate of utilization of counseling services, including religious counseling, psychological counseling, and psychiatry, but also is more clearly evident in its popular culture: its diet of soap operas, situation comedies, pop psychology books, and reality shows. It is here that the ordinary American absorbs models for analyzing his or her personal relationships and individual psychological characteristics. While, of course, things are changing rapidly and America's cultural tastes are widely exported, the fact remains that the ordinary American's cultural diet contains more in the way of professional and do-it-yourself amateur psychology and self-analysis than anyone else's. This long tradition of self-analysis may put Americans in a better position for certain kinds of end-of-life practices than many other cultures. Despite whatever other deficiencies U.S. society has, we live in a culture that encourages us to inspect our own motives, anticipate the impact of our actions on others, and scrutinize our own relationships with others, including our physicians. This disposition is of importance in euthanasia and assisted-suicide contexts because these are the kinds of fundamental choices about which one may have somewhat mixed motives, be subject to various interpersonal and situational pressures, and so on. If the voluntary character of choices about one's own dying is to be protected, it may be a good thing to inhabit a culture in which self-inspection of one's own mental habits and motives, not to mention those of one's family, physician, and others who might affect one's choices, is culturally encouraged. Counseling specifically addressed to end-of-life choices is not yet easily or openly available, especially if physician-assisted suicide is at issue—though some groups like Compassion in Dying and End-of-Life Choices (which merged in 2004 but later experienced some fission) now provide it—but I believe it will become more frequent in the future as people facing terminal illnesses characterized by long downhill, deteriorative courses consider how they want to die.

Finally, the United States population, varied as it is, is characterized by a kind of do-it-yourself ethic, an ethic that devalues reliance on others and encourages individual initiative and responsibility. (To be sure, this ethic is little in evidence in the series of court cases from *Quinlan* to *Cruzan,* but these were all cases about patients who had become or always were incapable of decisionmaking.) This ethic seems to be coupled with a sort of resistance to authority that perhaps also is basic to the American temperament, even in all its diversity. If this is really the case, Americans might be especially well served by end-of-life practices that emphasize self-reliance and resistance to authority.

These, of course, are mere conjectures about features of American culture relevant to the practice of euthanasia or assisted suicide. These are the features that one would want to reinforce should these practices become general, in part to minimize the effects of the negative influences. But, of course, these positive features will differ from one country and culture to another, just as the negative features do. In each country, a different architecture of antecedent assumptions and cultural features develops around end-of-life issues, and in each country the practices of euthanasia and assisted or physician-assisted suicide, if they are to be free from abuse, must be adapted to the culture in which they take place.

What, then, is appropriate for the United States' own cultural situation? Physician-performed euthanasia, even if not in itself morally wrong, is morally jeopardized where legal, time-related, and especially financial pressures on both patients and physicians are severe; thus, it is morally problematic in our culture in a way that it is not in the Netherlands. Solo suicide outside the institution of medicine (as in Germany) may be problematic in a country (like the United States) that has an increasingly alienated population, offers deteriorating and uneven social services, is increasingly racist and classist, and in other ways imposes unusual pressures on individuals, despite opportunities for self-analysis. Reliance only on withholding and withdrawing treatment and allowing to die (as in the United States) can be cruel, and its comparative invisibility invites erosion under cost-containment and other pressures. These are the three principal alternatives we have considered, but none of them seems wholly suited to our actual situation for dealing with the new fact that most of us die of extended-decline, deteriorative diseases.

Perhaps, however, there is one that would best suit the United States, certainly better than its current reliance on allowing to die, and better than the Netherlands' more direct physician involvement or Germany's practices entirely outside medicine. The "arm's-length" model of physician-assisted suicide—permitting physicians to supply their terminally ill patients who request it with the means for ending their own lives (as has become legal in Oregon)—still grants physicians some control over the circumstances in which this can happen (for example, only when the prognosis is genuinely grim and the alternatives for symptom control are poor) but leaves the fundamental decision about whether to use these means to the patient alone. It is up to the patient then—the independent, confrontational, self-analyzing, do-it-yourself, authority-resisting patient—and his or her advisors, including family members, clergy, the physician, and other health-care providers, to be clear about whether he or she really wants to use these means or not. Thus, the physician is involved but not directly, and it is the patient's decision, although the patient is not making it alone. Thus also it is the patient who performs the action of bringing his or her own life to a close, though where the patient is physically incapable of doing so or where the process goes awry the physician must be allowed to intercede. We live in an imperfect world, but of the alternatives for facing death—which we all eventually must—I think that the practice of permitting this somewhat distanced though still medically supported form of physician-assisted suicide is the one most nearly suited to the current state of our own flawed society. This is a model not yet central in any of the three countries examined here—the Netherlands, Germany, or (except in Oregon) the United States, or any of the other industrialized nations with related practices—but it is the one, I think, that suits us best.

Notes

From *The Journal of Pain and Symptom Management* 6(5), July 1991, pp. 298–305. © 1991 U.S. Cancer Pain Relief Committee. Revised and updated multiple times by the author, most recently in March 2004 for Bruce N. Waller, ed., *Consider Ethics: Theory, Readings, and Contemporary Issues,* Pearson Education and Longman Publishing, forthcoming 2004. Updated again in June 2004.

1. S. J. Olshansky and A. B. Ault, "The Fourth Stage of the Epidemiological Transition: The Age of Delayed Degenerative Diseases," *Milbank Memorial Fund Quarterly Health and Society* 64 (1986): 355–91.

2. In a study of end-of-life decisionmaking in six European countries, about one-third of all deaths were found to have happened suddenly and unexpectedly, ranging from 29 percent in Italy to 34 percent in Belgium. See Agnes van der Heide, Luc Deliens, Karin Faisst, Tore Nilstun, Michael Norup, Eugenio Paci, Gerrit van der Wal, Paul J. van der Maas, on behalf of the EURELD consortium, "End-of-life decision-making in six European countries: Descriptive study," *Lancet* 361 (August 2, 2003), 345–50, table 2, p. 347.

3. S. Miles and C. Gomez, *Protocols for Elective Use of Life-Sustaining Treatment* (New York: Springer-Verlag, 1988).

4. C. L. Sprung, "Changing Attitudes and Practices in Forgoing Life-Sustaining Treatments," *JAMA* 262 (1990): 2213.

5. T. J. Prendergast and J.M. Luce, "Increasing Incidence of Withholding and Withdrawal of Life Support from the Critically Ill," *American Journal of Respiratory and Critical Care Medicine* 155, 1 (January 1997): 1–2.

6. M. B. Hamel, J. M. Teno, L. Goldman, J. Lynn, R. B. Davis, A. N. Galanos, N. Desbiens, A. F. Connors Jr., N. Wenger, R. S. Phillips. (SUPPORT investigators), "Patient Age and Decisions to Withhold Life-Sustaining Treatments from Seriously Ill, Hospitalized Adults," *Annals of Internal Medicine* 130, 2 (January 19, 1999): 116–25.

7. John M. Luce, "Withholding and Withdrawal of Life Support: Ethical, Legal, and Clinical Aspects," *New Horizons* 5, 1 (February 1997): 30–7.

8. *New York Times,* July 23, 1990, A13.

9. Accounts of the use of Oregon's Death with Dignity Act (Measure 16) begin with A. E. Chin, K. Hedberg, G. K. Higginson, and D. W. Fleming, "Legalized Physician-Assisted Suicide in Oregon—The First Year's Experience," *New England Journal of Medicine* 340 (1999): 577–83, and are updated annually in this journal and at the website of the Oregon Department of Human Services. The 171 cases of legal physician-assisted suicide that have

taken place in the first six years since it became legal in Oregon represent about one-tenth of one percent of the total deaths in Oregon.

10. For a fuller account, see my remarks in "A Dozen Caveats Concerning the Discussion of Euthanasia in the Netherlands," in my book *The Least Worst Death: Essays in Bioethics on the End of Life* (New York: Oxford University Press, 1994), 130–44; John Griffiths, Alex Bood, and Helen Weyers, *Euthanasia and Law in the Netherlands* (Amsterdam: Amsterdam University Press, 1998), and the three nationwide studies of end-of-life decisionmaking mentioned hereafter.

11. P. J. van der Maas, J.J.M. van Delden, and L. Pijnenborg, "Euthanasia and Other Medical Decisions Concerning the End of Life," published in full in English as a special issue of *Health Policy,* 22, 1–2 (1992), and, with C.W.N. Looman, in summary in *Lancet* 338 (1991): 669–74.

12. G. van der Wal, J.T.M. van Eijk, H.J.J. Leenen, and C. Spreeuwenberg, "Euthanasie en hulp bij zelfdoding door artsen in de thuissituatie," pts. 1 and 2, *Nederlands Tijdschrift voor Geneesekunde* 135 (1991): 1593–8, 1599–1604.

13. P. J. van der Maas, G. van der Wal, "Euthanasia, Physician-Assisted Suicide, and Other Medical Practices Involving the End of Life in the Netherlands, 1990–1995," *New England Journal of Medicine* 335 (1996): 1699–1705.

14. Bregje D. Onwuteaka-Philipsen, Agnes van der Heide, Dirk Koper, Ingeborg Keij-Deerenberg, Judith A. C. Rietjens, Mette Rurup, Astrid M. Vrakking, Jean Jacques Georges, Martien T. Muller, Gerrit van der Wal, and Paul J. van der Maas, "Euthanasia and Other End-of-Life Decisions in the Netherlands in 1990, 1995, and 2001," *Lancet* 362, (2003): 395–9. A full account is available in Gerrit van der Wal, Agnes van der Heide, Bregje D. Onwuteaka-Philipsen, Paul. J. van der Maas, *Medische besluitvorming aan het einde van het leven: De praktijk en de toetsingsprocedure euthanasie* (Utrecht: De Tijdstroom, 2003).

15. L. Pijnenborg, P.J.van der Maas, J.J.M. van Delden, C.W.N. Looman, "Life Terminating Acts without Explicit Request of Patient," *Lancet* 341 (1993): 1196–9.

16. Onwuteaka-Philipsen et al., "Euthanasia and Other End-of Life Decisions," 2003. These figures are an average of the results of the two principal parts of the 1990, 1995, and 2001 nationwide studies, the interview study, and the death-certificate study.

17. G. van der Wal, P. J. van der Maas, J. M. Bosma, B. D. Onwuteaka-Philipsen, D. L. Willems, I. Haverkate, P. J. Kostense, "Evaluation of the Notification Procedure for Physician-Assisted Death in the Netherlands," *New England Journal of Medicine* 335 (1996): 1706–11.

18. Van der Maas et al., "Euthanasia and other Medical Decisions Concerning the End of Life," 673.

19. Van der Maas et al., "Euthanasia, Physician-Assisted Suicide, and Other Medical Practices Involving the End of Life in the Netherlands, 1990–1995," p. 1705.

20. Margaret P. Battin, Agnes van der Heide, Linda Ganzini, and Gerrit van der Wal, "Legalized Physician-Assisted Dying in Oregon and the Netherlands: The Impact on Patients in Vulnerable Groups," in preparation.

21. Kurt Schobert, "Physician-Assisted Suicide in Germany and Switzerland, with Focus on Some Developments in Recent Years," manuscript in preparation, citing "Grundsätze der Bundesärztekammer zur ärztlichen Sterbebegleitung," in *Ethik in der Medizin,* ed., Urban Wiesing (Stuttgart: Gustav Fischer, 2002), 203–8.

22. That is, it no longer sells or supplies such drugs. A scandal in 1992–93 engulfed the original founder and president of the DGHS, Hans Hennig Atrott, who had been secretly providing some members with cyanide in exchange for substantial contributions; he was convicted of violating the drug laws and tax evasion, though not charged with or convicted of assisting suicides.

23. See my "Assisted Suicide: Can We Learn from Germany?" in *The Least Worst Death*, pp. 254–70.

24. P. Admiraal, "Euthanasia in a General Hospital," paper read at the Eighth World Congress of the International Federation of Right-to-Die Societies, Maastricht, the Netherlands, June 8, 1990.

25. See the editorial "Doctors Must Not Kill," *JAMA* 259 (1988): 2139–40, signed by Willard Gaylin, Leon R. Kass, Edmund D. Pellegrino, and Mark Siegler.

26. Van der Maas et al., "Euthanasia, Physician-Assisted Suicide, and Other Medical Practices," 1705.

27. Govert den Hartogh, personal communication.

28. Margaret P. Battin, Agnes van der Heide, Linda Ganzini, and Gerrit van der Wal, "Legalized Physician-Assisted Dying," in preparation.

29. H. ten Have, "Coma: Controversy and Consensus," *Newsletter of the European Society for Philosophy of Medicine and Health Care,* May 1990, 19–20.

30. David Orentlicher, "The Supreme Court and Terminal Sedation: Rejecting Assisted Suicide, Embracing Euthanasia," *Hastings Constitutional Law Quarterly* 24 (1997):947–68; see also *New England Journal of Medicine* 337 (1997): 1236–9.

31. Physician-assisted suicide was briefly legal in the Northern Territory of Australia in 1997, and four were performed before the law was overturned, but these cases did not occur during the study period.

32. Helga Kuhse, Peter Singer, Peter Baume, Malcolm Clark, and Maurice Rickard, "End-of-life Decisions in Australian Medical Practice," *Medical Journal of Australia* 166 (1997):191–6.

33. Van der Heide et al., "End-of-Life Decision-Making in Six European Countries, 345–50.

34. Georg Bosshard, Esther Ulrich, and Walter Bär, "748 Cases of Suicide Assisted by a Swiss Right-to-Die Organization," *Swiss Medical Weekly* 133 (2003): 310–7.

35. Swissinfo, June 19, 2003, citing a University of Zurich study. Available at: http://www.swissinfo.org.

36. Institute of Medicine, *Unequal Treatment: Confronting Racial and Ethnic Disparities in Health Care* (Washington, D.C.: National Academy of Sciences, 2002).

3

Going Early, Going Late

The Rationality of Decisions about Physician-Assisted Suicide in AIDS

Introductory Note

This essay was originally written in 1993, eleven years after the HIV/AIDS epidemic had been recognized and just as the first effective drug therapy was beginning to be developed. In the decade that followed, the prognosis has improved dramatically for people with HIV/AIDS in the developed world, as protease inhibitors and other effective therapy have become available. Public education about the routes of transmission, the provision of anonymous testing, and publicly funded treatment, as well as the development of programs supporting clean-needle and safe sex practices, have all contributed to the slowed rate of new transmission. Better prophylaxis against transmission in pregnancy is now available, and where adequate maternal health care is available, the rate of transmission in pregnancy, delivery, and lactation has been reduced from about 21% in 1994 to about 2% or less in 2003. At the same time that the rate of new infections has slowed, the HIV virus subtype prevalent in the United States has been evolving into a comparatively chronic, less lethal form. Furthermore, genetic studies have revealed that some individuals in some populations are less susceptible to the HIV virus than others, potentially providing evidence about the likelihood of contracting the disease. Extensive research is underway in microbicides, vaccines, and other methods for reducing transmission. In general, much better information is available to physicians and to the public about the transmission mechanisms, natural history, and treatment possibilities of the disease. Despite a modest recent rise in new infections, the death rate from AIDS in the United States has been dropping rapidly, and the disease has declined as a leading cause of death.

Despite these dramatic advances, I have included this essay in its original 1993 form because I think its argument about choices for or against suicide is particularly instructive in the light of later developments. Some people with AIDS who did choose suicide in that decade might still be alive had they not done so; some people who did not choose suicide are still alive; some who did not choose it died very hard deaths; and others who made the same choice died comparatively easy deaths. Retrospective gainsaying is a problematic exercise; the focus of concern here is the nature of the choices made by people with AIDS given the information and treatment available to them at the time. Predictive guesses about the likelihood of cure or advances in treatment, including the many developments not foreseen at an early point in the history of the AIDS epidemic, are very much a part of the choice-structure that is discussed here.

This 1993 essay remains relevant for another reason: in much of the world, including southeast Asia, China, Latin America, and especially sub-Saharan Africa, access to effective treatment is not reliably available, either for financial reasons or political reasons or both. Global AIDS programs are being developed, but only after nearly 1/100th of the entire world's adult population has been infected by the HIV virus. Now a far more entrenched, widespread problem in many places in the developing world, especially sub-Saharan Africa, than it ever was in the United States or western Europe, AIDS has devastated personal social networks and entire societies on an enormous scale.

To say that AIDS in the developing world now looks somewhat the way AIDS did in the developed world a decade ago is thus misleading, in the sense that the scale of the epidemic in Africa and elsewhere in the developing world is far larger and exacerbated by poorer social conditions and health infrastructure. Yet there are fearsome parallels: a lethal, still virtually unchecked disease is ravaging the country. Similarly, to say that decisions made by people with AIDS in the developing world now are like those made by people with AIDS in the United States a decade ago is both misleading and accurate. On the one hand, the circumstances are vastly different: in the most desperately affected parts of the world, people with AIDS are unlikely to receive much in the way of health care at all, or to have a personal physician with whom decision-making might be done, or for that matter to have surviving family members or close friends. On the other hand, however, decisions in both the poor and the rich world are alike in one central respect: both involve facing a disease from which one is likely to die, and perhaps die a difficult death.

This is also not to say that were conditions better in parts of the world that do not have robust health-care infrastructures, decisions about suicide in the end-stages of AIDS would be identical to those in affluent parts of the world like the United States and Europe. Background assumptions about the moral permissibility of suicide in general or in circumstances of terminal illness are not always the same as those in the largely Judeo-Christian industrialized cultures of the United States and Europe. Considerations of stigma associated with the disease and financial implications for one's survivors may also be different in different regions of the world. Thus decisions about suicide in AIDS may look very different in different parts of the world. Nevertheless, in many respects, even a decade or more after the original appearance of this essay in 1993, decisions about suicide in AIDS in many respects still look the same in core structure: people in all cultures and in all health circumstances recognize choices that involve difficult tradeoffs in trying to maximize good life left while avoiding the worst aspects of a bad trajectory of dying.

This essay is framed about AIDS. But it also applies in many, many other conditions of which people die: cancer, heart disease, various neurological disorders and types of organ failure, and so on. However, the argument is not identical in all of them. For some conditions, the characteristic downhill course is far more predictable than that of AIDS; in others, pain and symptom control is much more effective; in some, stigma is less and social prejudice plays little role; and in some, physician-patient communication is easier. The expected downhill trajectory varies widely from one disease to another, and with very different degrees of reliability in prediction. Social and legal conditions relevant in decision-making also vary widely: in some places—the Netherlands, Switzerland, and Oregon, for example—assisted or physician-assisted suicide is legal, so that patients can openly discuss their choices with their physicians and also in the presence of family and friends, something much riskier in other places. Yet there remain difficult conditions where the structure of the choice may look very much like that discussed in this essay: for example, multiple myeloma, where the question may be whether to take a chance on a bone marrow transplant or allow oneself to die earlier from the disease; Huntington's, where the end-stages are predictable and grim; or Alzheimer's, where the final decade or more may have an unusually large impact on family caregivers. It will also be relevant in emerging new diseases, including some, like Ebola, already known, and others that have not yet appeared. In each of these conditions, different aspects of the decision structure outlined in the following essay may be highlighted, but they all remain relevant. Indeed, for all the conditions of which human beings die—at least all those in which the illness that will prove fatal is characterized by a long, foreseeable downhill course that could end in a hard death—the considerations raised here remain deeply, often painfully relevant.

* * *

Vigorous, often vitriolic debate over active euthanasia and physician-assisted suicide in terminal illness has occupied both the public and the medical profession in many countries in recent years. Comparatively little public and professional discussion, however, has focused on AIDS.[1] Rather, the examples raised in the euthanasia debates most often involve cancer and to a somewhat lesser extent neurological and other diseases—like ALS (or Lou Gehrig's disease), Alzheimer's disease, multiple sclerosis, stroke, and terminal organ failure—and only rarely involve AIDS, even though AIDS is like all these conditions in involving extensive deterioration in a terminal condition over a typically extended downhill course, the end-stages of which can be sometimes very difficult indeed.

This skewing of emphasis may seem odd, given that in the United States alone there are, as of this writing [1993], over a third of a million people who have been diagnosed with AIDS and more than a million are thought to have a precursor HIV infection. Worldwide, a million and a half people have been diagnosed with AIDS, and another ten to twelve million are thought to be HIV-infected. It is estimated that by the year 2000, now just a short six years away, the cumulative number of HIV-infected adults and children will reach thirty to forty million, including an annual number of new AIDS cases in women equal to that in men. Thus, AIDS is a major killer, with no known cure and an often dismal end-stage; given that this is so, why is there so little discussion of physician-assisted suicide in AIDS? No doubt there are several reasons. For example, in discussing attitudes among one affected group, gay men, Timothy F. Murphy points out that there is a kind of public philosophy among people with AIDS that is so dedicated to advocacy for increased research and social change that it in large measure rejects the possibility of failure.[2] Furthermore, Murphy continues, gay men with AIDS are often distrustful of the medical establishment, which after all had declassified homosexuality as a mental illness only eight years before the initial report of AIDS. I think there is also another reason for the comparative absence of reference to AIDS in the debates over the legalization of euthanasia and physician-assisted suicide, at least in the United States: among people with AIDS, especially those in the most cohesive gay communities of the major West Coast urban areas, assisted suicide and physician-assisted suicide, perhaps even physician-performed euthanasia, are already available—indeed, one might wish to say that they are effectively legal in the sense that their practice is not obstructed by law enforcement. In these communities, it is assumed, every AIDS patient knows how to get help if that is what he or she desires, and it is always possible to find the necessary drugs and a sympathetic doctor or friend. Indeed, it is said, in these communities where the death rate from AIDS has been so high, almost everybody who wants it has a hidden little stash, which doctors make it possible to acquire: a bottle of pills sequestered away, ready when one's own turn comes. Neither is there community disapproval of such preparations. There is no risk that one's stash will be discovered and taken away or that one will be committed for psychiatric care on the grounds of suicidal risk. To be sure, assisted suicide in AIDS deaths is not so nearly legal that it is possible, for instance, to consult an independent psychologist or counselor for an objective evaluation of one's motives[3] or to announce one's plans to a helpline or medical organization, but provided one is discreet, help is available with little risk. Everyone knows; no one talks.[4]

Even if assistance in suicide is virtually universally available in the West Coast gay AIDS communities in the United States and perhaps elsewhere, we still do not know how frequent the practice is. Adequate empirical information on the prevalence or characteristics of suicide, assisted suicide, physician-assisted suicide, or euthanasia among people with AIDS is not available in the United States or most countries. The only reliable data come from the Netherlands, where voluntary active euthanasia and physician-assisted suicide are openly available. According to a very large study completed in 1991, some 10–20% of all AIDS patients die by euthanasia or assisted suicide,[5] a rate higher than the 3% of all patients or the 6% of patients with terminal cancer whose deaths occur in these ways. Varying estimates in other countries more often reflect, one may suspect, the views of the observers and the policies of the institutions they are associated with rather than well-established fact. And there is an enormous range of informal estimates, ranging from nearly zero to 50%. Some physicians who treat AIDS patients say that virtually all of their patients raise the issue of suicide; other physicians say they have never been asked for assistance. Some Hospice workers claim to know of very few such cases; they claim that although many patients entering Hospice say they have plans for suicide, these plans are later abandoned. All agree, however, that if such cases occur, they are rarely reported as suicides, hence objective data on frequency would be difficult to obtain. Yet despite the lack of information and disagreement about the frequency of such choices in the United States and elsewhere, all parties also seem to agree that at least in the gay AIDS communities in some geographical areas, assistance in suicide is already available. One might even be tempted to say that assistance in suicide has become available in these areas in ways not unlike the situation in the Netherlands of several years ago—it is still a technical violation of the law and not reported to the authorities, but nevertheless not prosecuted, not prevented, and not subjected to social disapproval. Rather, it is generally understood and accepted, an option available to those who want it.

Thus, observing that assisted suicide is already an option available to some persons with AIDS, I shall not address the question of whether it should or should not be available, legally or otherwise, for persons dying of AIDS. This horse is long since out of the barn. Rather, I wish to consider what becomes of the much more pressing ethical question: *if* such assistance in suicide is already available, what should the role of those who assist be, and what should be avoided? Is everyone equally positioned to offer counsel and/or practical help?

I shall make one central assumption here—that *if* assistance in suicide is provided, it should protect as much as possible the rationality of the patient's choice. This is not to suppose that all such choices by persons with AIDS or any other terminal condition are rational but only to insist that, as much as possible, the conditions for rationality in these choices about suicide be preserved. To be sure, some patients "choose" suicide in panic, depression, or despair or in conditions of dementia, delirium, or psychosis; but some patients also make these choices in a thoughtful, reflective, reasoned, "rational" way. *If* assistance in suicide is available, our central assumption here runs, it should operate to favor the latter rather than the former sort of choice.

With this assumption in the background, we can then begin to identify the ways the conditions for rationality can be enhanced or undermined. To do this, what we must provide is an analysis of what we might call the "rational structure" of the choice faced by a person contemplating the possibility of suicide—what components it has, in what order they occur, and what types of problems can be addressed. This will be the first project here. In the second part of the essay, I will look at what sorts of assistance in suicide we can expect to find directed at what components of this choice, and how such assistance can enhance or undermine its rationality.

This analysis—part conjecture, part observation—of the "rational structure" of a choice about suicide in AIDS yields one possible schema of the ideal structure of a choice, without, of course, having anything to say about the content of the choice: a person with AIDS might equally rationally decide for or against suicide.

That it is possible to explore the "rational structure" of end-of-life choices is not to say that choices actually made by people about how their lives shall end are experienced in this structured way; nor is it to say that such choices are not sometimes (perhaps even often) distorted by internal or external pressures, psychopathology, institutional restrictions, and the like. Nor should developing such a schema be confused with depicting the psychological stages through which a person facing death actually passes. The schema proposed here is not the only possible account of these decisions; other plausible schemas might be constructed in quite different ways (as, for instance, if formal rational-choice or game-theoretic models were adopted as a starting point). But the background assumption of any schema remains the same: that it is possible to dissect out or exhibit the elements of rational choice, even though the person making such a choice may experience doing so as a unified event, in order to show where differing external influences and pressures should or should not be brought to bear. This analysis also helps to identify what sorts of considerations the person making the decision should not overlook. If, in keeping with the central assumption here, where assistance in suicide is already available it should operate to protect as much as possible the rationality of patient's choices, a look at a schematic account of the rational structure of end-of-life decisions lets us see what may obstruct or enhance rational decision making, and whose intervention can reinforce or undermine such a choice.

The Rational Structure of End-of-Life Choices in AIDS

Four principal levels of choice confront a person with AIDS. These levels of choice can be phrased as four questions, all tightly interrelated but each raising distinctive issues. Although these are phrased as four particular questions, they are actually question-types, incorporating a wide range of related and subsidiary questions. I shall phrase them as they might be asked by a person with AIDS or an HIV-infected person foreseeing future development of AIDS.

1. *Is assisted suicide an option I want to consider?* This question functions as a "gateway" question: it screens out cases in which the person does not want to consider suicide an acceptable alternative in any circumstances. A diagnosis of AIDS often leads a person to probe his or her own fundamental values, including ethical and religious views, and although the issue of suicide is not always raised explicitly, he or she may still consider whether he or she has any principled or absolutist objection to suicide. For people with AIDS who do have objections— and there may be many of them—there is no *decision* to be made about assisted suicide, even where it is widely available: it is already ruled out. To be sure, this may involve a deeper-level choice about whether to accept traditional religious or other values, but once this is made, there is no further issue about suicide. For many other people with AIDS, however, whether to consider suicide as an option in AIDS represents a major, life-defining choice.

Closely related to this is a further question of values: does one elect to undergo death in a comparatively passive way or attempt to assume control over the processes of dying? Of course, this distinction is not a bifurcating one between complete passivity and complete activity; on the contrary, many choices in death may have features of both, for instance the refusing or discontinuation of specific forms of treatment. To refuse treatment—say, antibiotics in an otherwise fatal infection or a ventilator in respiratory failure—may appear to be "passive" because it has the effect of allowing death to occur rather than physically causing it; but to refuse treatment may also appear to be "active" because it involves a deliberate step taken with the knowledge that death will occur as the outcome. Treatment can also be refused with the direct intention that death occur: this is to exercise a still greater degree of control that has death as its outcome. Seeking all available help, both curative and palliative, can also be regarded as exercising control, even though in a genuinely terminal illness this will nevertheless end in death.[6] The question here about assuming active control over one's own dying is very closely related to the question of whether one views suicide as acceptable at all: both are questions about what causal role one wishes to play in one's own oncoming death.

2. *Shall I hold out for the chance of a cure?* For the person with AIDS whose underlying values permit or encourage taking an active role in his or her own death, a next question presents itself: given that AIDS remains fatal, but also given that research efforts are very broad and aggressive, shall one hold out for the possibility of a cure (or, in the language of some patients, a miracle), whether it be a reversal of the condition or at least an effective, long-term treatment? This question may arise more forcefully than it did even just a few years ago, prior to the development of treatments such as AZT and ddI, whatever their efficacy, but the likelihood of developing a cure or long-term treatment is still unknown. Indeed, many researchers would say, in the wake of the discouragement of the 1993 Berlin AIDS conference, it is a long shot. That holding out for a cure is a long shot may be especially evident where what is at issue is the prospect of rescue from already advanced AIDS, as distinct from reversal of HIV infection or protection from exposure to HIV. On the other hand, virtually overnight discoveries of cures or effective treatments for previously fatal diseases do sometimes occur (for example, the discovery of insulin for the treatment of diabetes), and there is very active AIDS research going on in a wide variety of areas. A number of vaccines and therapeutic drugs are currently being tested, and there have been dramatic advances in the control and treatment of the associated symptoms. Futhermore, thanks in substantial measure to the activism of groups like ACT UP, regulatory procedures for new drug approvals have been vastly accelerated. Though it is of course an exaggeration to say that if a cure were developed today, it would be in one's hands tomorrow, hopes of rapid access if a cure or effective treatment were developed have increased dramatically. Hence the high priority of this second question of the schema: a patient might see suicide as a possible option; but also believing that a cure is just around the corner, this patient will reject suicide just as the patient answering no to the first question of the schema does, though not for moral or religious reasons. Thus, though it is also a predictive question like other components that arise later in the schema, this question too may function in a "gateway" role.

Of course, the question of whether to hold out for a cure is not merely a question of whether to take a long-shot chance that a cure may be discovered and save one's life; it also raises the question of whether to submit oneself to ongoing medical investigation and experimentation.[7] This also brings with it the possibility of iatrogenic damage from experimental protocols and thus, paradoxically, the possibility of still earlier death. Thus, the question of whether to hold out for a cure is a complex one. No doubt due to greater awareness among persons with AIDS of the hardships some experimental regimens have imposed, physicians are currently noting a sharp decline in the number of patients volunteering for studies—though this will no doubt rise again if some test drugs prove to have positive results. Whatever the background fluctuations in numbers of patients entering studies, however, the schematic question remains the same for all: *should I hold out for a cure?*

3. *How shall I time my suicide?* A person with AIDS, having already decided to assume a causally active role in bringing about his or her death by suicide, and having also decided not to hold out for a cure, faces a third choice: how shall his or her exit be timed during the foreseeable period of decline? This is not a gateway question about whether suicide is to be undertaken at all; it is instead a pragmatic question about when it is to be done. It is also a question that is, I think, particularly crucial in decisions about suicide in AIDS but is also rarely explored with respect to the question of how its rationality may be preserved.

Assuming that the person with AIDS who chooses suicide in preference to continuing life throughout the terminal course of the disease does so in order to avoid the worst elements of the end-stages of AIDS—presumably the loss of cognitive, sensory, and motor functions and the occurrence of painful or discomforting symptoms—the question of timing becomes crucial: how shall one's death be timed to avoid the worst but not lose any more than necessary of the remaining good life left? These are questions such a person may raise: *Shall I go early, or shall I go late? Or shall I not plan a time of exit at all, but rather wait to see what happens at the end, and initiate my suicide just when the time seems right?* These questions about the timing of a projected suicide are not questions likely to be asked by the person whose suicide is the product of despair, depression, or self-blame for having contracted AIDS; they are questions characteristic of rational choice, where the effort is to protect oneself from the bad things that may happen during the downhill course of AIDS but not lose the good.

Two sorts of ingredients are required in order to address this question. First, a person must be able to identify his or her own preferences concerning what conditions of life are unacceptable: blindness? pain? incontinence? being bedridden? memory loss? dementia? There may be social components as well: loneliness, social stigma, loss of communicative capacity, financial destitution. Does the person view these things as the worst elements of the end-stages of AIDS—and bad enough to be avoided by suicide? Identifying one's own preferences also involves recognizing what count as conditions worth living for: affection, communication, sensory pleasure, artistic projects, intellectual work, commitment to a cause, and so on. But identifying one's preferences must be accompanied by a second component: some way of predicting probabilities of the states of affairs that are the subject of these preferences. How likely is blindness to occur? How likely is pain?

What is the probability of becoming bedridden at the end? How likely is it that I will lose communicative capacity altogether or develop significant dementia? On the more positive side, how likely is it that I will reach more profound communication or deeper understanding or have experiences of new importance and beauty? Social conditions may be even harder to predict than medical ones, but their identification is not altogether impossible. In any case, it is only with these two ingredients, knowledge of one's own personal preferences about the medical and social conditions one might find oneself in and knowledge of the probabilities of their occurrence, that a person can begin to answer rationally the question of how to time a suicide he or she has already decided to commit.

To be sure, this third schematic question about timing one's suicide also involves basic value commitments about ethical and religious matters, like the first question of the schema, and issues about whether to take a long shot like the second, but because it is a pragmatic rather than a gateway question, it is different in an important way: it is a predictive question not about things that will most probably not occur (such as cure) but about things that almost certainly will. After all, we know what happens during the initial, intermediate, and final phases of AIDS. Some patients get Kaposi's sarcoma; many get *Pneumocystis* pneumonia; many get thrush. Later, blindness may develop; dementia is common; many lose the use of limbs. At the end, many can no longer communicate. To be sure, a few are symptom-free for many years and then die comparatively quickly, without sustained deterioration, but for most, there is an extended course of terminal deterioration marked by a range of predictable medical events. It is against this background information that a person with AIDS must make his or her choice about death.

A decision about timing is thus a prudential decision not so much to be made under uncertainty (when the probabilities of specific outcomes are not known) but a decision to be made under risk (when they are known). When making a decision under risk, that is, when the possible outcomes and their probabilities are known, the decisionmaker—the person with AIDS—adopts one of two decision strategies, maximax or maximin. (Of course, the decisionmaker may not be aware that this is what he or she is doing or be familiar with this terminology; he or she does so nevertheless in an intuitive way.[8] To decide what to do, one calculates a utility function by multiplying the value (or disvalue) of a given outcome by its probability; this is just to say that one's choice is based on one's preferences—the states of affairs, or medical and social conditions one could find oneself in—multiplied by the likelihood that they will actually materialize. To choose what to do, the maximax decisionmaker, on the one hand, seeks to maximize the best possible outcome that the terminal course of AIDS could bring—a longer life with less suffering. To adopt a maximax decision policy, thus, is to try to *maxi*mize the *maxi*mum outcome—that is, to shoot for the best that could happen. The maximin decision maker, on the other hand, seeks to preclude the worst possibility in the terminal course: a life of greater suffering; this decision maker tries to *maxi*mize the *mini*mum outcome. Thus, the maximax decision strategist, foreseeing that the end-stages of AIDS can sometimes be comparatively benign and may involve an extended period of life with comparatively little suffering, especially if good hospice or other care is provided, will probably decide to go later in the overall down-hill course of AIDS, postponing any active exit or choice of suicide until toward the very end so as not to miss any remaining moments of good life. The maximin strategist, on the other hand, foreseeing that the end-stages of AIDS can also in-volve severe incapacity, pain, social isolation, and dementia, chooses an earlier exit: suicide now, in order to *ensure* that these especially bad things cannot occur. Both decision strategies carry risks: the maximax decision maker, who tries not to miss any remaining moments of good life left, risks encountering the worst; the maximin decision maker, trying to avoid the worst, risks missing the best. But one cannot have it both ways: there is no decision strategy under risk that *guarantees* both getting the best and avoiding the worst.

4. *What weight shall I give to the welfare of others—my partner, family, friends, caregivers, community, and society?* In a recent documentary on euthanasia in the Netherlands, a Dutch physician remarked that it is much easier for the phy-sicians and the family if the patient chooses to have euthanasia later rather than earlier in the final course of the disease, since this allows physicians and especially family members to adjust to realities and give up unrealistic hopes for a cure.[9] This is only one of a myriad of considerations about the welfare and interests of others that might affect the choices about suicide to be made by a person with AIDS; these considerations can variously include such diverse elements as the fears, needs, religious beliefs, financial security, insurance status, education, research interests, or emotional needs of others, and may include other individuals, groups of persons, institutions, or even entire societies. Such considerations, it is crucial to understand, can operate either for or against a choice of suicide.

There are two related ways in which the interests of others may be relevant to choices of suicide during the downhill course of AIDS. First, others may have interests which run counter to one's own—as, for instance, when a person with AIDS wishes to exit sooner but the spouse will lose the disability payments that continue as long as that person lives; or when the person with AIDS wishes to keep going, but a loved one will be free to get on with the rest of his or her life only after that person is gone. Here, one's own interests appear simply to conflict with those of others. Second, however, it may be the case that because the person with AIDS cares about another, it is in both parties' interest that the disability payments continue or that the loved one be able to get on with the rest of his or her life. Despite the profound differences in these ways in which one person's interests may be relevant to another—whether these interests conflict, or whether one person's interests include those of another—in either case, preserving ration-ality in choice requires us to treat these as the fourth and last component of the choice made by the person considering suicide.

It may seem odd to place basic questions about the impact of one's death and the way one chooses to conduct one's dying on other individuals, on communities, and on social institutions at the end of this schema; indeed, it might be argued that they belong in first, not last, place, in the rational structure of end-of-life choices about AIDS. After all, the interests of others may be of profound concern to the person making a choice, whether those others be specific individuals or larger groups; and an individual may have duties and obligations to other individuals or groups even if he or she regards their interests as conflicting with his or her own. However, placing this consideration last rather than first has one central feature that contributes to protecting the rationality of the choice: while placing it first would control the other three elements, placing it last need not, but instead exhibits the character of the choice. For instance, the first question, *Is assisted suicide an option I want to consider?* may receive a quite different answer if one places the interests of others first rather than making one's choice and then attempting to minimize any negative impact on others. The second question, *Shall I hold out for the chance of a cure?* might also be answered differently if the interests of others are given principal weight. Placing the current question of what weight to give the interests of others last precludes pre-deciding the other questions in a way that favors the interests of others. This may seem to favor enhancing self-interest and minimizing any expected altruism in choices about dying. But it does not preclude the reverse: after all, the person who reaches this fourth element and answers it in favor of giving greatest weight to the interests of others rather than to his or her own interests—whether that is because he or she takes the interests of others to be part of his or her own or because he or she has obligations to respect these interests, even though they are contrary to his or her own—can of course review the earlier components of the choices he or she has faced and amend them accordingly. But in doing so, the character of this review and the amended choices it yields is exhibited: it may be altruistic in the milder sense that the decisionmaker takes another's interests as his or her own, or it may be altruistic in the stronger sense that one sacrifices one's own interests to serve those of others, whether this be a matter of choice or obligation. Making these choices last, not first, functions to keep a person making these difficult end-of-life choices from never really recognizing what his or her own interests really are and so operates to enhance the rationality of the choice. Rational choices can be self-interested; rational choices can also be self-sacrificing; but they cannot be fully rational when one does not recognize what is at stake.

Physicians, Friends, and AIDS Suicide

If this four-level model describes the rational structure of decisions about suicide in AIDS, then it may also invite us to see what sorts of influence by others might be appropriate and what would not. This is crucial in a climate in which assistance in suicide is widely available, whether or not technically legal. Assistance could come from many different parties: physicians, nurses, family members, spouses, lovers or partners, friends, children, work associates, psychologists, religious advisors, and many others, including individuals, groups of individuals (for example, support groups), and perhaps institutions and societies. For the sake of simplicity I shall discuss only two possibilities here, physicians and friends. Assistance can play a substantial role in choices about suicide, and it is essential to recognize the ways in which different parties can reinforce or disrupt the rational character of such choices.

Consider the respective roles a physician and a friend—a close friend, perhaps a partner, spouse, or other real intimate—might play in a person's choices about suicide. Of the various sorts of assistance a person with AIDS might seek, provision of a lethal drug or other means to be used in the suicide is clearly central: this makes the suicide possible, especially if the person with AIDS rejects violent means conventionally associated with suicide—guns, jumping, hanging, and so on—but would take a euthanatic drug guaranteeing an easy, painless death. Here, the roles of physician and friend are alike in certain respects—anybody can hand over a bottle of pills or help fit a plastic bag around someone's head—but they are clearly different in important informational aspects: the physician knows which drugs will be effective, how much of them to take, what their shelf life is, and how to prevent unwanted side effects like vomiting or convulsions.[10] The physician can also obtain the drug from a pharmacy or other reliable source guaranteeing their effectiveness. Unless the friend is also medically trained or has access to specialized information,[11] and also has access to reliable sources of drugs (so that, for instance, the shelf life has not expired), he or she will not be able to guarantee the easy, painless, foolproof death the person with AIDS may be seeking. Indeed, one study in Vancouver from 1980–1993 discovered that of the suicides assisted by friends, half were bungled, often increasing suffering contrary to all intentions.[12] Hence, the rational choice for a person with AIDS, other things being equal, would be to prefer to receive the euthanatic drug from a physician, not just a friend, unless of course the friend has obtained it directly from a physician; it would be irrational for a person planning suicide to prefer the street market or home-compounded drugs a friend might provide, or other more violent, potentially painful methods.

But handing over the drug, as I said, is not all there is to assisting in suicide. At least equally important is the influence others can have on the person's decisions about whether and when to do it. Here, too, the physician and the friend may play very different roles in protecting or undermining the rationality of the choice, and they play quite different roles in affecting different parts of the four-level schema I have identified. The physician's role is adapted to his or her medical competencies, beyond providing a drug. What the physician is best equipped to provide is information about the disease and about its end-stages. This is after all what the physician knows from both the medical literature and clinical experience. In particular, the physician can inform the patient about the various medical events a person dying with AIDS can expect to encounter along the way, thus providing information that is crucial for the patient at the third level of the schema—after he or she has decided to consider suicide in the first place and also not to hold out for a cure— when the patient is deciding how to time his or her suicide by picking that point in the downhill course of AIDS to go.

Indeed, the physician has two kinds of information that are relevant in this third stage of decision making: information about what conditions are likely to occur and information about their probabilities. The physician knows that the end-stages of AIDS can involve, among other things, blindness, loss of motor function, dementia, and pain, and knows how frequent these outcomes are. The conditions themselves are the foci of the patient's value-judgments: how does the patient value, or rather disvalue, say, being blind, bedridden, demented, or in pain? Some patients will regard these conditions as extremely undesirable—so bad, indeed, that it would be better to avoid them by death. Other patients will regard them as undesirable but not cataclysmically so; it would be better on the whole not to have these conditions, but life with them is still preferable, in these patients' views, than no life at all. It is these value-rankings about preferences regarding possible future conditions that the person with AIDS then uses in making decisions about suicide: if a maximax decision maker, the person will then try to maximize life free of these conditions or encumbered only by the least devalued of them; if a maximin decision maker, he or she will make choices about timing a suicide to preclude the occurrence of the worst.

But there is a second informational ingredient the physician can provide that is also crucial in these decisions: this is information about the probabilities of the various conditions that are the foci of the patient's values. How *likely* is it that a person in the end-stages of AIDS will lose motor function, or cognitive capacity, or go blind? This is not trivial information; it is information that the person with AIDS, whether employing maximax decision strategies to shoot for the best possible outcome or maximin strategies to try to preclude the worst possible outcomes, requires. For some, this will mean going early in the course of the disease, for others, it will mean going late. For a maximax decision maker, it would be irrational to go early, at least to avoid a state valued as bad but not very likely to occur; it would be equally irrational for a maximin decision maker to go late if that means risking a condition he or she views as unacceptably awful.

Considering the role such information must play in protecting the rationality of choices about AIDS, however, we must note with alarm the fact that the resources for making such decisions do not seem to be fully available and that the full range of crucial information is not always readily provided by physicians. For example, as far as I know, although there are several patient-centered, readable, accessible guides to the specific medical events in the downhill course of AIDS, they do not generally contain information about the *probabilities* of these events, despite the enormous group of people who have reason to be concerned with these facts and despite the huge body of information now available in the medical literature on AIDS. There is no such comprehensive body of information, easily accessible and readily understandable, to which a patient could turn. There are some sources—AIDS hotlines, for instance; although they usually list the various fungal, bacterial, viral, protozoan, oncologic, and neurologic opportunistic diseases and other conditions that can occur during the course of AIDS, they do nothing to provide information about the likely frequency or severity of them. Nor do they provide information about the types and probabilities of pain, even though, "contrary to popular belief" (as current researchers have put it), pain is a frequently encountered symptom, varying in prevalence from 50–60% in Hospice and hospital inpatients to 97% in patients close to death.[13] To be sure, many physicians or other caregivers involved in the treatment of AIDS will try to give their patients realistic accounts of what they can expect ahead, but this may often be skewed either by the inadvertent "hanging of crepe"—telling the patient the dimmer prognosis so that the patient will credit the physician and be stimulated by new hope if things turn out better than predicted—or the converse, the often paternalistic desire to shield the patient from profoundly discouraging reports.[14] I know of no information about the accuracy of prognoses given patients with AIDS, even though some AIDS specialists complain that nonspecialist physicians tend to underestimate both the length of life and the length of comparatively good health remaining to a person with AIDS. In short, what is not available is reliable probabilistic information that a person with AIDS, wishing to negotiate the final stages of the disease in a rational way, could use in deciding how to time a suicide he or she is considering. To be sure, this information might be quite complex—since the probabilities and specific natures of various conditions may vary among subpopulations of persons with AIDS (say, gay men, children, or IV drug users) and since it furthermore keeps changing over time, as the virus itself and medical treatments evolve—but it is still information essential for the making of a rational choice.

What often occurs instead is a generalization from familiar cases: the patient draws inferences based on the experiences of a friend or lover who has already gone through the terminal phases of AIDS and died. If the lover or friend has had a comparatively smooth course, terminal to be sure but not marked by severe suffering, the patient's own conclusion may be that the end-stages of AIDS are not to be feared. On the other hand, if the patient's closest exposure to death from AIDS has been with a person whose demise he or she perceived as really very bad, this patient may be tempted to generalize from this single case that the end-stages are at all costs to be avoided. It is, after all, what this patient knows best about AIDS, and the physician has not provided information that would set this single case within an overall framework of probability. To be sure, the same form of anecdotal reasoning is also prevalent in many other forms of illness, including both hereditary diseases like Huntington's disease, where the patient has typically watched a parent die, and widely distributed conditions like cancer or heart disease, but it is nevertheless a major risk in AIDS.

But, of course, this is not the way to make a rational choice about the timing of one's own suicide, either where the choice is motivated by the desire to optimize the enjoyment of good life or to avoid the worst of the end-stages, for it overlooks such matters as base rates of various events, predictive factors about one's own condition, or particular susceptibilities of the subgroup of which one is a member; hence this approach precludes any reasonably accurate assessment of the probabilities of the various possible events during one's own terminal course. Yet this is the very thing the physician conversant with AIDS is in the best position to provide—far, far better than the friend.

The friend, in contrast, has presumably little or no competence in predicting the medical events or their probabilities that characterize the downhill course of AIDS, beyond the kind of anecdotal predictions just described. On the other hand, if the friend is a friend in any robust sense of the term—not merely an acquaintance but someone with whom the person shares experiences at a much deeper level—then the friend will be much more in tune with that person's own basic convictions and background social, religious, and metaphysical beliefs. After all, the friend is someone who *knows* the person with AIDS, hence knows at least something of his or her personal and religious values, values that have central bearing on the question of suicide in AIDS. Larger cultural elements and institutions, which the friend may share with the patient, are likely to play a role here, for example, in stipulating whether causing one's own death is to be regarded as wrong, whether death can have meaning, and whether there is merit to suffering. There are things the friend is much more likely to know about the patient than the physician qua physician, especially if there are large religious, ethnic, or cultural differences between the physician and the patient.

It is clear, then, that it is the friend rather than the physician who is better positioned to help sort out the person's fundamental beliefs and associated value commitments. It is these matters that are of principal relevance to the first element in our four-part schema—that gateway question that addresses the issue of whether one wishes to consider suicide as an option at all, or chooses in any way to try to control one's own dying. Of at least the first three levels of this choice, this question is, I think, the most basic (though probably the least consciously and deliberately made), since it involves fundamental beliefs, often held at a pre-articulate, non-conscious level, typically inherited from religious traditions and heavily influenced by family and social expectations, about the nature of death and the appropriate role of the individual in facing it. To be sure, the physician can ask the patient about his or her underlying values and basic world view, but the physician cannot be expected to appreciate the answer—if indeed the patient can articulate it effec-tively in the first place—in anything more than a superficial way, especially if there are large cultural differences between them. In effect, then, the ways in which the physician qua physician can help the person with AIDS are quite unlike the ways friends can help: the friend helps best with first-level concerns, the physician with third-level ones.

Second-level choices pose perhaps a different problem. Neither friend nor phy-sician is better qualified with respect to second-level, intermediate choices about whether to hold out for a cure. This is because this choice involves a classic de-cision under uncertainty, where there is no way to calculate the likelihood of the desired possible outcome. Neither information from a physician about events of end-stage AIDS or their probabilities, as they are currently known, nor values-insight from a friend can have much force here, since neither party has any basis for saying how likely it is that a cure or treatment will materialize, or if so, what kinds of outcome conditions it might produce. Might a "cure" lift the death sentence but leave the patient permanently respirator-dependent? Might effective therapy lengthen the overall time-to-death, but not by very much? Or might a treatment be a real cure, producing complete reversal of the disease and a return to full health? Lessons from previous longshot cures and therapies are not much help here: given the enormous differences in the nature of the diseases, the research situations, and many other factors, it is impossible to extrapolate from past research except perhaps to say that longshot, overnight cures and therapies have been rare, but that they do occur. Of course, in deciding about suicide in AIDS, one could adopt some sort of combination policy—say, for instance, that one would hold out for a cure until a certain point in one's decline and then switch to a more active role in one's death—but this is just a miniversion of the original problem: at what point does one quit holding onto hope, and how does one time one's end?

Not only does deciding whether to hold out for a cure look different from the point of view of the person with AIDS and from the point of view of both physicians and friends, but since both physicians and friends often involve themselves in these choices, we must insist that responsibility for the outcomes of such choices be appropriately assigned. It is one thing for a person with AIDS to adopt a long-shot strategy in holding out for a cure; it is quite a different thing for someone else, whether friend or physician, to *advocate* a longshot strategy by urging the patient: "There's always hope of a cure!" To be sure, there *is* always hope of a cure or a long-term treatment, even if it may be extremely small: this is what it means to say that the climate in which such choices are made involves uncertainty. We do not and cannot know whether or when a cure will be found, whether it will be effective for those already ill, and what residual devalued conditions it might produce. The most negative outcome is that no cure materializes, and the person holding out for it who would otherwise have exited earlier endures end-stage conditions he or she regards as very, very bad—conditions he or she otherwise would have preferred to avoid. When the person with AIDS adopts a decision strategy under uncertainty, it is he or she who assumes responsibility for accepting the negative outcome, should a negative outcome be what occurs (as, in a longshot choice, it most likely will). But when other parties advise a person with AIDS to hold out on the grounds that there is always the chance of a cure, it is to them that we must assign at least partial responsibility for the negative outcomes that (most likely) will occur, for they have in effect encouraged the person to decide in a way that makes it *likely* that he or she will suffer these especially bad things.

Of the four levels or components sketched here in articulating the rational structure of end-of-life decisions, I have argued that friends have the most appropriate input into the first, physicians into the third, and that neither is better qualified for input into the second. The story is still different at the fourth level—the question of what weight to give the interests and welfare of others—for neither friends nor physicians, I think, may appropriately influence decision making at this level at all. This is because influence from physicians or friends so strongly invites self-interest on their part. Since the choice the person with AIDS faces in reflecting on how his or her life shall end is a choice about whether to prefer the interests of others to his or her own, any influence from parties directly affected risks biasing the choice. Physicians have interests in their standards of care, in their professional reputations, or in their research projects, not to mention their fees or the demands of their cost-containment boards; intimate friends have a huge range of emotional and practical needs. Of course, a patient's choices about whether to respond to the interests and needs of others may still be shaped by the expectations of ethnic, cultural, or religious groups, but this is not the same as being swayed by specific, potentially self-interested other persons.

Thus the difference in suicides assisted in decision making and performance by physicians, those assisted by friends, and those not assisted at all is not a trivial one, since although either physician or friend can discuss the issue and supply a drug, their influence in the choice of suicide may be of quite different character. Appropriate assistance from friends and physicians may well enhance the rationality of suicide choices; in fact, however, it may not work in this ideal way at all. While it is currently impossible to generalize about the behavior of physicians or friends in giving advice about suicide or providing the means, it is my guess that these parties often do it wrong, especially where the practice continues to be legally prohibited. Some physicians (perhaps many) do just the opposite of what they are qualified for: they pronounce on the first-level issue—whether or not patients may choose suicide or request physician assistance in doing so—but are reluctant to provide details about the actual character or probability of specific medical events of the terminal decline, lest that disturb the patient or undermine trust and hope, especially if it is clear that the patient intends to use this information in planning his or her own death. Indeed, in the debates surrounding legalized euthanasia and physician-assisted suicide, and in the disputes over figures like Jack Kevorkian, the medical profession as a whole has occupied itself primarily with what is a first-level question—whether suicide and physician-assisted suicide should be allowed—but has not sought to identify for patients the actual probabilities of what they can expect, including both negative matters such as pain, incapacity, blindness, and dementia, and positive ones signaling a smooth and easy course. Thus the problem is not just individual physicians who sometimes exceed the physician's proper role in providing input into the choices of AIDS patients considering suicide, but that collectivity of physicians referred to as the medical profession.

Similarly, the friend, whether partner, spouse, close associate, or significant other, unless also medically trained, has no special knowledge of the likely medical events of the terminal course, yet people in these roles often volunteer anecdotal information about the end-stage experiences of various other friends and acquaintances with AIDS: they thus similarly exceed their appropriate role in influencing decisions about suicide. Providing anecdotal information in this way may reinforce the patient's tendency to generalize from single-case examples and hence too may undermine the rationality of the choice. Of course, some patients might not succeed in comprehending probabilistic information about possible outcomes even if they were provided with it, but this does not change the fact that the kind of anecdotal information about AIDS typically available to the nonphysician friend is not the kind of information the patient needs in order to to make his or her choice in a rational way.

Of course, some physicians almost become friends of their patients as they explore deeper values in facing AIDS, and some friends—especially in the well-informed gay AIDS communities—are as well or better informed about the medical aspects of AIDS than many nonspecialist physicians. And some people with AIDS are both superbly well informed and supremely capable of articulating their own deepest values. But where these things are not the case, we should distinguish between the roles of physician and friend more carefully than we often do when a person with AIDS is deciding how his or her life shall end, and discourage each from encroaching on the area in which only the other can provide that sort of help that enhances the rationality of a person's choice.

Is AIDS Really a Special Case?

One further issue complicates this picture. Throughout this discussion of the importance of specific types of information in decisions about suicide in AIDS, as well as information about their probabilities, it may have seemed that these probabilities could be reliably known, especially information about end-stage medical conditions and the way the person with AIDS values them. They can; but the pattern of that occurrence is a much more tumultuous one than that characteristic of many other terminal conditions. AIDS—even in its last phases—is characterized by wild swings, from critical illness to fairly good health. There are high fevers, periods of delirium, episodes of noncommunication, but interspersed with periods during which the person may feel and function reasonably well. Other terminal conditions, such as many types of cancer, neurological diseases, circulatory diseases, or organ failure, are more likely to exhibit a steady, predictable pattern of decline, and while there are often exacerbations and remissions or periods of greater or lesser activity of the disease, they do not exhibit such broad swings as AIDS. This is because most of these other terminal conditions involve increasing deterioration of specific tissues or bodily functions, not a series of opportunistic diseases made possible by decreased immune status. This is not to say that other terminal conditions are not variable, but that the variability is not likely to be as wild as that characteristic of AIDS. What makes the problem of deciding rationally about coming to the end in AIDS so difficult, where suicide is the option under consideration, is the certainty of the decline but the unpredictability of its exact course. Maximin decision makers are more likely to go early and maximaxers much later, but neither decision strategy can be very reliable in achieving what both sorts of decision makers in general want: as much good life as possible, but with little risk of truly adverse states.

Among the reasons physicians have not preferred the kind of information that would enhance the rationality of patients about dying, it may be that they understand how particularly difficult rational choice must be in a volatile condition like AIDS. Nevertheless, this does not mean that it is not morally imperative to protect the rationality of these choices as much as possible, especially in communities where it is feasible for patients to make them, or that either the physician or the friend can be excused from reflecting carefully on what assistance to offer and what not to offer someone facing death from AIDS.

Notes

From *The Journal of Medicine and Philosophy* 19:571–594 (1994). An ancestral version of this article appeared as "Physicians, Partners, and People with AIDS: Deciding about Suicide," *Crisis: The Journal of the International Association for Suicide Prevention* 15 (1994): 15–21; used by permission of Hogrefe & Huber.

I would like to thank Ad Kerkhof, Timothy F. Murphy, and my colleagues in the Division of Medical Ethics, Department of Internal Medicine, University of Utah Medical School and LDS Hospital—Jay Jacobson, Jeff Botkin, David Green, and Leslie Francis—for comments on earlier drafts on this essay.

1. One exception of which I am aware is Stephen K. Yarnell and Margaret P. Battin, 'AIDS, psychiatry, and euthanasia,' *Psychiatric Annals* 18 (1988): 589–603. See also Jan E. Beskow, ed., HIV and AIDS-Related Suicidal Behavior: Report on a WHO Consultation. Bologna, Sept. 22–23, 1990 (Bologna: Monduzzi Editore, 1991); and James L. Werth, 'Rational Suicide and AIDS: Considerations for the psychotherapist,' *Counseling Psychologist* 20 (1992): 645–59.

2. Timothy F. Murphy, *Ethics in an Epidemic: AIDS, Morality and Culture* (Berkeley, Calif.: University of California Press, 1994) 28–51.

3. Except perhaps in the State of Washington, where the new organization Compassion in Dying now openly offers assistance in suicide to the terminally ill together with extensive counseling. According to Thomas Preston, M.D. (personal communication), Compassion in Dying believes it has prevented more suicides among terminally ill people than it has aided.

4. Things may be changing. Beginning in San Francisco in July 1993, Derek Humphry, past president of the Hemlock Society and author of *Final Exit* (1991), has held a series of well-publicized open discussions with people with AIDS in various cities in the United States.

5. P. J. van der Maas, J.J.M. van Delden, L. Pijnenborg, L.: "Euthanasia and other medical decisions concerning the end of life," [English edition of the Remmelink report] *Health Policy* 22 (1991).

6. As David Hume pointed out, there is an asymmetry in the way we regard active control over dying: for example, traditional religious thought regards active control that brings about death, as in suicide, as impermissible interference contrary to divine plan, but does not regard medical or other efforts to prolong life as interfering with divine intention in a similar way. David Hume, "On suicide" (1777), in *The Philosophical Works of David Hume* (Edinburgh: Adam Black, William Tait, Charles Tait, 1826).

7. Murphy, *Ethics in an Epidemic,* 28–51.

8. The reader who is not familiar with this terminology may wish to consult the classic exposition (R. D. Luce and H. Raiffa, *Games and Decisions* (New York: Wiley & Sons, 1957), especially chap. 2). 1 have not followed Luce and Raiffa's terminology, however, in describing the decision maker who attempts to minimize the maximum loss when facing negative consequences as adopting a "minimax" strategy (p. 279), though what I have said here could be easily translated into that terminology.

9. Roger Mudd, "Choosing Death," PBS Frontline documentary, The Health Quarterly, WGBH (Boston, Mass: WGBH Educational Foundation, 1993).

10. The assumption that the physician knows these things may not be warranted in a culture in which physician assistance in suicide or performance of euthanasia is illegal. When these practices were becoming effectively (though not technically) legal in the Netherlands, the Royal Dutch Pharmaceutical Association mailed a brochure identifying suitable drugs and their appropriate doses to every physician in the country; this was intended to prevent the sorts of poorly informed experimentation with means of euthanasia that could otherwise be expected to occur.

11. Derek Humphry, *Final Exit: The Practicalities of Self-Deliverance and Assisted Suicide for the Dying* (Eugene, Ore., The Hemlock Society, 1991), might be considered an example of such a source.

12. These results were reported by Russel D. Ogden in a thesis submitted for a master's degree at Simon Fraser University. See C. H. Farnsworth, "Bungled AIDS suicides result in increase of suffering," *New York Times* (June 14, 1994), C12.

13. W. O'Neill and J. S. Sherrard, "Pain in human immunodeficiency virus disease: a review," *Pain* 54 (1993): 3–14.

14. M. Siegler, "Pascal's wager and the hanging of crepe," *New England Journal of Medicine* 293(1975): 853–7.

4

Is a Physician Ever Obligated to Help a Patient Die?

Physician-assisted suicide will probably soon become legal on a state-by-state basis, culturally tolerated, and openly practiced. But while this change will resolve some moral issues, it will raise others. One particular question which, I suspect, covertly fuels many physicians' anxieties about legalization of physician-assisted suicide is this: Is a physician ever *obligated* to help a patient die? If physician-assisted suicide were to become legal or legally tolerated, would the patient have a right to assistance, a right held against the physician for performance of this duty?

It may seem obvious that physicians can never be obligated to do something they regard as morally wrong—especially not something that may seem to them to be as profoundly morally wrong as contributing to the self-killing of their patient. Whatever the law says, for some physicians, conscience still may not permit it. All proposals for the legalization of physician-assisted suicide that have been proposed to date take this stance: that the physician may elect to help, but is not obligated to do so. In voter initiatives in Washington, California, and Oregon, in state legislative initiatives, in model statutes such as that of the Boston Working Group,[1] and so on, all proposals have opt-out provisions, or "conscience clauses," that permit the physician to refuse to participate in a suicide. Oregon's Measure 16, which passed at the polls in November 1994 and withstood a repeal measure in 1997, and is now its Death with Dignity Act, is representative. It says: "No health care provider shall be under any duty, whether by contract, by statute or by any other legal requirement to participate in the provision to a qualified patient of medication to end his or her life in a humane and dignified manner."[2]

But the basis of opt-out clauses—the ubiquitous assumption that a physician's scruples provide adequate justification, legally and morally, for excusing him or her from assisting in suicide—is rarely challenged. Furthermore, there is little challenge to the informal understanding that if the practice of assisting suicides were to remain extralegal but still become widely accepted, physicians could nevertheless choose to opt out, based on their conscience or any other personal consideration. It is just this assumption that I wish to examine here. It is my view that even the physician with the most profound moral scruples against physician-assisted suicide can, in certain circumstances, incur an obligation to provide this assistance. But when this turns out to be the case, it is almost always the product of that physician's own doing, and thus could have been avoided.

I hasten to add that I support the legal recognition of opt-out provisions in legislation concerning physician-assisted suicide. But that does not mean that a physician has no *moral* obligation to help, even if there is no legal one. Opt-out clauses, whether explicitly stated in legal documents or informally embedded in culturally understood social expectations, cannot always provide moral protection, even if they do shield a physician from legal action or social blame.

This paper has two principal parts: a long background section that examines the argument over physician-assisted suicide and shows how a positive right to assistance is generated from two basic moral principles, and a more sharply focused applications section that examines how a patient's right to assistance in suicide can impose an obligation on the physician to assist, even if the physician has scruples against doing so.

To address the question of physician obligation, we must first review the principal arguments for and against physician-assisted suicide in terminal illness, since these arguments establish whether the dying patient has rights to assistance in suicide. These rights would at a minimum include the "negative" right not to be interfered with or prevented from committing suicide if the means are available from a willing physician, and they might also include the "positive" right to require a physician to provide such help if requested.[3] If there are such rights, do they impose obligations upon physicians, even when as physicians they do not want to participate and even when the law provides opt-out clauses protecting them from any legal obligation to do so?

The Case for Physician-Assisted Suicide

The moral argument in favor of permitting physician assistance in suicide is grounded in the conjunction of two principles: self-determination (or, as bioethicists put it, autonomy) and mercy (or the avoidance of suffering). The moral right of self-determination is the right to live one's life as one sees fit, subject only to the constraint that this not involve harm to others. Because living one's life as one chooses must also include living the very end of one's life as one chooses, the matter of how to die is as fully protected by the principle of self-determination as any other part of one's life. Choosing how to die is part of choosing how to live.

The second component of the moral argument in favor of physician assistance in suicide is grounded in the joint obligations to avoid doing harm and to do good (the principles of nonmaleficence and beneficence, as bioethicists often put them). In medical-ethics discussions, some writers call this the principle of patient interests or patient welfare, but in the specific context of end-of-life questions, I like to call this the principle of mercy—the principle that one ought both to refrain from causing pain or suffering and act to relieve it.[4] The principle of mercy, or avoidance of suffering, underwrites the right of a dying person to an easy death, to whatever extent possible, and clearly supports physician-assisted suicide in many cases. Suicide assisted by a humane physician spares the patient the pain and suffering that may be part of the dying process, and grants the patient a "mercifully" easy death.

The principle of mercy is relevant in two general classes of cases, one comparatively unproblematic, the other far more disputed. In the first case, the dying patient is currently enduring pain or other intolerable physical symptoms (such as continuous breathlessness, nausea, vomiting) or is suffering from emotional and psychological anguish. In the second case, the patient with a terminal illness anticipates and seeks to avoid pain and suffering, knowing that they are highly likely to occur in the future course of the disease. Narrow constructions of the principle of mercy are typically interpreted to support just the patient's right to avoid current pain and suffering; the requirement that the patient be undergoing "intolerable suffering" is often read in this way. Broader constructions support preemptive strategies intended to avoid anticipated pain and suffering before they begin.

Of course, with modern pain-management techniques—especially those pioneered by the hospice movement for treating pain before it develops, on a regular schedule, rather than as needed after the patient already experiences it—most pain in terminal illness can be avoided. Other symptoms caused either by the disease itself or by the treatments employed to arrest it (including diarrhea, itching, restlessness, confusion, hallucinations, and many others) can also be controlled at least to some extent with adequate management. And suffering—that constellation of emotional and psychological factors often described as anguish, despair, hopelessness, fear, and dread—can be greatly relieved by sensitive counseling and plain old-fashioning caring.

But not all pain, symptoms, and suffering are amenable to treatment or actually receive treatment. The 1995 SUPPORT study, for example, showed that about half of patients dying in five major teaching hospitals were reported to have experienced moderate to severe pain at least 50 percent of the time during their last two or three days of life.[5] Many other studies both in the United States and worldwide document inadequate treatment of pain from cancer and other causes. Sometimes this failure is due to fears of creating addiction to narcotics, sometimes to ignorance of contemporary escalating or "ladder" methods of pain management, and sometimes to lack of adequate drugs, facilities, personnel, and other resources. Whether or not nearly all pain *could* be controlled, the reality is that much pain in dying patients is not effectively treated.

It is always possible to relieve pain, other symptoms, and suffering by producing partial or complete unconsciousness through sedation. But some patients do not want this sort of relief, even if it could be effectively managed over time. They regard as repugnant programs that stress the heavy use of analgesics, especially opiates, because this treatment does not accord with their conceptions of death with dignity, or with the sort of easy passage they wish for themselves and for the family members who will be close observers of it. They do not want a medicalized, drugged dying process; they do not want "terminal sedation." They want a death they can meet consciously, in the company of their family, at a time and place and in a manner of their own choosing.

It is these two basic moral principles, self-determination and mercy, in which the right to suicide in terminal illness is grounded. Like rights of self-determination generally, the right to suicide in terminal illness is initially the negative right (sometimes called a liberty right) not to be interfered with; patients retain the right to control what is done to them in the sense of preventing what they do not want. That is what liberty, in the negative-right sense of the term, is. In the circumstances of terminal illness, however, self-determination may become a positive right as well—a right to require someone to help, a right to request or demand what one actively wants. This transformation can occur because endstage terminally ill patients, dying of degenerative processes in a long, debilitating illness, may not be able to exercise their right to influence the circumstances of their death without assistance from another person. They are often institutionalized in a hospital or other facility or bedridden at home, with constant surveillance ("care"), perhaps in pain or with other disturbing symptoms. And while some terminally ill patients do find alternative means of committing suicide—shooting themselves or jumping from buildings—for most of them this is completely unrealistic or utterly repugnant. The right to control one's own dying as far as possible in order to avoid suffering or pain is the right to seek an *easy* death. It is not merely the "right to die"; it is the right to try to die without suffering and with what is often called dignity, in a way, perhaps, that underscores the importance of the very end of life. But this is a right nullified without the assistance of someone who can provide both technical and emotional support.

The most plausible party for providing such assistance is the physician. It is the physician who has access to drugs, who has specialized knowledge of appropriate dosages, and who knows how to prevent side effects such as nausea and vomiting.[6] Equally important, the physician can be a source of emotional support for both patient and family. Seen in this light, the right to assistance in suicide is plausibly construed as the dying patient's right to help from his or her own physician, at least where there is a personal physician who knows the patient well, who has been directly, extensively, and intimately connected with and responsible for that person's care, who may know the family, and who understands, better than any other physician or other party able to provide assistance in suicide, that person's hopes, fears, and wishes about how to die.

The realistic physician also knows how the sort of death the patient seeks is likely to contrast with the expected course of events if assistance is not provided. Not only is the right to suicide in order to achieve an easier, more acceptable death not much of a right if one cannot exercise it by oneself, but it is only fully supported where such help is provided by the most effective person in this role, the patient's own physician, or, if there is no such arrangement, the physician currently responsible for providing the patient's terminal care.

It is important to recognize that in serving as the basis for the rights of dying patients, self-determination and mercy do not function as independent principles, each sufficient in itself. A mere request for physician-assisted suicide by a perfectly healthy person does not justify a physician's assistance. Similarly, the mere fact of pain or suffering in a terminal patient does not license a physician to end that person's life, if the person does not seek physician-assisted suicide.[7] Fears that legalization would license assisted suicide for a healthy person without pain or suffering, or involuntary or nonvoluntary mercy-killing, are often expressed by those who oppose it, but this is to misunderstand what the bases of a patient's right would be under any of the current proposals. *Both* principles, self-determination and mercy, must be applicable for the patient to have any substantial claim on the physician's help.

In practice, these two principles do not always function in independent ways. The principle of self-determination may play a large role in what constitutes acceptable and unacceptable forms of pain relief to the patient. The principle of mercy likewise plays a role in what the patient conceives of as an easy death, taking into consideration both his or her own comfort and the comfort of family members or others who will be observers of the death or directly affected by it.

A person's background views about the significance of the final parts of one's life—the last months, weeks, days, hours—may also influence how patients exercise their rights. In a contemporary secular view, perhaps borrowed from medieval theology but often (though not always) cleansed of its religious underpinnings, these last moments are given special weight in a way that makes the physician's role particularly important. In medieval Christian theology, the final moments of life were the last chance for repentance, perhaps made in the religious ritual of extreme unction but in any case held within the conscience of the dying person. Repentance and complete acceptance of God in the last moments of life were held to be crucial, in that they might pave the way for salvation. A lot rode on these last moments.

The modern secularized version of this scene recognizes, at a minimum, that the very last part of one's life can be of paramount emotional, reflective, and social significance; it can be viewed as the conclusion, the resolution, the culmination of a life now completely lived. That is the reason some people choose to end their lives directly, so that they can finish their lives as themselves, able to think, communicate, and (for some) to pray, rather than be overtaken by pain or sedated into oblivion.

Thus we begin to see the basic structure of the argument about physician-assisted suicide. The side favoring physician-assisted suicide argues from the conjunction of the moral principles of self-determination and mercy to establish the right to direct assistance in dying—a right which in turn generates obligations on the part of the physician. At a minimum, the physician is obligated to refrain from attempting to prevent the suicide, whether by threat, force, or involuntary hospitalization. And insofar as the patient's right becomes a positive claim to assistance, the physician, as the party most knowledgeable in medical matters, must provide help in doing what the patient seeks. And because the patient's trust and comfort with a familiar caregiver is also crucial in seeking an easy death, the obligation to assist is particularly strong for the patient's own physician.

To be sure, relabeling might take some of the sting out of this obligation. Were the physician's role redescribed as "attending" in a "patient-directed" or "self-enacted" death, rather than "assisting" a "suicide," it might not seem so controversial or so difficult for physicians with scruples against "suicide" to comply with.[8] That is why the practice is often called "aid-in-dying" or other less freighted names, and why legislative measures, including Oregon's Death with Dignity Act, can insist that what is authorized "shall not constitute a suicide."

But relabeling is not the point. The point is that if the patient has a right to physician-assisted suicide, aid-in-dying, or whatever the act is called, the two underlying moral principles clearly show that at least in some circumstances, the patient's personal physician may have not only a negative duty not to interfere, but also a positive obligation to provide the assistance the patient seeks—despite whatever opt-out legal clauses or social expectations may be available.

The Case against Physician-Assisted Suicide

If the patient has the right to seek an easy, merciful death, including death by means of physician-assisted suicide, the corresponding obligation on the part of the physician to provide assistance can be overridden only by other relevant considerations of equal or greater weight. The two basic arguments most frequently used to oppose physician-assisted suicide are the slippery-slope argument, which points to the likelihood of abuse, and the principled argument, which points to the intrinsic wrongness of killing.

The slippery-slope argument, backbone of the literature opposed to physician-assisted suicide, claims that legal and societal recognition of physician-assisted suicide will lead by gradual degrees to outright abuse: from a few sympathetic cases of suffering, we will move to the coercion of dying patients by malevolent family members who harbor long resentments or fragile ones who cannot bear the stress, to the callousness of cost-cutting insurers and health-maintenance organizations, and the greed, arrogance, or impatience of physicians who for a variety of reasons do not take adequate care of their dying patients. Finally we will reach the point where patients with disabilities or chronic illnesses or other conditions requiring extraordinary care are forced into "choosing" suicide when that would otherwise not have been their choice.

Focusing on physicians, the slippery-slope argument points to inadequate training in terminal care, fatalism about patients who are dying, overwork and severe time pressures in clinical settings, endemic racism, prejudice against the elderly, the disabled, those who have mental illnesses, and those who do not speak English, frustration with patients who are not improving, and many other factors which, it claims, will lead physicians to nudge, push, or force their patients in this direction. In its extreme forms, the slippery-slope argument predicts that we will end with medical holocaust: widespread involuntary killing, disguised only by the fact that its victims are not herded into concentration camps but remain dispersed in various hospitals, nursing homes, long-term care facilities, and bedrooms of their own homes. Patients will be killed against their will, it is argued, once we open these floodgates.

Slippery-slope claims have been the focus of most objection to legalization of physician-assisted suicide. But claims of this type are notoriously difficult to defend, since they require both adequate evidence of causal factors that will lead to the feared future circumstance and reasons for thinking there are no adequate ways to prevent the predicted slide. But while cost pressures within a currently chaotic medical care system may provide reason for expecting manipulative pressures on terminally ill patients to choose suicide (in addition to or in spite of equally manipulative pressures to extend treatment), there are many resources for erecting barriers to abuse—waiting times, documentation of requests, prohibition of fees, mandatory counseling, and the analysis of records after the fact to identify deviant patterns of physician practice.[9] Certainly, we must be continuously alert to the risks of abuse. But this risk, like most risks in slippery-slope arguments, is not predictable with sufficient probability to warrant the undercutting of terminally ill patients' basic rights to a physician's assistance—especially their own physician's assistance—in suicide if they choose.

The second moral claim of the opposition to physician-assisted suicide, that killing is intrinsically wrong, is often presented with religious defenses. This argument is not so much concerned with future abuse but with the very fact of killing that physician-assisted suicide involves right now. Killing, it is argued, has been repudiated by religious codes from ancient times to the present; killing violates the sanctity of life; killing destroys the Creator's work. That killing is wrong, it is asserted, is a basic moral principle, regardless of whether it is set in a religious context or not and regardless of whether one kills another or kills oneself. While the argument concerning the wrongness of killing is more often used against active euthanasia, it is also employed against physician-assisted suicide.

Most religious and ethical systems recognize some forms of killing as justified: killing in war, killing in self-defense, killing in capital punishment, and so on. In discussions of physician-assisted suicide and euthanasia, the claim that killing is intrinsically wrong is often transmuted into the claim that *doctors* should not kill. Though it might be permissible for soldiers in combat, jailers acting at the orders of the justice system, and innocent persons defending themselves from aggressors to kill in specific circumstances, it is never permissible for doctors, acting *as doctors,* to kill. It is simply outside the physician's role, a basic violation of it, in fact. Healing, the doctor's professional task, precludes killing.

But does the physician's role really preclude direct involvement in a patient's death? Clearly the physician's role centers on healing, but when healing is no longer possible and the patient is dying (after all, everyone must die eventually), what is the physician's role in this circumstance? Historical precedent will not resolve the issue: while physicians in some time periods have at least officially rejected assistance in a patient's suicide, physicians have at other times accepted it. For instance, the mainstream Greek physicians of ancient times regarded it as part of their role to provide patients whom they could not treat with a lethal drug, either at the patient's or the family's request; hemlock was developed for this purpose.[10] At the same time, the Hippocratic school of medicine held that the physician ought not to do this; this view is the one incorporated in the Hippocratic Oath. Indeed, there has been dispute about this issue throughout Western medical history.

But the issue here is not just whether doctors throughout the ages do or do not agree about their roles in caring for a dying patient and whether that may include direct killing. Such a determination would hardly answer an issue about *rights*. It is possible that physicians throughout the ages have rejected any involvement in ending life; it is also possible—and there is much evidence to suggest this—that they have been quietly willing to do so in sympathetic circumstances. One thinks, for instance, of Freud's physician, who promised and delivered a lethal drug at Freud's request after Freud had endured many years of oral cancer. But that possibility is changing as physician roles vis-à-vis the dying become a matter of broad public concern.

In the late twentieth and early twenty-first centuries in the developed world, most people face death from diseases with characteristically prolonged downhill courses (cancer, cardiovascular conditions, organ failure at various sites, neurological diseases, and so on), and these often involve extended pain, limitation of function, and suffering. Physician-aided death has always been an issue, but not a frequent one, since previously there were not many cases in which dying took this extended, more difficult form; now, at the end of this century, it is becoming an issue of massive scope.

It is also important to observe cultural differences in notions about the proper duties of physicians. Doctors in the Netherlands, where physician-assisted suicide and euthanasia are broadly accepted and legally tolerated, take direct aid-in-dying to be among the duties of the conscientious doctor. While many physicians report that performing euthanasia is personally difficult, they say they believe it to be part of the physician's role, and expect one another not to desert their patients at the end. As the Remmelink Commission, which examined the practice of euthanasia and physician-assisted suicide in that country, reported, under certain circumstances, "a large majority of physicians in the Netherlands see euthanasia as an accepted element of medical practice."[11]

Nor is the religious conception of "innocence" of much help in explicating the principle of the wrongness of killing. Especially within Catholic teaching, this principle holds that it is wrong to kill the innocent, not that it is wrong to kill altogether. But not only is it difficult to separate the innocent from the guilty in any nontheological sense that could be used in public policy (aside from singling out convicts, enemy soldiers, and assailants of nonaggressive people), it would also mean, applied in the context of assisted suicide in terminal illness, that it was just the guilty, not the innocent, who could hope to have their pleas for assistance in suicide answered. But this, of course, seems backwards: if anyone is to be forced to suffer when they choose not to do so, it should not be the innocent but the guilty.

Are these arguments—the slippery-slope argument concerning abuse and the argument from the wrongness of killing—sufficient to undercut the patient's rights of self-determination and mercy that jointly support a moral right to physician assistance in suicide? It is crucial that the arguments favoring physician-assisted suicide and the arguments opposing it are of different structures. The arguments in favor of assisted suicide appeal to the conjunction of two fundamental moral principles: self-determination and mercy. These two basic moral principles are acknowledged by all parties, including physicians, patients, and observers (both opponents and proponents of physician-assisted suicide), as just that: basic moral principles. Even physicians who oppose physician-assisted suicide accept the principle of self-determination—it is, after all, what underlies the opt-out conscience-clause provisions in legislation concerning physician-assisted suicide.

The same principle is also recognized by the patient seeking help as the basis of his or her own right of self-determination. Physicians and patients alike also recognize obligations of mercy: relieving pain and suffering is a central part of the physician's task, as well as what the patient seeks from the physician.

Furthermore, opponents of physician-assisted suicide also appeal to both these principles: autonomy or self-determination is the basis of the right not to be killed against one's will (feared as the consequence of the slide down the slippery slope) and mercy is the basis of the patient's right to avoid the fear and emotional pain that the prospect of being killed against one's will would involve. All sides, then, recognize these two fundamental moral principles, though they may differ about their relevance in the issue of physician-assisted suicide.

The arguments *against* physician-assisted suicide, however, have a different structure; they are not based on fundamental moral principles. The principle "do not kill" cannot be directly defended without qualification, it is widely assumed, since it would also prohibit killing in war, self-defense, and capital punishment. Even the more limited principle of not killing the innocent, though defensible elsewhere, backfires in terminal-illness contexts. The more focused application "doctors should not kill" is not usually treated as an argument in principle, since it would run afoul of historical and contemporary cross-cultural variation, but as a form of slippery-slope argument. Why shouldn't doctors kill? The answers characteristically point to the bad consequences that would ensue if doctors were to kill or assist in the suicide of even those patients who asked for this help. Patients, it is said, would no longer be able to trust their doctors. Doctors would overstep the bounds of legally permitted assistance in suicide, moving on to killing that is in no way sanctioned by law. Perhaps the law, too, might expand its scope, permitting doctors to kill patients, especially patients with disabilities, where there were no acceptable moral grounds for doing so. Furthermore, the integrity of the medical profession would be threatened.

But when the question is pursued in this way, a principle-based argument is thus transmuted into a consequentialist one that points to the harms killing might cause. Unless it is held that *all* killing causes harm sufficient so that it cannot be permitted (a view almost never consistently advanced by opponents in the current public discussions of physician-assisted suicide), it is difficult to show why, if their dying patients earnestly request it in preference to irremediable suffering, physicians in particular should not kill, without appealing to a consequentialist argument. But this is not an argument in principle; it is an argument about possible future practice.

Given this difference in the structure of the arguments for and against physician-assisted suicide, we may conclude that the burden of proof runs in favor of recognizing dying patients' rights to physician-assisted suicide if they are suffering intolerably or if they anticipate intolerable suffering. Only principle-based claims of equal or greater weight, or predictive proof that widespread bad consequences and medical holocaust would really ensue, can override this right. Moreover, claims about possible harms cannot be merely conjectural, speculative guesses about what could happen but must provide clear, incontrovertible evidence of genuine threats that can be avoided in no other way. Slippery-slope arguments against rights succeed only if they can provide good evidence that the projected future harm is really great and truly inevitable.

Claims about abuse in Holland are often used to try to make this point, but many of those given broadest circulation in the United States involve substantial distortion of the facts. Despite claims about the notorious "1,000 cases" (actually about 900) in which suffering patients were euthanized without a current explicit request, there is no evidence of abuse that would be sufficient to prove that allowing physician-assisted suicide and euthanasia leads to medical holocaust.[12] Indeed, many observers think protections for patients in the Netherlands are improving as legal regulation and social recognition of a formerly underground practice increases. There is no sound evidence of a pattern of generalized abuse.

The overall structure of the argument invites (though does not require) proponents of the physician-assisted suicide to show that widespread, serious abuse will not result, and this, I think, they are able to do. Certainly the possibility of abuse should always be taken seriously, by proponents and opponents alike, regardless of the structure of the argument. Even with the weight of principle on their side, proponents have been working to show that it is possible to devise adequate barriers against abuse. No compelling case has been made by opponents that legalizing or otherwise accepting physician-assisted suicide will cause overridingly great harms, sufficient to override the patient's basic rights of autonomy and mercy in the first place, and much of their argument has involved the kind of diffuse threat often employed in slippery-slope argumentation but without real corroboration. But if the opposition cannot reasonably establish that substantial harms would ensue, it has not produced a case strong enough for overriding a right.

The error many interpreters of the physician-assisted suicide debate have made, sizing up the arguments concerning self-determination and mercy on one side and the arguments concerning the wrongness of killing and the possibility of abuse on the other, is to treat these as equal, not just in content but in structure. But they are not equal in structure; the self-determination and mercy side is logically stronger, being grounded in basic moral principles, while the argument from the wrongness of killing (which is focused in practice, as we have seen, on the wrongness of *doctors'* killing and is argued primarily on slippery-slope grounds, or grounds of projected consequences) and the slippery-slope argument itself function as challenges to it. This structure of rights grounded in basic moral principles and correlative obligations (articulated by proponents) and reasons for overridings (articulated by opponents) captures all the elements of both sides of the argument.

The Physician's Obligation

This elaborate analysis, based on the structure of the arguments for and against physician-assisted suicide, may seem entirely irrelevant to the practicing physician. What bothers the physician is the claim that patients have a *right*—a right "against" the physician—for performance of an "obligation" to help patients kill themselves. Actual clinical situations in the real world are often not simple, and the relevance of ideals such as self-determination and mercy are far from clear. Even among physicians who recognize a moral obligation to assist dying patients with suicide, putting that policy into practice in actual situations is often problematic.

For example, a patient may seek help in suicide because of anticipated pain and suffering that lies in the future but has not yet occurred. Honoring this request is likely to be a problem where statutes define eligibility for physician-assisted suicide in terms of time to projected death. Oregon's Death with Dignity Act and most other U.S. proposals make eligibility for assistance a function of expected outcome (death within six months), but they do not specify what degree of medical deterioration must already have occurred. What if the physician cannot be certain that death will occur in six months? Or what about a suffering patient who articulated a wish for suicide in the past but has since become incompetent? This is the problem with more than half of the notorious 1,000 Dutch cases, where wishes for euthanasia had been expressed but there was no current explicit request. What should physicians do about conscious, competent patients who earnestly wish assistance in suicide and are enduring irremediable pain or suffering but cannot administer the means of death to themselves—for instance, patients who are unable to take oral drugs, or who are too disabled to use other means of administration such as self-injections or suppositories? Here, if the physician feels a moral obligation to provide assistance, it must be by physician-administered euthanasia, not physician-assisted suicide.

Of particular relevance is the situation some Dutch physicians report in assisting patients with suicide. Though the suicide may begin with the patient's self-administration of a lethal oral solution, suppository, or pills, if the effect is not complete or if vomiting occurs (as sometimes happens with oral drugs not preceded by an antiemetic), or if the effect cannot be complete because the volume required for one-time administration would be too large (as with patients who have difficulty swallowing), the physician must be prepared to perform euthanasia at the end.

Other situations also make things far less clear, as is the case with patients who are chronically but not terminally ill, or who suffer from paralysis, or who have some but not overwhelming pain, or whose suffering is exclusively anticipatory, at some distant and undetermined point in the future, and so on. Each of these mixed, difficult cases presents a different challenge.

The obligations of physicians in these situations are best expressed in terms of a double axis of continuums: the stronger the patient's current wish for a physician-assisted death (this is the self-determination axis) and the greater the patient's experience of unrelievable pain and suffering in the process of dying (this is the mercy axis), the stronger the dual basis of the patient's right, and hence the stronger the physician's correlative obligation to provide the patient with assistance in dying. At the other end of this double axis of continuums, where the patient does not want to commit suicide and is not suffering from a terminal illness, the physician has an obligation *not* to assist the patient's death. Intermediate points yield a range of somewhat weaker to somewhat stronger claims on the physician. In many of these, a physician may choose to respond to a patient's request for assistance but is not morally required to do so. Only toward that end of the continuum, where earnest request and a real need for mercy coincide, where the patient seeks an easier death but cannot accomplish this with ease or dignity acting alone, does the possibility of obligation to the dying patient arise. Thus, obligation to assist a patient in suicide may be a comparatively rare thing, but it nevertheless can arise. It is this obligation which, I think, physicians' scruples are too easily assumed to defeat.

What about the physician who objects? Even where physician-assisted suicide has been fully legalized and no legal penalty or other harm to the physician, family members, or others is anticipated, and where there are no issues about borderline cases like those above, a physician may still have scruples against participating in this practice. The opt-out clauses that are part of all current public initiatives and legislative proposals permit the physician to decline to participate. But in order to evaluate the moral weight of these opt-outs and determine whether they outweigh a patient's rights, we must know something about the reasons for them.

Consider the sorts of explanations various physicians might provide for declining to meet a patient's request for assistance in suicide. Some explanations involve doubts about the psychological and medical appropriateness of ending life in the specific case, such as "The patient is ambivalent" or "The patient's pain could still be alleviated." These reasons, in effect, challenge the criteria of eligibility by asserting that self-determination and mercy do not in this case fully apply. Other reasons could involve points of self-interest or self-protection, such as "It's too time-consuming," "I'll lose respect around the hospital," or "I don't want to dirty my hands." Reasons of self-interest may include both reasons of trivial concern, like "It takes too much paperwork," and concerns about more substantial personal risks, as in "I don't want to subject myself or my family to social ostracism or legal risk."

But some of the reasons a physician might offer, if being truthful, for not wishing to participate are rooted in more basic moral scruples: the beliefs that it is contrary to the physician's religion, that it is sinful, that it is a violation of the law, and that it is profoundly morally wrong. These are not trivial or merely self-interested excuses but serious, earnest reservations. It is important not to minimize the force of some physicians' objections or the range of behaviors such objections might proscribe. Kevin Wildes, a Jesuit, points out that because suicide is held in the Roman Catholic tradition to be inherently evil, so is assisting in a suicide.[13] But Wildes also argues that for a physician to refer a patient to another, more compliant physician would likewise be complicity in evil, and hence evil itself. A conscientious believer not only would make use of an opt-out clause but would refuse to have anything to do with the suicide at all, not even providing advice, confirming a terminal diagnosis, or transferring a patient's records to another physician (as most opt-out clauses, including that of Oregon's Death with Dignity Act, would require), for this too would be tantamount to complicity in evil itself.

It may seem self-evident that scruples of this intensity should be honored without reservation, perhaps especially where they have a religious basis. Clearly, it would do substantial psychological, emotional, and spiritual harm to physicians to force them to violate their own consciences, and under most circumstances this would be unnecessary: after all, patients may be easily able to find other physicians willing and prepared to provide the aid they seek. In such cases, the patient's rights of self-determination and mercy would still be satisfied, though by some other physician, and real harm to the physician with scruples would be avoided.

While genuine scruples on the part of the physician should be honored whenever possible, there are circumstances where the patient's right overrides these scruples. The patient may have a particularly strong relationship with the original physician, and may find it impossible to achieve such a relationship with another. Or there may be no other physician available with equal technical skill in terminal care or similar specialization in the patient's particular disease. Or there may be no other physician available at all. Or there may be no other physician available who is willing to assist in a suicide, a circumstance particularly likely in a practice area or facility where physicians tend to share the same values and views. If all physicians were to decline to participate, this would render the patient's right to assistance nil.

While in many situations it will be comparatively easy for a patient to find a physician willing to assist in suicide, especially if full legalization has occurred, there still may be circumstances in which a particular physician is the only one who could reasonably be called upon to provide assistance. Because in these circumstances the patient cannot find an alternative, the case for expecting this physician to cooperate, despite his or her scruples, is far stronger.

This may seem to be a rare circumstance, but it is closely related to another, far more common situation in which the physician does not tell the patient about his scruples until quite late in the downhill course of the disease. By this time the patient is often seriously incapacitated and in substantial need of ongoing medical care. As the patient deteriorates, it becomes increasingly difficult for the patient to transfer to the care of another physician—with whom, in any case, there would be no longstanding relationship or pattern of mutual understanding. By not informing the patient of his or her scruples in a timely way, the physician has in effect made himself or herself the only one available to this patient.

Nor can it be supposed that it is the patient's responsibility rather than the physician's to bring the matter up early on (though the prudent patient will certainly do so). The patient cannot be expected to understand the probable course of the disease, the likelihood of pain or other symptoms that are inherently untreatable, possible limitations of the physician's capacity to relieve pain and suffering (whether because of a lack of skill, a lack of information, or institutional priorities), or other factors in the medical course that lies ahead. The effect of delay is compounded if the physician—perhaps seeking to avoid "dirty hands" or any complicity in "evil"—refuses to consult, refer, confirm a diagnosis, transfer records, or cooperate in any way.

In short, because it has become too late for the patient to switch to another doctor to receive that aid to which the patient has a right, it has likewise become too late for the doctor to announce any principled reservations he or she may have. Although the individual physician with serious reservations may not have an obligation to assist in the suicide of a patient where it is easy for the patient to transfer, in this case it is the physician's own behavior that has led to a situation in which that physician has become the patient's only choice.

Furthermore, the patient may have come to rely on expectations that the physician will help. Consciously or unconsciously, physicians often foster a patient's trust in their capacity to negotiate a peaceful, dignified death. Especially if physician-assisted suicide is legal, patients may come to expect that their physician will provide assistance in suicide if asked to do so. Furthermore, the physician may even believe there is some medical reason to encourage this expectation, since evidence suggests that when patients believe they can count on the physician to provide aid-in-dying on request at a later date, this expectation allows them to extend their lives longer.[14] The patient who believes that help will be available whenever it is finally needed will often hang on until the very last minute.

Of course, the obligation may be different when the patient's terminal condition is of sudden onset or could not be foreseen: for instance, in unexpected, massive stroke, in accidental trauma, and in various other conditions. But the majority of cases are not like this. In the contemporary world, at least in developed countries, most dying involves a downhill, deteriorative trajectory, the general outlines of which the experienced physician can readily foresee. This includes virtually all cases of cancer, much cardiovascular disease, most neurological conditions, most organ disease or failure, virtually all end-stage AIDS, and so on. It may be particularly true when the patient is hospitalized or institutionalized in a nursing home or other health care facility (as is the case for the vast majority of deaths occurring in the United States) or otherwise under close surveillance. The physician *can* foresee what is coming and how the patient is likely to die; by remaining in a position of care for the patient, the physician incurs a growing obligation, as the patient's capacity for independent action diminishes and the need for mercy grows, to assist in easing the patient's death in the way that the patient desires.

To put this in another way, the physician's obligation to help arises primarily within a relationship that develops during the course of providing care for a dying patient. As time goes on and the patient's condition declines, the patient's rights grow stronger both on grounds of self-determination and of mercy, and thus the physician's obligation grows correspondingly more difficult to evade.

Nor is it adequate to argue that the patient's death can always be softened by either of the two principal means of negotiating death that are already legal and already widely employed: first, the withholding or withdrawing of treatment without which the patient will die, such as respiratory support or artificial nutrition or hydration, and second, the over-ample use of pain-relieving drugs, especially morphine, which, although ostensibly used with the intention of relieving pain, also decrease respiration and thus hasten death. These two strategies, now ubiquitous in U.S. medical practice, are not adequate means of satisfying the physician's obligation to the dying patient who seeks assistance in suicide, since the physician's obligation is rooted not just in the principle of mercy, which these means of negotiating death might provide, but also in the principle of autonomy or self-determination. Of course, if these strategies are satisfactory to the patient, then the physician's obligation to assist the patient in dying can be met in this way. But to repeat, some patients find these strategies distasteful or repugnant and, as an expression of their basic right of self-determination, seek means of dying they perceive as more dignified and more humane, more in keeping with their own basic values. They reject a form of dying they perceive as drawn-out, overmedicalized, drugged, undignified, and cruel, and they are not willing to settle for this, even to salve the physician's conscience—especially if they believe the physician's conscience or religious commitment is being used to trump their own rights.

Many physicians try to avoid such situations with promises like "I won't let you suffer," seeking to reduce the patient's fears and to give the patient the courage to continue. But the physician's obligation is *strengthened,* not relieved, by such tactics. If the physician proves unable to treat the patient's pain or suffering adequately, this simple, consoling phrase actually reinforces the obligation the physician now incurs. It is mercy that is promised in that little phrase, and it is the need for mercy that is part of the basis of the patient's right to assistance in dying.

"I won't let you suffer" may covertly promise something else as well—a period of dying that is not only pain-free but lived in a conscious, alert, still-autonomous way. This promise is certainly not explicit; but to at least some patients, "not suffering" does not suggest the absence of conscious experience, as in terminal sedation, but rather the enjoyment of conscious experience in which suffering does not occur. To some, at least, "I won't let you suffer" will seem to mean "I'll see that you can remain alert, still capable of emotion, communication, and other things that may be important to you, like final goodbyes or prayer, in a way that is not distorted by suffering."

The development of increasingly stronger rights on the part of the patient as the patient's condition declines and correspondingly stronger obligations on the part of the physician caring for the patient during that decline is exacerbated by medicine's tendency to delay decision making as long as possible, waiting until a crisis or change of status to raise most questions about withholding or withdrawing treatment, using opiates for pain management, or addressing other elements of terminal care.[15] This may reinforce patients' tendencies to evade and delay discussion of issues they find it painful to think about, especially if denial is part of their defense against bad news. But it is not only hesitation, fear of raising painful issues, or perhaps even cowardice on the part of both the patient and the physician that favors postponing discussion of these issues. Longstanding institutional practice contributes as well. Despite legal requirements like those imposed by the Patient Self-Determination Act, which requires hospitals and other institutions to ask patients if they have advance directives, and despite other recent changes, the institutional ethos of medicine tends to put decision making about end-of-life situations off as long as possible, until virtually the last minute at which an effective decision can be made. Not only do these patterns of delayed decision making tend to displace responsibility away from the patient onto the physician, family members, and others, as the patient becomes increasingly incapacitated and less and less capable of genuine participation in them, but these patterns also tend to put physicians into an increasing moral bind and make them still more vulnerable targets for moral blame—though blame of a different sort, and even harder to see for a physician who objects in principle.

If decision making is postponed long enough, the patient who would perhaps have requested the physician's assistance in suicide may become incompetent, delirious, or comatose. As these final stages of deterioration occur, self-determination and mercy—the principles that formed the basis of the patient's original right to aid—cease to be relevant in any direct way. The incompetent or delirious patient is no longer capable of current, self-directing autonomous choice and cannot effectively request assistance in suicide, and may not be able to carry it out even if assistance were provided; and if unconscious, the patient is no longer capable of experiencing suffering or feeling pain. Since neither autonomy nor mercy is relevant any longer, the patient's original right to assistance in suicide may seem to evaporate, and with it the physician's obligation to assist. Thus, it may seem, if the physician with scruples delays long enough, he or she is home free.

But I think not. There is a new basis for moral blame here, and blame of a stronger sort. The physician no longer merely fails to meet the obligation a patient's right to assistance generates, but now is blameworthy for suppression of that right as well. If the singular importance of this right is rooted in the secularized medieval view that the last moments of life can be of particular significance, it is not a trivial right that is being suppressed, and the physician's blameworthiness in doing so is greater than it would be for suppressing other rights, such as rights to information about a prognosis, or informed consent to procedures, or access to certain treatment. If the kinds of rights suppressed in caring for a patient near death are far more substantial than those that might be violated during other periods of caring for a patient who is temporarily ill but will recover, then a physician does a particularly grave moral wrong in delaying, prevaricating, and eluding the patient's claim.

Conclusions

That physicians may come to have obligations to provide direct assistance in the matter of dying does not mean that they are required to honor any patient request. It is still up to the physician to assess as carefully as possible (preferably in consultation with others, especially those with expertise in diagnosing depression or other psychologically confounding states) whether the request is stable, unambivalent, uncoerced, fully informed, and reflects the patient's most basic values—in short, whether it is a rational request, rationally made. It is also up to the physician (again, preferably in consultation with others, especially experts in the treatment of pain) to ascertain that there are no alternative ways acceptable to the patient of relieving the current pain and suffering or that which is about to occur.

But where the patient's request really does originate in autonomy and in the claim to mercy, it does mean that the physician is obligated not to entrap the patient into compliance with the physician's values rather than the patient's own values, which is what happens when choices are ignored or decision making is delayed. This will be the particular temptation (though it would not be phrased in this way) of those physicians who have the strongest reservations and scruples against killing or assistance in suicide. After all, these are the physicians who are most likely to want to avoid the issue, to delay any discussion of dying, to promise not to let the patient suffer at the end so as to avoid having the patient raise the question of suicide assistance in the first place, and to delay assistance until the patient's own deterioration renders the issue moot. Perhaps these physicians will signal, albeit unconsciously, that physician-assisted suicide is not a topic open to discussion. But in doing so, especially if physician-assisted suicide is legal or broadly accepted in the culture, they become the physicians most likely to have generated for themselves a strong moral obligation, one they will most bitterly resent. Paradoxically, it is physicians with the firmest moral scruples who may be the most likely to find themselves in this profoundly unwanted situation.

This conclusion is not a palatable one, especially for physicians who have the strongest moral reservations but who are not alert to the moral consequences of their own behavior. Physicians who entrap patients into compliance with their own values paradoxically also entrap themselves into having moral obligations they do not want. Even if the law protects these physicians from being forced to honor them, the moral obligations they have brought upon themselves will remain. Opt-out clauses may provide legal protection, but they do not guarantee moral protection too. Of course, a patient's right to assistance from a particular physician may be overridden where both the psychic damage to the physician's conscience would be genuinely grave and the disruption to the patient of transferring to another physician comparatively small, but it is not always the case that both these conditions are met. There may be little moral sympathy for physicians whose own behavior creates the dilemma they seek to avoid.

This conclusion applies not only to physician-assisted suicide but to any mode of life-ending assistance to which a patient has a right but to which a physician has scrupled objections, be it withholding or withdrawing of treatment, the overuse of opiates, the cessation of nutrition and hydration, the induction of terminal sedation, and so on. The irony is that in most situations it is fairly easy for physicians to protect themselves from such obligations. All it requires is announcing in advance—*well* in advance—what scruples one has and whether these would preclude one's willingness to assist, so that the patient can seek care somewhere else and not become dependent on aid from this physician. Ideally, such a discussion might occur at the beginning of a continuing relationship between a physician and patient, long before any evidence of terminal illness might arise, so that both physician and patient would be aware of differences in individual values that might some day be relevant in the matter of terminal care. After all, if the vast majority of people in the developed world die of diseases with characteristically long downhill courses, there is a substantial chance for any individual patient that the issue will eventually arise. Of course, in the comparatively transitory climate of contemporary medicine, the possibility of such conversations between patients and their personal physicians so far in advance may be wishful thinking; but there is no reason they could not occur far, far earlier than such conversations ordinarily do.

Physicians must also be careful not to lean too heavily on assertions of scruple by the institutions in which they practice. Catholic hospitals, some networks of Hospice, and the VA system, for example, have all articulated opposition to physician-assisted suicide, as have other organizations. Although institutional announcement of scruples in effect involves institutional refusal to honor patients' particularly important rights, the patient cannot assume that the physician's scruples track those of the institution or are significant to the physician to the same depth or degree. It may be easier for institutions than for physicians to announce scruples about physician-assisted suicide; for an institution, announcing scruples requires merely issuing a position statement or policy directive—and making sure the patient is informed of this. Physicians, by contrast, have to talk clearly, directly, even intimately with their patients—their *own* patients—who are dying. Prior, clear announcement of their own personal scruples will perhaps be less difficult for doctors in a future in which physician-assisted suicide is legal, but only if the current climate of medical decision making also changes.

But physicians' own behavior is not the only culprit in engendering moral obligations they do not want. Public attitudes and practices contribute to this as well, paradoxically reinforcing obligation-producing behavior on the part of physicians. Believing that physicians' objections to assisted suicide excuses them across the board, the public has not demanded full, compelling evidence for any claim that would have the effect of overriding a patient's principle-based rights. Society leads physicians to assume that trivial, self-interested objections will trump patients' rights as easily as profoundly held scruples (though the Boston Working Group's model statute would not do so), and society does not notice the way in which the legal structures now being developed to protect genuine, profoundly held scruples invite this. Society does not require physicians with either trivially or profoundly held scruples to own up to them in advance, and to put them forward for the patient's inspection. And society lets physicians and institutions delay decision making so long that the patient's rights, and the physician's corresponding obligations, are effectively eclipsed. We think that we have solved the moral problem in this way. We haven't. On the contrary, we have only made it worse.

Notes

From Linda L. Emanuel, ed., *Regulating How We Die: Ethical, Medical, and Legal Issues Surrounding Physician-Assisted Suicide,* Harvard University Press, 1998, pp. 21–47. © 1998 President and Fellows of Harvard College. Reprinted by permission.

1. The Boston Working Group's model statue provides: "No individual who is conscientiously opposed to providing a patient with medical means of suicide may be required to do so or to assist a responsible physician in doing so." Charles H. Baron, Clyde Bergstresser, Dan W. Brock, Garrick F. Cole, Nancy S. Dorfman, Judith A. Johnson, Lowell E. Schnipper, James Vorenberg, Sidney H. Wanzer, "A model state act to authorize and regulate physician-assisted suicide," *Harvard Journal on Legislation* 33, no. 1 (1996): 1–34.

2. Oregon Death with Dignity Act, Section 4.04. The Act does require, however, that

if a health care provider is unable or unwilling to carry out a patient's request under the Act, and the patient transfers his or her care to a new health care provider, that the prior health care provider shall transfer, upon request, a copy of the patient's relevant medical records to the new health care provider (Section 4.04). To be sure, a health-care provider would be legally obligated to transfer the patient's records at the patient's request in any case.

3. Many of these arguments can also be made for and against physician performance of active euthanasia, though since that is no longer the focus of most legislative proposals in the U.S., I won't discuss it further here.

4. For example, Dan Brock uses the term mercy in his *Life and Death* (Cambridge: Cambridge University Press, 1993). I've discussed at some length the relationship between the principles of nonmaleficence and beneficence, now canonical in the bioethics literature, and what I like to call the principle of mercy. The former are comparatively narrow principles, requiring not doing harm and doing good, respectively. The latter, the principle of mercy, is a broader principle that amalgamates both in the context of suffering. Thus the principle of mercy requires not just refraining from causing pain or suffering, which the principle of nonmaleficence would require, but also acting to relieve pain or suffering, as the principle of beneficence would require.

To call this principle the principle of mercy, then, is to use shorthand for much more cumbersome terms, but it is also to invoke traditional conceptions of the physician's role in the matter of pain and suffering. See my account "Euthanasia: The fundamental issues," originally appearing in *Health Care Ethics,* ed. D. Van De Veer and T. Regan (Philadelphia: Temple University Press, 1987), reprinted in Margaret P. Battin, *The Least Worst Death* (New York: Oxford University Press, 1994).

5. The SUPPORT Principal Investigators, "A controlled trial to improve care for seriously ill hospitalized patients," *JAMA* 274, no. 20 (1995): 1591–1598. Objections to the methodology of this study include the fact that these reports were taken from family members or other survivors, not the patients themselves.

6. When the practices of euthanasia and physician-assisted suicide first came to light in the Netherlands, it became clear that some physicians did not know the appropriate drugs or dosages to use; some attempted to use wholly inappropriate drugs, such as insulin or morphine. In response, anesthesiologist Dr. Pieter Admiraal published the appropriate information in a booklet sent to all Dutch physicians; this information has been revised and updated repeatedly. See Gerrit K. Kimsma, "Euthanasia and euthanising drugs in the Netherlands," *Journal of Pharmaceutical Care in Pain and Symptom Control* 3, nos. 3/4 (1995), and 4, nos. 1/2 (1996), also published as *Drug Use in Assisted Suicide and Euthanasia,* ed. Margaret P. Battin and Arthur G. Lipman (Binghamton, NY: Haworth Press, 1996).

For information on methods of physician assistance in suicide used by Compassion in Dying, Seattle, see Thomas A. Preston and Ralph Mero, "Observations concerning terminally ill patients who choose suicide," in the same volume. Derek Humphry's *Final Exit: The Practicalities of Self-Deliverance and Assisted Suicide for the Dying* (Eugene, OR: The Hemlock Society, 1991), has also provided drug information to the general public.

7. Some authors argue for the legitimacy of directly caused death on grounds of mercy in the absence of patient request when the patient is no longer competent and cannot make a request or express any wishes but is suffering severely. No contemporary writer with whom I'm familiar argues for directly caused death where that is contrary to the patient's wishes.

8. The term "patient-directed" is from Totie Oberman, personal communication, American Association of Suicidology, May 1995. The term "self-enacted" is from Stephen Jamison.

9. Actual cost savings from physician-assisted suicide may be far smaller than generally

believed. See E. J. Emanuel and M. P. Battin, "What are the potential cost savings from legalizing physician-assisted suicide?" (*New England Journal of Medicine,* 339 (3): 167–172 (July 16, 1998), where we estimate that the cost savings from patients who would choose physician-assisted suicide or euthanasia, were these legal, would be less than 1 percent of the total U.S. healthcare budget. For a more detailed discussion of safeguards against abuse, see Battin, "Voluntary euthanasia and the risks of abuse," in Battin, *Least Worst Death,* pp. 163–181.

10. Ludwig Edelstein, "The Hippocratic Oath: Text, translation, and interpretation," in *Supplements to the Bulletin of the History of Medicine* no. 1 (1943), and in *Ancient Medicine: Selected Papers of Ludwig Edelstein,* ed. Owsei Temkin and C. Lillian Temkin (Baltimore: Johns Hopkins University Press, 1967). Also see Danielle Gourevitch, "Suicide among the sick in classical antiquity," *Bulletin of the History of Medicine* 43 (1969): 501–518; Darrel W. Amundsen, "The physician's obligation to prolong life: A medical duty without classical roots," *Hastings Center Report* 8, no. 4 (1978): 23–30; Margaret Pabst Battin, *Ethical Issues in Suicide* (Englewood Cliffs, NJ: Prentice-Hall, 1995); and Ezekiel Emanuel, "The history of euthanasia debates in the United States and Britain," *Annals of Internal Medicine* 121, no. 10 (1994): 793–802.

11. Paul J. van der Maas, Johannes J. M. van Delden, Loes Pijnenborg, and Caspar W. N. Looman, "Euthanasia and other medical decisions concerning the end of life," *The Lancet* 338 (1991): 609–674. The first Remmelink report is available in full in English as a special issue of *Health Policy* 22, nos. 1 and 2 (1992); the follow-up report is available in condensed form in Paul J. van der Maas et al., "Euthanasia, physician-assisted suicide, and other medical practices involving the end of life in the Netherlands, 1990–1995," *New England Journal of Medicine* 335 (1996): 1699–1705.

12. See Loes Pijnenborg, Paul J. van der Maas, Johannes J. M. van Delden, and Caspar W. N. Looman, "Life-terminating acts without explicit request of patient," *Lancet* 341 (1993): 1196–1199. This more detailed examination of the approximately 1,000 cases of euthanasia without explicit request uncovered in the original Remmelink Commission report shows that in about 59 percent of them the physician did have some information about the patient's wish, though short of a full, current request; in nearly all of the other 41 percent of cases, the patient had become no longer capable of discussion, was suffering unbearably, there was no chance of improvement, and palliative possibilities were exhausted. While the Dutch do not seek to defend every case that occurs, it is clearly not the case, as outside observers often insinuate, that in the Netherlands patients are routinely killed against their will.

13. Kevin W. Wildes, S. J., "Conscience, referral, and physician assisted suicide," *Journal of Medicine and Philosophy* 18, no. 3 (1993): 323–328, a special issue entitled "Legal Euthanasia: Ethical Issues in an Era of Legalized Aid in Dying," ed. Margaret P. Battin and Thomas J. Bole, III.

14. Thomas A. Preston and Ralph Mero, "Observations concerning terminally ill patients who choose suicide," *Journal of Pharmaceutical Care in Pain and Symptom Control* 3 (1995): 3–4; also in *Drug Use in Assisted Suicide and Euthanasia,* ed. Battin and Lipman.

15. See Margaret Battin, "The eclipse of altruism: the moral costs of deciding for others," in Battin, *The Least Worst Death,* pp. 40–57.

5

Case Consultation

Scott Ames, A Man Giving Up on Himself

Case Report by John T. Maltsberger

Scott Ames was at the peak of his career when the sky fell on him. At 38 he was a highly successful television executive in New York. His wife, Elaine, was a glamorous and intense mutual fund manager. Together, they were a much-admired couple. Their friends were shocked and horrified when Scott was urgently admitted to a psychiatric unit on the West Coast after he tried to asphyxiate himself with a poisonous gas.

Scott and Elaine had lived together for 4 years before they married in a fashionable church ceremony followed by an elegant and large reception. But a short time after the wedding Elaine fell ill; in the course of her medical work-up it was found that she was infected with HIV. Scott was promptly examined and to his horror discovered he was not only HIV positive, but that he had early symptoms of AIDS.

These calamities threw their lives into turmoil. Elaine blamed Scott for infecting her, but he maintained that he had been faithful to her throughout the time they were together, and that he had had a negative HIV test some time before the marriage. Scott in turn blamed Elaine for their infection. They kept their tragedy a secret for fear it would compromise their careers. Scott's health deteriorated, however, and 3 months before he tried to kill himself he became so sick he could not continue his work. In shame and desperation his family and a few close friends were told the truth about his health.

At first he accepted treatment for AIDS, but after a month, unable to tolerate the nausea, diarrhea, fever, and headache, he stopped the treatment though Elaine begged him not to.

He began to plan his own "euthanasia" from the time he received the AIDS diagnosis, and, keeping no more secrets, talked openly about his plans to die. He studied the web page of The Hemlock Society on the Internet, and visited other sites of a similar nature. He decided to use a plastic bag and toxic gas. On the morning of his attempt, he checked into a hotel without telling anyone, and tried to asphyxiate himself.

His suicide attempt failed. He lay in a coma in a hotel room for several hours before regaining consciousness. Disappointed to have survived, he telephoned his friend Roger, who immediately came to help. Roger contacted Scott's parents on the West Coast. Flight arrangements were made, and Roger drove Scott to the airport and helped him fly off. Scott's parents met the airplane and drove him to the emergency room of a large general hospital where he was promptly admitted to the psychiatric unit.

During the admission physical examination, a brain mass was discovered. A biopsy confirmed he had a tumor, and a diagnosis of lymphoma was made. A few days later he was further torn emotionally—in the psychiatric unit he learned Elaine, who had remained back home, was filing for divorce.

Scott cooperated in his medical workup, but he refused all treatment for AIDS and for the lymphoma. He believed that his prognosis was poor, and that he had only a few months to live. This was a fairly realistic estimate, if he refused treatment. His doctors urged him to accept treatment, which they believed could extend his life, but he rejected their advice and said he would be better off dead.

The nurses in the psychiatric unit found him difficult. Aloof, sullen, and irritable, he avoided conversation with everybody, except for a motherly older nurse who worked on the weekends. She felt she knew him better than the staff members and the other patients; only to her could he disclose his anguish and despair.

He was evasive when asked what he planned respecting suicide. He said he just wanted to live out his days with his parents and to die in peace, sooner rather than later. He accepted his doctor's prescription of antidepressant medication, but insisted that he wanted to leave the hospital.

The inpatient psychiatric team grew discouraged. They felt drained by Scott's hostility and his rejection of treatment, and feared he would kill himself if discharged. Some believed it might not be such a bad outcome, given his circumstances. In addition, the staff was under pressure to keep hospital stays brief, and they feared Scott might require an inpatient stay that could go on for months.

Scott wanted to be discharged to his parents' home, which was not far from the hospital. His father had retired at the close of a distinguished civil service career, and his mother, an outstanding teacher, had given up her work at the same time. They were politically conservative people, active in their church and in local politics. Their social life was focused in their country club.

Scott was raised in privileged circumstances and attended private schools, and graduated from a prominent university before moving to New York. He had good relationships with his three siblings, a sister and two brothers, who lived not far away from the parents. Though he described his parents as "good natured, hard working, educated, and loving," they impressed the ward staff as emotionally cold and angry about what had happened to their son.

Scott denied any previous psychiatric history, but he was evasive about previous drug and alcohol abuse. He had never before attempted suicide.

A suicide risk consultation was arranged. The psychiatrist described Scott as a slim, fit, attractive man who was uncomfortable and tense through the interview. He answered questions reluctantly and sparingly, plainly feeling that they were intrusive, though he denied it. There was no evidence of delusions, hallucinations, or thought disorder. He acknowledged feeling depressed, and his affect was constricted. He was in some postbiopsy discomfort, and seemed unenergetic, slowed down, and moved about little.

The psychiatrist asked him about suicide. Scott replied that he only wanted "a place to rest," but was otherwise evasive. He said he just wanted to go home with his family.

The psychiatrist noticed that Scott had moved from horror and shame at the time of the original diagnosis to a depressed hopelessness. His privacy had been exploded, his wife was sick, she had rejected him, and he had a brain tumor. Plainly he was a ruined and dying man. The consultant thought that there was a considerable risk the patient would take his life if he were discharged, but his parents appeared loving and supportive (even if horrified). Scott was willing to see a psychiatrist on an outpatient basis, and accepted antidepressant prescriptions.

Though questions about his competency were raised, the prospect of a forced prolonged hospitalization seemed more likely to worsen the situation than to make it better. The patient and his parents would be certain to resist. Any course other than discharge seemed not only unwise but also meddlesome.

Case Discussion by Margaret P. Battin

To begin, suppose all the facts asserted or implied in this case are true: Scott Ames does have AIDS, he does have a brain tumor, he did infect his new bride with the HIV virus, he is angry, hostile to treatment, and isolated, and he is highly likely to kill himself if he is released from the hospital. Here's the dilemma: Discharge him—to his death—or keep him hospitalized indefinitely against his will, in order to prevent the suicide. What to do?

This case comes from a major teaching hospital, where the patient was given a very extensive workup and the diagnoses were not in doubt. If there were space here to present all these details, we would have full access to the entire range of professional opinions concerning Scott's diagnosis and the prognosis for his HIV infection, his response to treatment, his lymphoma, and his depression, details it is important to know but which cannot be presented in a necessarily brief sketch of the case like that presented here. To fully understand Scott's case, we'd also want the opportunity to examine him in person, in part to see what he understands of what he has been told. We'd want to ask him questions: Why did he have an HIV test prior to his marriage? What risk behaviors, if any, occurred between the time of his test and the marriage, and is he willing to talk about them? Why exactly does he experience the diagnosis of AIDS with such shame? Why has he refused to continue treatment for his AIDS—is it really a matter of the side effects? And we'd want to ask his treating physicians questions as well: Given that Scott has blamed his wife for the HIV infection they share, has any attempt been made to confirm with laboratory studies who infected whom, or whether each of the new spouses had been infected independently? What were his early symptoms of AIDS, and what about the complaints associated with his treatment? After all, the complaints sound more like symptoms of HIV infection than adverse reactions to the drugs used to treat it. We'd also want to know what type of lymphoma Scott has; most lymphomas are treatable and many are curable, though his may be different. In what ways can his type of tumor be expected to impair his emotional experience and cognitive functioning? Could it be a physiological cause of his depression? And, finally, we'd want to know whether or not the antidepressant Scott was taking was an appropriate choice, since it's not clear that sufficient time had elapsed to evaluate its effectiveness.

These are the medical questions. There may be institutional issues as well, about funding, bed space, and the like. And we'd want more information about social issues: What about the siblings with whom he spent a happy childhood; how do they understand their brother's "giving up on himself," and what help can they offer now? Does the motherly older nurse have any special insight to offer into Scott's refusal of treatment?

Yet even if we had full access to all the information gained in Scott's very thorough workup and psychosocial investigation, it seems, nothing really changes the picture: He still has AIDS (now quite far advanced); he still has the brain tumor (a bad one, progressing rapidly), and he still clearly intends to commit suicide if he can escape to his parents' house. Scott's case poses what seems to be a compelling ethical dilemma: Honor his wishes and thus consign him to suicide, or keep him in the hospital and violate his moral, if not legal, rights to liberty.

To discharge him, or to keep him hospitalized? This is no easy choice. But part of what makes it difficult is the very way it is framed, as a choice between two stark alternatives. Indeed, clinical choices in suicide-risk situations often look like this: discharge to death, or continue incarceration (as Scott might put it) against the patient's will and not clearly in the patient's interests. Yet I think there is a third alternative: Take Scott's interest in suicide as perhaps reasonable, certainly as an understandable choice for someone in his predicament, and work *with* him, not against him, in planning for it.

This may seem to be heresy, but in this case it seems far preferable to the other two alternatives. How to do it? Let someone volunteer (we hope it will be the sympathetic, motherly nurse) to work with Scott, help him explore his options, help him see his choices not from the panicked position he feels himself to be in, but as objectively as possible. For example, explore with him whether he really does have in mind to kill himself at his (loving, supportive) parents' house—is that what he wants for them? Where might he want to go instead? Would he plan to let his parents know in advance? What about his (ex) wife—would he like a farewell visit with her, perhaps facilitated by a neutral but understanding party? After all, she too has HIV. What about Roger, the friend who came to his rescue after his previous suicide attempt? How about other old friends—would he like help in contacting them and some idea of how to say a meaningful goodbye that does not blame them for his misfortunes or implicate them in his suicide? Does he need prescription drugs for his suicide, or more information from the Hemlock Society, or what? What about funeral arrangements, his will, the obituary for the newspaper? And would he like to have someone nearby, if not in the same room, when he finally ends his life, someone to accompany him the last few steps?

There is no way to predict the outcome of a strategy like this. My guess is that if Scott were really offered help in thinking through his plans for suicide in a straightforward, non-disapproving, non-duplicitous way, he would be much less likely to kill himself, at least not right away. With time, it might be possible, in working with him to explore his options, to put him in touch with that underground network of people with AIDS (including many physicians) who provide help to each other in dying. Should he happen to live in Oregon, he could even seek *legal* physician-assisted suicide, complete with counseling and medical support. If it is true that his life is ending—if it is true that he has reached the end stages of AIDS, and that the brain tumor, though palliable, is ultimately untreatable, lethal, and sure to disrupt his cognitive functioning—then in such grim circumstances the most loyal, respectful way to treat this person, this suffering human being, is to support him in a choice that may be truly his own about how his life shall end. Perhaps his choice will shift away from suicide if he finds that he really is offered genuine understanding and loyal support; perhaps it will not, but we will have helped him in his misery rather than thwarted him in what he now sees as the only solution to his desperate situation. We can realistically hope to make him less desperate, even if we cannot presume to change his mind.

With this answer, we can see what made the original dilemma so hard—to discharge him to his parents' house and let him kill himself, or to keep him hospitalized indefinitely against his will to prevent the suicide. *Both* these options are bad choices, and though I realize that it is heresy in circles dedicated to traditional ways of thinking about suicide prevention, both of them are I believe far less realistic and humane than the one I am suggesting here: To offer this patient support and help with the solution he sees. Of course, I wouldn't recommend this for just any suicidal person, but assuming that Scott really is facing death from AIDS compounded by a brain tumor that will destroy his capacity for cognitive function, it is appropriate to support what in these circumstances may be a reasonable choice and that is a choice of his own.

Of course, paradoxically, this support may be just what enables Scott to live a little longer, and certainly a little better, despite the conditions that afflict him.

Notes

From *Suicide & Life-Threatening Behavior* 33(3): 331–337 (Fall 2003). Case statement by John T. Maltsberger. © 2003 Guilford Press. Used by permission.

For a helpful discussion of this case, I thank Brooke Hopkins, and for a medical review, Jay Jacobson.

6

Robeck

One

For days on end, you think nothing.

For days on end, you think nothing.

For days on end, you think nothing. Then small thoughts intrude: "Where is the hammer?" "It is time to pay the bills." "How warm and unusually dry it is for July." These thoughts are only small disturbances, however, in the vast flat sea of your mind.

Then one moment the man catches your eye. He has been there all along, but you have not noticed him. The people one lives with are like that, just *there*—you do not always see them. But now you notice this man: you suddenly see the skin that has grown loose on his arms, the pale brown patches on his hands, an underbrush of coarse, yellowed beard beneath his chin. He has become old.

Other thoughts intrude: you examine your own hands, flattening them out on the writing-desk before you. They have the same loose skin, the same telltale brown patches; the knuckles are enlarged and the fingers permanently bent in the same characteristic way. You have become old, too.

But if you are old, then it is time. *Time.* This thought, larger than the rest, invades your consciousness; it surrounds the little thoughts that have gained toeholds in you, and establishes itself as a permanent guest.

You move to communicate this thought to your mate. "John," you say, and the old man turns to listen to you. "John. It is time."

The old man is startled by the large, unexpected thought; he had thought you would bring him only the smaller, everyday ones. But he seems to understand, although his mind moves only slowly to greet it.

"Yes," he says.

It alarms you to think you had almost forgotten. You see how your thinking-parts have begun to subside, and that you are beginning to merely respond, sometimes to the words of others, to the television, to your sons when they visit or the nurses who help you bathe, with responses that are acceptable, polite, even affectionate, but almost wholly automatic. You are not sure where you learned them; they have been there for years, but it is only now that you have ceased to think along with them.

Almost forgotten! The thought strikes you as an emergency of the most urgent sort, and you survey again your hands, your arms, the gnarled protrusions of your fingers, to see if you are equal to the task. It will not be easy; you have let it slip too long, and they will all be eager to thwart you. "She must be watched," they will say, "do not leave her alone."

"John," you say, urgently. "Do you remember?"

"Yes," he answers, and you watch him rise from the old flowered-brocade armchair, lift himself up on his gaunt forearms, propel himself in cautious steps across the floor. He makes his way to the bureau that stands in the hallway. He opens one drawer, feels inside with his hand, then opens another drawer, feels inside, moves away, leaving both drawers open; then he turns toward you in the room, simply standing, his back partly bent and his eyes staring vacantly ahead.

"There's nothing in there," you tell him. Your mind drifts back to an old problem, one which you and he had never solved. *When the time comes,* it had begun, but you and he had never been able to specify concretely what would occur, when the time had come.

"There's nothing in there," you repeat, but you see that he has already forgotten the purpose of his search. He stands aimlessly in the middle of the room, bent, unthinking, unimaginably old. After a while, you pull yourself to your feet, move unevenly across the room to meet him, and guide him slowly across the room to the couch. He sits, slowly, first marking out the spot where he will place himself, then guiding himself by slow degrees into it. Carefully, you sit beside him. Your hands meet, but the knuckles of them both are arched like pyramids, and the fingers so inflexible they no longer intertwine.

"I've dreamt that over and over again," Annis Robeck tells her husband. She has begun the packing again; she lifts a limp flannel nightgown from one of the drawers of their dresser and holds it up by the shoulders to the light.

John Robeck shifts uncomfortably on the small chintz chair.

"In the dream, you're a hundred and five years old," Annis tells him. She runs her fingers through the frayed lace on the yoke of the nightgown. "It used to be *my* mother's," she says absently of the nightgown, "it was supposed to be for Luel."

Then she returns to the subject of the dream. "I'm a hundred and seven."

"Luel wouldn't have worn it."

"Do you know what a hundred and seven feels like?" she demands. "It feels like an airtight glass case, or a cocoon." Annis spreads the nightgown out on the bed, next to the chair in which her husband is sitting. "At least that's the way it is in the dream. Only it's your mind that can't move, not your limbs." She folds the nightgown into careful thirds. "I suppose it can be for Luel's kid."

"She won't wear it either," Robeck says insistently. "She'll throw it away. I don't know why you bother." He moves uncomfortably again on the little chintz chair. He watches his wife take another nightgown from the drawer of the dresser they have shared for so many years, and hold the garment up to the light so that it falls open. She inspects it without much interest, and drops it by a sleeve into a large paper bag. He can see the interior of the drawer now: ever since he has known her she has been a rampant saver of everything, and her drawers are jungles: knots of sleeves and the isolated legs of stockings, tangles of miscellaneous underwear, clutches of odd handkerchiefs and gloves and unmatched socks. He has always found it somewhat mysterious, as if these drawers held secrets to her person he had not yet discovered. But now she is bringing a severe order to the chaos, and he sees that doing so is giving her an extraordinary pleasure.

"I'm glad it won't happen to us," she says, and he realizes she is still thinking about the dream. He watches her take the items from the drawer one by one, examine them, and drop them in the charity bag or fold them carefully for the boxes labeled with the names of their children. He studies the boxes: they are large brown cardboard cartons, lined with tissue. He sees how boldly she has labeled them: *Roddy, Evan,* and the name of Luel's child. There are more boxes like them in the closet, in the cellar, in the attic.

"Anyway," Annis is saying, "I think she ought to have a chance." She is thinking, he decides, about the nightgown and the recalcitrant child.

He says nothing; he focuses his mind clearly on the girl, but he cannot decide how old she will be by now.

"A bit of a sense of the flow of generations wouldn't hurt her," Annis continues. "You know, great-grandmother's nightgown, grandmother's nightgown, now it's mine. Maybe she'll save it for her own daughter."

"She won't. And she won't have a daughter, either."

"Well, perhaps you're right." But Annis does not seem to be disturbed by this thought; she continues packing with the same quiet explorativeness as before.

"It's like treasure-hunting," she once said to him. He watches the way she moves, and the remarkable grace of her body for a woman of her age. Now and then she holds an old scarf to her cheek, or slips a forgotten glove onto her hand, holds it up, admires it. There is no hurry in her actions.

But she stops, turns, studies her husband, as if she has suddenly noticed something.

Robeck's eyes follow the outlines of the enormous dresser they share: five copious drawers on the right, which are hers; his three on the left, containing his thin, carefully stacked piles of undershorts, handkerchiefs, two pairs of folded trousers, and several rather harshly laundered shirts. He wonders briefly why he has not thrown the shirts away; they are too big for him now, and quite out of style; he wears mostly small flannel blouses. But his eyes follow the rims of the drawers that are his, those that remain against her ever-encroaching collections; she has already usurped two drawers on the left, and only these three are his.

"No," he answers after a time. "No. Not yet."

Two

Robeck sits forward at his desk. In front of him is a pad of narrow-ruled paper; his pencil lies at an angle across the pad, and a few lines of irregular handwriting cross the top of the page. His hand twists the pencil in an idle circle. There is a mug of lukewarm coffee on the desk; he lifts the cup to his mouth, and watches uneven concentric circles form on the surface of the coffee. He looks away from the paper that confronts him; with some satisfaction he notes a large pile of orderly manuscript pages at the back of his desk. It is the bulk of his opus terminus, *A Defense of Ending*. The *Defense* has become much longer and more substantial than he had thought it would be; he had thought of it originally as a terse little note, to be published at the appropriate moment in the principal journal in his field; but somehow, during the year he had been at work on it, it had become a major treatise. Then, it would merely have attracted a bit of curious attention; now, it will accomplish something more.

He sits forward, picks up a random portion of the manuscript, and reads it:

> . . . indefinite or infinite individual survival would, of course, spell disaster for the species. This is as true for humans as it is for other groups. We observe that in animal groups, when a population begins to exceed the carrying capacity of the site . . .

He smiles; it is a subtle argument, firmly rooted in the biological sciences, but one he knows is persuasive. He flips forward through the manuscript; he finds to his pleasure that it grows less pedestrian in its science, more eloquent in promoting its argument: *Bury the old,* he has written,

> . . . initiate the new. No man can be loyal to his kind who fills a world with used ideas, disintegrating practices, an outworn mind . . .

An objective admiration grows in him, the kind of distanced admiration he has always felt for work that is good, whether it is his own or someone else's. He is pleased, and pleased too that he has managed to keep all the little personal hopes and humiliations out of it: there is not a word in the *Defense* about the discomforts of insistent and accumulating arthritis, or about the indignities of superannuated status, or any of the other consternations that defeat the old. It is an argument from responsibility, from an ultimate concern for the condition and future of one's world.

But the conclusion is somehow difficult. He takes up the pencil, puts the manuscript portions back in the pile. He places the lined pad at an exact forty-five-degree angle on the surface of his desk, poises the pencil to write. He studies the lines he had just been writing, but he sees that his handwriting has become crabbed and uneven, not at all like the bold strokes in which he had composed the earlier parts of the *Defense*.

One ought perhaps feel oneself obliged by these considerations to attempt a step
which . . .

He puts the pencil down, stares off across the little room. He has never really
noticed how complete his office has become: the walls are entirely covered with
bookcases, and each bookcase is now precisely filled with books, neatly aligned,
all of them carefully alphabetized and entered in a little card file kept in the drawer
of the desk. Robeck allows his gaze to slip slightly out of focus; he is thinking
about the conclusion he has begun to write for his *Defense,* and he knows there is
something wrong with it. But what he notices among the blurred outlines of the
books that line his room is the way some of them stand out: hot red, chrome yellow,
startling shades of green. It is an extraordinary, delightful effect; the spines of
almost all his books are undifferentiated brown-gray, except for these few. He
begins to understand: they are the new books, printed in the recent, garish years
of textbook marketing; most of his books are half a century old. He realizes: it is
an old man's library.

He returns to the paper; he holds the pencil on its side and draws a broad,
irregular *X* through the lines he has written. He tries again:

One must feel obliged by these considerations . . .

But he does not finish; there is a knock at the door. Robeck can tell from the
humility of the knock that it is Liller, his coworker on the rat studies. Liller has
been knocking in his humble way for all but two of the nearly twenty years Robeck
has known him; Robeck still remembers when the knock changed. It was aggressive
when Liller first came, almost offensive, as if the knock were intended to dislodge
the occupant of a room rather than merely summon his attention; but when it
became apparent to all, and finally to Liller himself, that he would not assume
Robeck's position as the head of the unit, the knock had become easier, less stri-
dent. But it did not become servile, and Robeck inferred from this that Liller had
not actually wanted the position; he had somehow simply thought he ought to try
to get it. Since Robeck's official retirement a dozen years ago, they have been
intimate colleagues, and in the last three years have been working together on a
study of overpopulation behavior in rats. Liller is almost two decades younger than
Robeck, and sees this work in a very different way.

"Defending yourself again?" Liller asks, as he sees Robeck's new sheets at the
top of the pile of manuscript.

"Not from you," Robeck laughs. Liller knows about the *Defense,* and he knows
what is to accompany it. But Liller is the only one of the staff who does know;
Robeck had told him at a moment when he had to tell somebody, and had sworn
him to a secrecy he knew Liller would keep.

"The rest of the world, then?"

"Heroically," Robeck says. "Up to the end. It may be done quite soon."

"Just the manuscript, I hope," Liller says, alarmed.

Robeck laughs. "The act doesn't happen until the word has gone forth," he
says pontifically, "and publication will take another month or two."

Liller says nothing; his face grows ambivalently serious.

"I've asked them to save thirty pages in the September *Reports,*" Robeck confides.

Liller knows what this means. "It's February now," he says.

But Liller has come with other news, though it is not especially good. "The institute wants to know when you'll be ready to move to the emeritus suites in the Berkeley Building."

"I never said I'd be ready."

"They didn't give you a choice."

Robeck remembers the letter, but not very clearly; he opens the only drawer of his desk that is not perfectly ordered, into which he stuffs the miscellaneous correspondence and memoranda he does not want to confront. He finds the letter; it speaks of "reassignment" to "more suitable office space," though it does not mention the absence of laboratory facilities, or the fact that all one's office-mates would also be old. The emeritus suites, thinks Robeck, and he pictures a bald hallway in a disused wing of the old administration building, where they farm out the aging researchers into a kind of geriatric scholars' nirvana.

"Tell them I won't be ready."

"They've already reassigned this office to somebody else," Liller says. "They just want to know when they can schedule the move. I thought you knew."

Robeck surveys the nearly completed manuscript, the rows of books, the laboratory paraphernalia, the office he has occupied for nearly fifty years. "Tell them I won't need to move. They can have this office in September."

Robeck sees Liller wince. But Liller, he knows, will communicate what he has said to the administration as an absolute insistence on staying here. Liller worships him now, but only half-believes his plan.

Robeck turns back to the manuscript again, and addresses himself to the conclusion:

I take a step which . . .

But he does not write. He finds his fingers playing with a paperclip; he discovers himself staring at the spines of the new-colored books, idly reciting the titles when he sees them. He leafs back through the manuscript: *Bury the old,* he reads; *outworn minds can entertain but one real thought: it is time to go.* A few pages further on: *One must not always think of oneself; there are others in one's world, and it is one's final obligation to make way for them.* The old arguments for senicide, recast for suicide: the old and finished man has an obligation to rid the world of his parasitic life.

Robeck puts the pencil to paper again; he needs only to remark on his personal conviction that the arguments are right, that they are to be exemplified in action. The *Defense* will be published afterward, or better, at the same moment as his deed; it will work to change the way human beings live—and end—their lives.

But he is not writing. Again he finds himself toying, this time penciling convolute designs around the letters of his earlier sentences, while some other part of his mind wonders whether, when his books are packed, the bright new ones will be sorted out from the old. He stares at the paper. He feels an uneasiness in his stomach, a shortness of his chest. Perhaps rest, or a little exercise—

He raises himself slowly to his feet, moves back from the desk, and takes his overcoat down from the peg on which it hangs. He thinks deliberately about the overcoats he has hung on that peg, and tries to remember the sequence of them, but succeeds only in attaining an amalgamated image of them when they begin to wear thin: dark wool overcoats, some dark blue, some brown, all growing threadbare at the sleeves and behind the collar, losing a button here and there.

He puts one arm into the current overcoat, and then, with difficulty, the other. Nothing at all is in his mind now, and he is grateful for the relief.

Three

Annis Robeck sits on the floor in front of the ancient desk in the hallway, searching for a packet of letters. The letters are not in the top or the second drawers, she knows; over the past several months she has already cleared these drawers of their entire contents, packed them in boxes, labeled the boxes like those in the bedroom with the names of their children, or tossed things easily away. But the next drawer will be harder; though no filing system has determined the contents of these drawers, this third one seems primarily given over to the artifacts of a generation of children: Roddy, Evan, dear lost Luel. At the top of the drawer are recent letters, photographs of Roddy and Evan in middle age with their own assorted children, announcements of Rod's promotions and Evan's exhibitions and copies of two thin books of poetry Luel had published, just before her death. There is a carpeting of postcards from various travels. A little further down in the drawer there will be letters from all of them in early adulthood, and while they were still in various degrees of school; still further down will be the artifacts of their childhoods. But the letters Annis is searching for will be close to the surface; they were written only a couple of years ago, one from each of the three.

"What are you going to want," Annis and John had written to each of them, "when the time comes?"

Roddy had said he wanted the house; Luel, renouncing the world for a garret and a purely poetic life, had answered hotly that she did not wish to possess anything; Evan had telephoned in alarm.

"Why do you want to know now?" he had asked.

"We're writing our wills," they had answered. "We thought you might like to have some say in what you get."

"Now?"

"No, not now. We'll let you know when the time comes. Plan to come and spend the summer."

Annis finds the letters; she takes them out, rereads them, and considers whether she has satisfied their requests. She cannot bear the thought of one's own children stooping to squabble among the untidy bits of one's own leavings: no, it would not be so, and she would see that all the little whims—"I want the antique desk!" "I want the silver grapefruit spoons!" "You be the one to take the car!"—were satisfied well in advance. It would be so easy, that way, so pleasant, so fully maternal. She puts the letters back in their jackets, opens the upper drawer of the desk. There is almost nothing in the drawer now: the title to the car, an old copy of their will, a packet of insurance policies. Taped to the bottom of the drawer is a short but growing list:

    discontinue milkman
    utilities
    check insurance
    cancel newspaper
    close accounts at bank

It is like going on a trip, Annis thinks; you always have to remember to find someone to feed the cat.

But this trip she will forget nothing. She will see Collings, the lawyer, tomorrow, the tax accountant Tuesday; next week the district attorney, so that there need not be even the slightest legal question about these events.

She thinks ahead for a moment to the appointment with Collings; she knows him well, and knows exactly what he will say. He will sit in the formal chairs in the living room; he will place his briefcase on the small side table and open it so that the inner pockets fan out; he will wait to say anything at all until she fully explains why it is that she has called him to come. He will hear it all, not interrupting and not reacting in any way, his bland young face entirely impassive, though he may in this case allow himself one cigarette from the dish on the coffee table. In this case, indeed, he will pause much longer after she has finished telling him what she wants, and he may even accede to a glass of soda or a cup of tea. When he has summoned himself he will finally speak, and address himself only to the question.

"If your husband predeceases you, the insurance benefits will go half to you, and half jointly to your two surviving children and the daughter of the child who is deceased. When you die your half of the insurance will form part of your estate, and be taxable at the usual inheritance rates. If, on the other hand, your husband predeceases you, the . . ."

"We want it to be simultaneous," she will say.

The young man will stiffen almost imperceptibly, sit forward on his chair, crush the cigarette out in the ashtray. "I see," he will answer, "in that case, the various insurance benefits will . . ."

Annis already knows about the insurance; she has studied the small print of each policy they've bought, and has been careful in the ones they've bought. They will forfeit nothing; the policies will have been in force for more than the required two years.

Even were it otherwise, she will tell Collings, it would not dissuade her. After all, insurance is for unforeseen and calamitous circumstances, not those one knows are coming; calamity is just what she wishes to avoid.

But Collings comes tomorrow, not today. Annis finds herself further down in the last drawer that swims with memorabilia of the children; she is down below the layer of recent, adult correspondence, and even down below the layers of late adolescence. At the bottom of the drawer they are children again, Roddy, Evan, and Luel, and she finds yellowed photographs of childish smiles, tediously crayoned drawings, valentines, an envelope with a small course lump in one bottom corner, bearing the notation "Evan's tooth" and a distant date in his own proud hand, locks of retroactively blonder hair, the silver rattle an old-fashioned aunt had presented, and all the children had used. Annis pauses: she will pack the things in boxes, again labeled with their names, but she is caught for a moment by an extraordinary sense of receding time, as if the lives of the children were unfolding backward. She starts: she can begin to see the inner secrets of their early being; it is as if she can see the shapes of their lives, all at once, reducing backward to an early infancy in which their characters are already fully formed. Now she can see back even before these infancies to a moment of tremendous pregnancy, in which she can contain these three future people perfectly and entirely. Even in their birthing— though she sees already that they will become imperfect, ordinary beings, who grow fat and cross, or die—she is overwhelmed with a sudden sense of the inestimable preciousness of them, and the unspeakable wonder of containing them all.

This retrospective pregnancy is an experience of some profundity, and Annis sits for a very long time, motionless, on the floor. When she finally rises, it is with some difficulty; she finds that she is stiff and a little chilled. But there are still things of this world to think about, she remembers; she has promised Max and Polly a last chocolate mousse, and if it is to be ready in time she must begin. She walks toward the kitchen, more freely now.

Four

Each arm, as he brings it down alongside his body, releases its own distinct wave of bubbles; Robeck works to make them as symmetrical and rhythmical as he can. It is a curious stroke he has devised, a kind of geriatric backstroke with certain affinities to a reverse dog-paddle; he knows it is awkward, but it works. For one thing, it succeeds in keeping his head out of water, now that age makes his eyes increasingly sensitive to the chlorine. And it accomplishes something else as well, though he wishes he did not need to have recourse to it: his awkward, flailing stroke marks him as an aged and feeble man, and even when the pool is at its most viciously crowded, grants him a berth of relatively undisturbed space. The pool is alive today with huge and heavy swimmers doing brutal sets of laps in cutthroat time; the surface of the water is cut to a froth, and the wake of one swimmer slaps the next in the face. Even so, Robeck is granted a berth of relatively undisturbed space, and he can perform his old man's swim without fear. Still, they are glad when he leaves; the lifeguard sits back from the edge of his chair, and the small, quiet space he had occupied quickly closes over with the chop of competition.

Robeck walks loosely across the tiled deck, eased by his swim, and goes into the locker rooms. It is a wonderland of freely sweating youth: young glistening men unlace their tennis shoes and strip off their shirts and lie limp and fiercely breathing on the benches, or slump into showers; near his own locker, a boy winces gratefully while another binds tape around a freshly injured ankle. Robeck pushes down his trunks, and hangs them in a clot over the door of his locker; he takes a towel from it, and enters the sauna.

Here it is crowded too; a row of glistening bodies lines the wooden bench bank, in various postures of collapse and contemplation; Robeck hesitates as the door closes solidly behind him, but the bodies move aside, and make a space on the bench for him. He sits, and the warmth closes in around him like an embrace; he feels the nearness of the bodies on each side of him, and it is comfort. Every muscle in his body seems to individually relax. He sees the knees and thighs of the bodies on each side of him, knees that project unequally out into the tiny room, muscled thighs flattened against the wooden bench. These men do not talk much, here in the heat, and Robeck studies all the angles at which a man's shoulders can slope, the outlines of their breasts, the shapes of their shoulders, the differing luxury of the hair in their groins, and the random way their penises hang to the side. He can see these bodies without moving his eyes, and his wonder and admiration for the variety of human shapes is increased by looking at them; it is the biologist in him. But they can see him too, he knows, without moving their eyes or betraying their curiosity, and he knows that they are examining the hunched slope of his back, the rippled skin on his chest, the wrinkled confusion of his thighs. They will notice the fact that he is missing the two small toes from his right foot, and will invent myths of how it could have occurred. He feels the heat invading his shoulders, his knees; he feels the precariously frail thinness of the skin covering his skull, and the way the hot dry air sears his lungs. Some of the people beside him have left; there is room now to lie down, and he does, and the heat closes in on him again. His eyes close, and his thin legs flatten against the wood. The heat is overwhelming. It is as if his limbs no longer work, as if his circulation ceases, as if all his reflex muscular systems no longer respond, and he cannot swallow, or breathe, or move the lids of his eyes. It is as if the remote appendages of his body, his toes, his fingers, curl in the heat; as if the sinews soften and melt, as if the soft inner tissues slowly liquefy. It is absolute inertia, unmovingness.

—He does not know whether he has groaned, or choked, or screamed, but they are over him now, quick, efficient: one of the glistening men raises Robeck's head, feels his breath, slides his arms beneath Robeck's back as another takes his feet; still another holds open the door into the cool outside air, and they carry him quickly efficiently glisteningly out into the room. They place him lying down on a bench; they wring towels out in cold water and place them on his forehead. But Robeck sits up, pulls a dry towel around his groin. One of the men brings another towel soaked in cold water; but Robeck gets to his feet. He can walk now; he holds the towel around him, and heads towards his locker. Two of the youths amble casually beside him, as if they were going that way; they will allow him to shower and dress himself, he knows, but they will keep him under their eye.

"Thanks," he admits.

"Nothing to it," one of them answers. "Heat makes terrible dreams. It's not a place for falling asleep."

Five

The clutter from the dinner is enormous: Empty dishes and empty glasses and empty bottles of wine litter the table, and it is clear that the meal that has taken place here has been a significant one. But there is evidence of something else too: the fringe of Polly's napkin has been braided, loosened, and rebraided during the meal; the silverware at Max's place has been rigorously, meticulously aligned, as if these dear friends had listened to a long and difficult tale. Even Robeck has fingered a row of breadcrust particles into an unintended design, though when he noticed what he had been doing he had dispersed them with an irritated flick of his hand. Now, however, the dishes have been pushed aside, and Annis has reached over to a drawer in the sideboard: the hard part is over, and they are ready to laugh now. The drawer is what Annis and John have always called their "Golden Years" drawer, and from it she produces all the retirement literature that has been forced upon them in the last ten years or so—handfuls of slick Golden-Living brochures, charter airline advertisements for islands of unending sun, glossy folders trumpeting in ornate tones the elegance and security of this rest home or that one.

"For instance," she laughs, " 'Magnificent seaside residence for the youthful elder.' " She pronounces the words with the coaxing whine of a vacuum-cleaner salesman: "The active liver." The brochure displays tanned, athletic couples playing doubles on a palm-fringed tennis court, and the only hint of age lies in the fact that their hair is gray. *Youthful elders,*" Annis mocks, "in fact, nine out of ten people in places like that are widowed women, not couples, and one in every four has trouble walking."

"Thirty-six percent of noninstitutionalized people over 65 have rheumatoid arthritis," says Robeck, who has clearly recited these figures before. "One in two is missing all their teeth. By 75, one in five can't hear. By 85, one in four can't see well enough to read a book." He says these figures automatically, as if he has learned them by rote.

"We don't want that," Annis says.

But now they have moved into the living room: brandy glasses by a receding fire, a light wool blanket that Polly and Annis had drawn up over their knees. The way the furniture is drawn up together suggests a kind of strong and sentimental intimacy, rare and prized and lasting well into the night. Here, all secrets are un-done; all past experience relived, all future hopes explored.

But there is a paler, rectangular patch on the wall above the fireplace. The large and treasured painting of Mont Blanc that has always hung there has been removed, and Robeck is in the kitchen swathing it in paper.

"We want you to have it," Annis had been saying, "You always loved it too." It is true; they have loved the painting. Robeck and Max, both climbers in their earlier years, had been members of a Mont Blanc expedition, now forty years before. It was a difficult though not disastrous expedition: no one reached the top, and Robeck lost the two small toes of his right foot to frostbite; still, the mountain has represented something special in their lives. They have often sat in the evening of the quiet living room, swirling coffee around the surface of a cup, following the contours of the south col, the north face, the traverse they were unable to make.

"We want you to have it," Annis had repeated, but Max was overcome: it is a tainted, premature, grave-robbing thing, and he cannot bring himself to touch it.

"If we willed it to you would you be glad?" Annis asked, and Max was brought to admit that he would be extremely proud.

"Then be proud now," Annis said, "while we can still see it," and she motioned to Robeck to take it off the wall. There was a legacy too for Polly, a bracelet of Annis's she had always admired, a gold-link chain that clattered delicately as she moved. Polly slipped it on, faltering a bit and clearly overcome with both admiration and an emotion too large. She enclosed Annis in a desperate embrace, and wept.

"Don't," she said. "Don't do it."

But Annis stroked her head, comforting her. "It is what we want."

Six

Robeck has been sitting with his pen poised above the surface of his *Defense* for fifteen minutes when there is a loud and agitated thump at the door, a noise that is part curse, part cry. It is Liller, coming from the rat lab.

"Air," he yells, "it was the air."

Robeck hurries behind him into the rat room. Yesterday two of the fifty rats were dead, though they showed no evidence of wounds: Liller had been excited, as it had seemed to show some evidence of a process whereby overcrowding produces not merely antisocial behavior but an inability to live.

Now Robeck peers through the Plexiglas cover into the rat environment: all the rest are dead.

"Look at this," Liller says, and he holds up a part of the tubing that serves the environment's air supply. There is a large kink in the tubing, where it has gotten caught between the environment and a heavy chair. Liller swears angrily, and in his frustration smashes a huge chemical reference text down on the thin Plexiglas cover. His research is ruined. He turns and strides in fury out the door.

Robeck bends forward over the rat box, and moves a large piece of the fractured Plexiglas out of the way. The box is littered with prostrate rats, their small eyes bulging, their small thick tongues protruding, and their small nailed claws drawn up in a primitive reflex. He and Liller will eventually remove the Plexiglas lid and shovel the dirt and the dead rats together into thick plastic bags, and take them off for disposal, but now Robeck stares down through the Plexiglas, at the litter of dead rats. He has seen hundreds of animals dead in the years he has spent in biology laboratories, most of them dead more cruelly than these, but he has never quite noticed the deadness before. He stares down into the cage at one particular random rat, observing the stillness, the unbreathingness, the absolute motionlessness of it. He knows he should stay, console Liller, begin the unattractive and discouraging task of cleaning up, but he cannot; there is a pressure in his chest and that now-familiar knotting in his abdomen. He needs to get out, away.

"Sorry, Liller," he says as he passes Liller's door, but then he is out, gone, with the hurried, awkward, slightly bowed gait that is now his, and takes with him the alternating visions of the dead rats and the despairing Liller, weeping in fury with his head buried on his desk.

Seven

Toward morning, Robeck has the first of his terrors. It is like a dream, he tells Annis, only more so—a kind of unreasoning, violent compression in the chest, as if someone were squatting upon it, and you can't breathe.

"Do you think you should call a doctor?" Annis asks.

It wasn't that, Robeck tells her, *it was something worse.* Like an earthquake in the earliest part of morning, when you are sure you're awake, but the world sways as if in a dream. Only in this earthquake the world is being swallowed up, he says, not just moved around.

Annis moves herself closer to him in the bed.

It was worse than a dream, Annis, he says.

Eight

By morning Robeck is chilled, and breathes with a wheezing sound. He moves only slowly from the bed; he ignores his usual exercises, wraps himself in a heavy bathrobe, makes his way slowly toward the kitchen. Annis is already there, soaking the dishes from last night's dinner; she is startled by the illness in Robeck, by the stoop in his shoulders, his paleness, the shuffle of his gait, the listlessness of his face. A rasp of gray stubble appears around his chin; his breathing is rough. She pulls a chair out for him at the table; he sits uncomfortably in it. She heats the coffee again; she cuts toast into the triangles he would have made himself, and brings them to him.

"I'm sorry about the dream," she says.

"It wasn't a dream."

But he will not, or cannot, talk about it. The next day is the same, only when he rises the vagrant gray stubble on his chin is a little more unsavory, and the stoop and shuffle in his gait more pronounced. The appointment with Collings is a disaster; Robeck sits impassive on a chair, saying almost nothing, and Collings says that he cannot represent them or even advise them in any such endeavor. He suggests psychiatric help, but Annis urges him toward the door.

"We are old," she says. "That's what you don't seem to understand."

"That doesn't make it any different," answers Collings. "What you have in mind is wrong."

"We don't think so," says Annis, closing the door.

In the afternoon and in the evening and again the following morning, Annis watches Robeck sit in the little chintz chair, not moving, wheezing slowly as he breathes, the fingers of his old gray hands knotted around the ends of the chair. She begins to bring him some of the things she has uncovered in her relentless, unceasing packing: a corsage he had given her, now brown and papery, pressed between the pages of a book; a lacquered eyeglass case that had belonged to his mother's mother's aunt; an address book from almost fifty years before. She opens it to random names; Robeck says he can remember none of them. Somewhere in the attic she finds a box of photographs; she sorts out one of him, dressed in knickers and holding a coil of rope and an ice axe; she brings it to him because she has found the knickers too, among the contents of a chest of discarded clothing the children had used for costumes. She can remember the summer, she says, they had spent in the Canadian part of the Rockies, and she describes the idyllic late-summer evenings, camped on a high plateau, watching their fire surrender to the night as the stars overwhelmed the sky.

"That was too long ago," he says. "I don't remember."

She finds the ring he had worn in college, and a box of trophies from the swimming team. "Get those out of here," he says, "I don't want to think about them." He looks at her with disbelief, and watches the way her hands clutch these old, forgotten objects: the ring, the photograph, the small bronzed statues. He begins to realize what he has been seeing, as he has watched her month by month pack away all the objects of their lives: she is turning inward now, into a past she thinks they both still treasure but that he has no wish to remember. Suddenly, he sees her as an old and failing woman, closing off a future, feeding more and more on the things of the past. If he were to suggest a trip, she would remind him that they had been to India and Australia and had spent several years in Europe; she would say she'd seen as much of the world as she thought reasonable, and did not see much point in distracting herself by trudging through more. If he were to suggest a literature course or a craftsmaking hobby or initiating a new friendship, she would say she'd had as much of these enterprises as she required, and would not want to clutter up the closing moments of her life with any more. She would resist any suggestion he might make to decorate their future; she did not think there would be one. He watches her, sitting perfectly still, cross-legged on the floor, her hands cupping the tiny locket she wore as a child, and sees the way she is imposing an end, deliberately bringing their lives to a close.

That is what they have planned, he knows. But he wonders why he cannot pick himself up out of the chair. He should go back to his office, he knows, to finish the *Defense;* space is still waiting in the September *Reports.* He should begin his packing—though he does not think it will take him long to dispose of his own belongings, and he has no desire to sort through them, cherish them, divide them up among his heirs in the way that Annis is doing; all he will need is a couple of cardboard cartons and the telephone number of the Salvation Army. But he cannot move, it is as if his arms have adhered permanently to the arms of the chair, as if his legs and lower body are glued to the seat, as if he is an upright Gulliver, tied to the chair by the ropes of tiny invisible beings. The image invades his mind: himself motionless, entirely motionless, unable to do or initiate anything, unable to smell, to breathe, to hear see think—

—and then images come of those who still do move, ragged children creeping

through war-torn European streets, sailors in shipwrecks, clinging to a bit of float-
ing board with a grip tighter than death, Ann Boleyn screaming for her life as she
is dragged along the Tower, silent Jews peering out of hollow hungry eyes in the
concentration camps, but still breathing, injured mountain climbers dragging themselves across icefields with fingers frozen up to the knuckles, people moving
through fires, withstanding falls, pushing their lungs again after they are pulled
from the water, the desperate community of those who resist death, who survive.
He thinks of the fierce old heart and gizzard of Franco, thumping on long after
death might have claimed him, of men lost in wells or caves or mines, unearthed
forty-eight hours after earthquakes, and he knows that he, Robeck, is one of them,
not one of those limp pale creatures whose slim hands slip from the edge of the
lifeboat or whose pulse is too weak to survive the shock, or who lie down in
hospitals, nursing homes, rented rooms, and refuse to get up, not because they
cannot but because they see no point in continuing on. He has always been one of
the stubborn ones, cantankerous, argumentative, rebellious; that is why he has defended his position with as much zeal as he has in his *Defense,* but he cannot let
its conclusion fall upon him.

"No," he says aloud. It is a hesitant, blurted sound, but it brings with it the
beginnings of a surge of relief, and again he says it, "No," louder this time, and
the relief is great and greater, and he feels opening out around him a vast new
open world, in which he can go any distance, in any direction. "No, no," he yells
wildly, "No. No. No."

Annis sees that something is happening to her husband; she rises in alarm from
the floor, sits by him. She puts her hand to the inner surface of his wrist, touches
his forehead for fever.

"I can't do it, Annis. I won't."

"What?" But she knows what, and she is silent a long time, as she always is
when something earnestly troubles her. It is one of the things he has always loved
about her, her care and caution in trouble, the collectedness with which she acts.
After a very long time, in which no transition or emotion can be seen upon her
face, she speaks.

"I do not want to force you to do anything," she says. "Especially not this."
She turns, and looks at him in a fully matter-of-fact way. "I am willing to wait."

"Annis," he says, earnest. "I can't do it now. I can't do it *ever.*"

She is silent again, for another long time. "Then I will have to think about
me."

Nine

Now the pain begins. In the days following Robeck's confession, his humor is
restored; he putters around the house as if cured of a long illness; but Annis's
tranquility is destroyed, and she retreats into the corners of the house. Robeck
spends more time at home, less time in his laboratory, now that he senses something
is wrong. But he sees Annis less often. He does not find her moving about the
kitchen, or reading enormous piles of books, or writing voluminous stacks of let-

ters; he does not have that warm sense of her presence that has always filled the house. There is a small, rather dark extra room, hidden behind the bedroom; she has always used it as a study, but now he sees that she spends much of her time there, noiselessly, seeming to do nothing. The door stands only slightly ajar.

He knocks.

"John? Come in."

He opens the door gradually, slides himself in. He has always been careful not to disturb his wife when she is here, and to respect the privacy of this small space of hers, but she has welcomed him into this room often before, and he remembers it as an enthusiastic outward display of her characteristic clutter: it is small, warm, stuffed with notices, postcards, pictures taped to the walls. Clippings from newspapers protrude from the leaves of books, half-finished letters spill from the typewriter, and everywhere plants thrive, long lush luxuriant vines that grow up from pots at the base of the windows, over the lintels, and track across the ceiling. He has always seen her as a creature of inexplicable mystery, lurking here in a fertile jungle of her own creation.

He stops, struck: all that is gone now: the walls are bare, the surface of the desk uncluttered, and the vines have been pruned back to severely disciplined size. The room seems large, stark, empty. The telephone book is closed, and there are no messages or reminders taped to the handset; all that he sees of the familiar clutter are three small, framed pictures of their children: recent photographs of Roderick and Evan, an old one of Luel. Annis is sitting in her chair, wrapped in a plain white cotton dressing gown, but she says nothing. Robeck sees a thin book lying open on the table beside her; he walks toward her, picks it up, examines it. It is a collection of poetry, by a poet whose name he does not recognize.

"Reading?"

"No. Just thinking."

"Is it all right with you if I come in?"

"Yes."

Robeck studies his hands, twisted together in a tight, nervous knot. He knows he is responsible for her distress. "I'm sorry," he says.

"So am I."

His eyes travel to the small framed picture on the desk; he cannot understand why she keeps a picture of the dead child among the live ones, as if nothing were changed. "You must be very disappointed," he says.

She is silent a long time. "When you've lived a lot of your life toward a single moment, and that moment disappears," she finally begins, but she does not finish the sentence. She stares distractedly out the window, into the trees. "It's been important to me to live my life with you, John. I wanted to end it with you."

Robeck watches his old, stained hands knot, but says nothing; he is caught in a curiously ambivalent, difficult moment, where on the one hand he seems to be rediscovering the young, mysterious, idealistic girl he had married, but on the other hand finds the gulf between himself and this old woman she has become increasingly vast. He realizes that he has humored this fantasy of hers, but he cannot see why she does not give it up now.

But Annis rouses herself from her reverie: she is suddenly wholly matter-of-fact, and the dreamy quality of her voice is gone.

"John," she says, "Look. I can't force you to anything. And I don't want to force you to do anything, especially not this."

"You said that before," he says.

"But I still have to decide what I want for myself, you know, *alone*. That's what I'm doing in here—trying to figure out whether I should do it without you."

His immediate impulse is to say *Don't, please don't,* but he catches himself in midsentence. All these compassionate years he and she have attempted to keep from influencing each other when they could, from requiring, admonishing, manipulating each other, so that the one would do what the other chose; instead, they have sought to leave each other as much leeway and freedom as possible. It is old habit, not inclination, that restrains him now.

"I understand," he says, and it is only partly a lie.

He bends over her as she sits in the chair, and places a kiss on the smooth surface of her forehead. Then he moves backward out the door, leaving it just as much ajar as when he came.

But in the kitchen, he flattens his hand against the slick sterility of the formica counter, inspects the merciless surface of the glass pan. He turns the gas on furiously to boil the water for coffee; he watches the flame writhe beneath the underside of the pan, and watches the boiling water dance. He watches it for a long time after the water begins to boil, but eventually he turns the gas off, pours the water onto a dark heap of coffee powder in the bottom of a cup, watches it fill, foam up, and then subside.

Ten

Robeck sits forward at his desk, the surface of which is now perfectly clear except for the manuscript of his *Defense*. The order in his office is now reestablished after the demise of the rat project: the books have been reshelved, files reinserted in their proper drawers, and even the adjoining laboratory facilities have been cleaned, so that no miscellaneous glassware or unsterilized surgical tools or odd scraps of paper are left lying around. Robeck riffles his fingers through the stacked pages of the manuscript.

"Have it typed for me," he is saying to Liller. Liller leans across the desk, fingering the tails of his limp necktie, but now Robeck sees a smile break out across Liller's face.

"I thought you'd stopped working on it," Liller says, "You've hardly been here at all. I was afraid . . ."

"You were afraid I'd given up. Well, you're right. I'm not going to publish this thing after all."

"Not publish it?" Liller drops dismayed into the chair beside Robeck's desk. The chair is not a standard chair, but one that stands a little lower to the ground than an ordinary chair. It has the odd property of exaggerating, to anyone who sits in it, Robeck's unusual height and size. Even now that age is beginning to make him slightly stooped and hollow, Robeck is still a large, imposing man, a figure who suggests both brilliance and power.

"I've made one of the most significant discoveries of my life," Robeck says, elevating his voice for mock-dramatic effect, though even Liller can see that he is in earnest. This is a man who has made many significant discoveries, and Liller leans forward in the chair.

"I've discovered I was *wrong*," Robeck says. "Thoroughly, entirely wrong." He skims his fingers across the edges of the manuscript again. "Look, Liller, what would you do with a book you'd written and then decided was wrong?"

"I guess I'd try to fix it," Liller says stupidly.

"You can't just fix it. The whole thing is wrong, through and through."

"Then I guess I'd have to throw it away."

Robeck picks up the pile of manuscript, drops it in Liller's lap. "Throw it away, then."

"But John," Liller protests. "It *can't* be wrong." Liller has studied the argument of the book carefully, and finds it irrefutably plausible, entirely correct. And he also finds it important. He begins to recite the central argument: "In the species *homo sapiens* as in other species, various natural forces, including disease, predators, and disability, have always served to eliminate the aging members of the population . . ."

Robeck joins him in unison:

". . . thus freeing resources for the consumption of the younger, reproducing members of the group."

Liller is startled to have its author make fun of this serious thesis. But he continues:

"Disease, predators, and disability are no longer effective . . ."

"—thanks to modern medicine—" Robeck intones.

". . . in eliminating the aged, and resources that are crucial for the younger, reproducing members are now consumed by the old."

"—and the very old. And the very very old."

Liller begins to see the humor of the skit, and begins to cooperate with the appropriately theatrical delivery:

"It might seem that the solution is to eliminate the old—"

". . . and the very old. And the very very old."

"But this would infringe upon"—and here Liller assumes a tone of cataclysmic seriousness—"*human rights.*"

"Right," peeps Robeck.

"So it clearly becomes the obligation of the old—"

". . . and the very old. And the very very old—"

". . . to eliminate themselves. A remarkably responsible arrangement. It saves the world—"

"protects human rights—"

"conserves resources—"

"spares pain—"

"and gets all those nasty old folks to get themselves out of the way. Listen, Liller, there's something terribly wrong with that argument."

"What?"

"I don't know. But if there weren't, I'd have to kill myself, and I just can't do it." The troubledness of his remark is evident even through the continuing attempt at humor, and Liller too becomes serious.

"That's what you were planning to do. Publish this, and then show the world you were right."

"Well, I can't publish it. But I can't throw it away, either," Robeck says, mostly to himself. Then he turns back to Liller, suddenly somewhat impatient. "Just get this typed, will you? And tell them I'm staying in this laboratory, whether they like it or not. I've given them a damn lot of years of my life, they can give me a few square feet of reasonable working space a couple of years longer." He opens the drawer of his desk, takes out a clean yellow pad, thwacks it down on the surface of the desk, and before Liller has even escaped through the door with the manuscript, has begun to write.

Eleven

When Robeck arrives home, Annis is in her little room, but is not silent in there as usual. The glittering sound of the typewriter greets him, and he rushes to the door.

"Annis," he says overjoyed, as she opens the door to greet him. He looks at her, filling himself with the soft round contours of her body, the way she ties her hair back in a bun that is time-honored and ageless. Age seems somehow so peripheral to her, as if it were a mere accident of her person, and not something central, inevitable, and wrong.

"What are you doing, my love?" he asks, and he asks it entirely naturally, as if he is not in the least surprised that she is not still sitting silently in her darkened chair.

She explains that she is writing letters; she leads him into the room, and shows him a large map of Britain spread out on the floor. He notices that the absence of the vines allows more light into the room, and that the bareness of the walls makes the room seem brighter than he'd remembered. He sees an old address book, something she must have uncovered in all her earlier packing around the house, lying open on top of the map.

"Going somewhere?"

She smiles, eases herself to the floor, flattens out the map with both arms outstretched. Robeck squats beside her; the map, he sees, is confined to southern England, and he watches as she traces a complex route through the countryside, from one small village to another, bypassing anything that might be regarded as a standard tourist sight.

"Would you like to go?" she asks, and he finds that he has taken her hand, is holding it gently in his.

"That's where your family's from, isn't it?" He pauses, thinking. "We've never been there."

She smiles again. "Just the people on my father's side. He was born *here*." She points to an infinitesimally tiny village on the map. "There are relatives here"— she points to another village—"and here, and here. I'd like to say goodbye to them."

"Goodbye?"

"Do you want to come with me?"

He turns away. "You don't know those people," he says. "I don't see the point of it."

She tries to explain, but he does not understand, and in the end he rises up from the position in which he has been crouching beside her on the floor. He goes quickly out of the room, leaving the door ajar.

Twelve

In another, distant city, two middle-aged men are having lunch; they are the two men whose small, framed photographs stand, together with a picture of the third, dead child, on the desk in Annis's room. One is a tall, large, imperious man, with thick dark hair and piercing eyes; the other looks very much like him but is small, softer, with a more gentle manner. They meet erratically, whenever one of them happens to be in the city where the other one lives, and they continue the same conversation from one meeting to the next.

But the waitress interrupts with the check; she is a plump middle-aged uninteresting woman, whose short flounced skirt reveals middle-aged legs, but her breasts are pushed up into a taut imitation of an eighteenth-century wench.

"My turn again, Evan," says Roderick, the larger, imperious one. It is he who has selected this restaurant, and it is he who will pay. He slides his wallet out of the breast pocket of his coat, folds it open. It is the wallet of a banker, filled with bills that are stiff and new. He selects several, places them in the coin tray on the table.

"Makes you look more prosperous than ever," the younger one chides.

"More prosperous than Evan, anyway," the older one jokes, but then they return to the conversation that has been continued over months, from one city to another.

Roderick starts it: " 'What shall we do when the institute kicks him out?"

"I didn't know they were going to."

"I don't think they can keep those old ones around forever. Besides, last time I saw him he said they were trying to get his laboratory space away from him. There's some pretext like putting all the emeriti together in one building."

"He won't stand for that."

"He may have to."

Evan leans forward across the table, serious now. "But he shouldn't have to. He's a well-known man, they can't just push him aside. Don't you think they owe him something?"

"There's no point in being sentimental about it, even when it is your father.

An old man is an old man; that's the way they'll look at it, so we might as well look at it that way too."

"Did they ever talk to you about that 'responsible-ending' stuff?" asks Evan.

"A couple of years ago," Roderick growls. "He was going to get cyanide from the lab, they were going to take it together. When they got old. I think he was even writing an article about it."

"I didn't know about the article," says Evan.

The waitress returns with the change: it is a pile of loose one-dollar bills. Roderick Robeck takes out his banker's wallet, places it on the table. He picks up the first dollar bill almost disdainfully, flattens it out, places the second one squarely across it, so that it is aligned perfectly with the first and the figures and faces are all pointing in the same direction; he does the same with the third and fourth bills. He puts the disciplined bills into his wallet, and places the wallet back in his pocket. Then he speaks:

"I told them it was disgusting. I told them not to ever mention it again."

Thirteen

When he discovers the plane ticket lying on the desk in her little room, Robeck cannot believe it: he had assumed somehow that she had changed her mind, and abandoned the plan. She had not mentioned the trip again, and now that he was spending less time in his office, they had been going for drives, for strolls in the country, drinking tea in the afternoons of roadside cafes. Annis had suggested that they walk along the ocean; they had picked their way among the rocks at the water's edge, and watched the surf swirl in to catch itself in caverns, then leave itself behind in tranquil pools. They had bent together to study the anemones spread out in alluring polyps beneath the surface of the water. They had sat on rocks that (as nearly as they could remember, they confided to each other) they had each sat on fifty years before, before they had met, or married, or had their children.

"I'd do it all again, John," Annis had said happily, and they had sat among the rocks arousing in their memories the intense, eager moments of their earlier lives.

"How did we get so old?" he had said once, genuinely puzzled, but it was only a momentary complaint, and they had moved arm in arm along the beach, to rediscover other times.

But later, after they had returned home and Annis had settled into a bath, he had happened to catch sight of the ticket. He had not meant to enter her room, but somehow he had found himself in there, as if teaching himself in small bits at a time to accept its unaccustomed bareness, the new austerity with which she was choosing to live.

He grabs the ticket and races into the bathroom, enraged, waving the ticket. "What is this?" he explodes.

She shrinks back, involuntarily and futilely attempting to cover the indiscreet folds of her body with the single washcloth.

"What did you use for money?" he demands.

She is astonished; in all their years together they have never quarreled over money, and she is startled that he should think of it now. She removes the washcloth from her body, wrings it out, drapes it carefully over the edge of the tub. With effort, she lifts herself out of the water, stands at full length before him, so that he sees the way her used breasts sag, her skin lies loosely across her fallen belly, and the hair between her legs has grown sparse and pale. She pulls a towel around herself.

"Money," she says. "Well, I will tell you," and she explains something he has known all along but avoided remembering. When they had first agreed to end their lives together, years ago, she had suggested that they start a little "final fund," so that whatever expenses would need to be paid could be drawn from it, and not from the pockets of their heirs and children. He follows her into the study.

"There was a lot left over," he watches her say, and she shows him an envelope in the drawer of her desk. In the envelope is a formal-looking document, printed like a certificate; Robeck finds his eyes travelling across the name of a funeral company, the legend "prepaid plan."

"It was the cheapest I could find," says Annis. "It's all paid for." From the folder she produces a little card: there is a telephone number printed on it.

"All you have to do is call them," she says. "They know what I want."

Robeck stares at the card. Above the telephone number is an italicized phrase: *in time of need.* He crushes the card in his fist, stuffs it into his pocket. He shoves his hands into his pockets, walks rapidly back and forth across her empty little room. He feels like a child, when his mother deserted him again and again, appearing in smart business suits or sleek party clothing, to tantalize him with the briefest of kisses, and be gone. He looks at the ticket again.

"Will you come back?" he asks finally.

She is quiet a long time, sensing his distress, his needfulness, his new, uncharacteristic dependence, and struggling with her own new feelings of confinement, restriction, her longing to go.

"Yes," she answers.

"Good."

But she cannot resist trying once more. "Will you come with me, John? I would like you to."

"No." She watches him put his hand into his pocket again, find the crumpled funeral-service card, extract it from his pocket and flatten it out in his hand. He looks at it again, crushes it tightly, and heaves it across the room. It falls behind the dresser she has been so carefully clearing out. "I won't have anything to do with that," he says, and she sees his hand grip tightly as he steadies himself against the edge of her desk.

There is a new petulance in her voice, which she does not like but cannot avoid. "But John, you used to understand . . ."

"Things change," he says, his eyes narrow and his fist still clenched. "The answer is *no.*"

Fourteen

Annis arrives at the airport in an ancient, cavernous Checker cab, whose sullen driver deposits her suitcase on the sidewalk without ceremony. She finds herself inside; it is a large, old airport; various other wings of it have been redecorated with brightly painted walls and equally bright carpets, but this particular portion has not. She checks her ticket near the entrance to the plane; the noise of the passengers and the engines of the planes in which they will depart echoes hollowly against the grimy walls, and her back begins to ache with standing. Ahead of her in line, an enormously old and nearly blind woman is lifted from her wheelchair by two efficiently trained attendants onto a mechanized loading chair, and the wheelchair itself is folded and carried up the ramp. Parents carry babies who will begin to squall when the plane's engines are revved up; honeymooning couples and middle-aged retirees slouch in line, impatient to spread themselves out in seats and unfold their tourist maps of London.

It occurs to her that she may be the only one on the plane both content to go, and content to return.

Fifteen

Robeck sits in the low chair beside his own desk, and Liller leans across its edge.

"I think I know what to do," Robeck is saying, and he gestures from the chair with great excitement. He thumps his hand down on the pile of manuscript pages. "This is the *first* part," he says, "just as it is. Now I'll write a refutation, to show what's wrong with it." He stands up behind the desk, takes out another yellow pad, puts it down on the surface of the desk.

"The *Reports* will have to give me another thirty pages," he says with a twinkle.

But Liller does not move. "I don't see what's wrong with it," he says, primarily to himself. Then he turns toward Robeck, wholly guileless, like a pupil seeking praise for an unexpected piece of work. "I was going to do the same thing myself," he says, "you know, the cyanide. When the time came."

Robeck looks at him, with the unrestrained, urgent stare that had intimidated so many other researchers, and had won him such wide respect. "That's certainly part of the problem," he says. "I have to figure out the rest."

Sixteen

They have all assembled to meet her, five generations of the same southeast England sheep-farming family, an assortment of children in whom the giggles are barely suppressed, middle-aged pink-cheeked women given largely to gossip, sturdy young men, red-complexioned from the constant wind and the occasional sun and the continuous pints of ale in the local pub, and even the patriarch figure, now past ninety, is here: an ancient quizzical old man with stark-white hair who is virtually unable to hear. But his eyes are alert, and they follow Annis; it is clear that the family has explained to him who the visitor is: the daughter of his oldest brother.

Annis greets her uncle, and realizes with astonishment that it makes her feel like a child. Her own parents have been dead for years, and without them, she has felt fully adult; but this ancient man is her uncle, her father's brother, a man of her parents' generation, not her own, and she discovers that it makes her feel as if there were some part of life she had not yet discovered, through which she still might go. She wishes it were possible to talk with him, this ancient man, that he were not so hard of hearing, but she cannot, and in the end she can only sit beside him, smiling from time to time, feeling the attention and affection of his continuingly alert gaze.

But after the meal, the women of the family slide back into their gossip, and the men sit, infrequently speaking, with large mugs of ale and their strong cigars, and Annis realizes again that she is only remotely related to these people, by blood perhaps but not by more. In the morning, she gets into her car; she says the cheerful goodbyes of ordinary hospitality, but with her larger farewell she is silent. She does not see the old man, who is almost twenty years older than she, or any of the rest of this large family again.

There are other branches of the family to visit as well, equally eager to greet her, but equally involved in their own intertwined interests. She cannot tell them what she has really come to say, for that would somehow affront the workings of these families, and constitute a breach of that rural decorum they so carefully preserve. Increasingly frequently, she finds herself driving alone through the countryside, through the narrow lanes, barely wide enough for a single car, in between the hedgerows. She studies their composition: at their root lie ancient stone walls, upon which moss has flourished and seeds have sprouted; here a soil has formed, and now large bushes, sometimes full trees, grow from the tops of these old stone walls, their roots reinforcing, anchoring them ever more firmly into the English country-side. In the country with which she is familiar, fields are divided by a single rail fence, sometimes a clean stone wall; these are replaced when they fall, but here in the land of her ancestors the barriers between one field and the next show centuries of growth, decay, continued growth.

She drives further into the countryside, stopping when she is tired at old coun-try inns, small, low-ceilinged, wooden-beamed buildings, where exhausted travelers have recovered themselves since 1190, or 1377, or 1537. At one, she orders a pitcher of tea and drinks it alone, thinking back of the people who have sat on this same bench as she, warming themselves at this same hearth as she, not only last week, or last year, not even in the previous decade or anytime within the small memories of those still alive, but backwards four, six, nearly eight hundred years, and she feels the absolute insignificance of her own remarkable presence on this bench. Someone else will occupy it tomorrow, still someone else the following day, and still others will continue to come for future hundreds of years, small ephemeral individuals supplanted by new equally ephemeral ones, who will take their imper-manent seats on this bench just as she has.

She pays the bill; for some entirely extraneous reason, she realizes that half the time has elapsed until she has planned to go home. A small irked feeling rides up inside her, but she does not resist it, and it subsides of its own accord. She sees no reason to worry yet, though somewhere, somehow, she knows what is coming.

Seventeen

The emptiness of the house is almost as great in the day as in the night; Robeck is alone now, where there are no noises of his wife, not even the heavy, full silence when she sits in her room. He had not known that an empty house could become emptier, but each day it is more so, and his very breathing seems to grow less audible, his movements to cease. Occasionally, he tries calling friends; he spends an evening or two at dinner, explaining that Annis is out of town, but afterward there is the cavernous emptiness of the uninhabited house, where even the memories are packed away in boxes, or have vanished. He tries to work on the new portion of his manuscript, but does not succeed: he spends hours twisting paperclips between his fingers, or wandering idly through the animal labs; he cannot bring himself to write, and finds that he has nothing to say. In the evenings he returns home, opens one can of vegetables and fries an egg, or puts a single frozen dinner into the oven. He sits stupidly in front of the television, drugged by it but not amused. He eats the same things again and again, watches the same programs every evening, and he always finds it hardest of all to put an end to the light when he goes to bed. Sometimes he cannot bring himself to do so, but leaves it burning.

By the midpoint of Annis's absence, he begins to hunt through the house. He does so slowly at first, looking idly into a cupboard here, opening a single closet there. But everywhere he finds the same thing: the drawers are empty, the contents of the cupboards packed, and in the attic what he finds are stacks of cardboard boxes, one stack for Roderick, one stack for Evan, a small stack labeled with the name of Luel's kid. He opens one or two at random: they are wildly filled like the insides of her drawers had been, with all the minutiae and little sentimental objects that compose a life and might conceivably be passed on. The cartons are ready, he sees, to be removed to other houses, and then the great parental house, except for the barest essentials, will be almost entirely empty.

He goes fast, then: he sorts fearfully through the contents of the desk, the dresser, the drawers in her little room. He finds her calendar: there are no dates on it, no committee meetings scheduled, or bridge tournaments, or even garden shows, beyond the following month. He finds a pile of correspondence from various far-flung friends, all recently arrived, all bidding farewell in a variety of styles and penmanships and stationery. Some of the responses are more awkward and uncertain, some easeful and understanding. New letters arrive in the mail; he opens one:

> It is odd Anny how the news that you're about to bring your life to an end disturbs me and yet causes me this funny satisfied joy i think i am much too afraid of death even now remember i am a year older than you are Anny but it does make me remember all those brilliant days when we hiked in the Tetons and the Rockies

and the huge blisters and the professional size of the mosquitoes But do you also remember Anny lying out there under all those stars you used to always talk about the meaning of life i guess you know it now. You were always such a hero to me Anny i will miss you but i am clapping for you now

He remembers the card she had given him: *In Case Of Need,* and fishes behind the dresser to find it. He dials the number:

"Yes, a Mrs. Robeck has made pre-need arrangements with us. Who, may I know, is calling?"

"Mr. Robeck."

"Well, Mr. Robeck, how nice to talk with you. Mrs. Robeck is very eager to save you worry and concern and additional expense, you know, at the time of need." It is a female voice, brittle, but well trained in professional sympathy. "May I ask you, is she in her final illness now?"

"No," he says uncertainly. Then, instead, "yes."

"I'm very sorry, Mr. Robeck. But might I suggest to you that it would be a great comfort for your wife if you were to make pre-need arrangements as well, perhaps the simple cremation like the one she has ordered, or perhaps something more elaborate, so that . . ."

"No," he protests, and hangs up.

He calls the police. The man who arrives is also graying; a large, affable man who has handled domestic cases for years, and stayed well away from the blood and public gunfire of the street. But he has seen deaths and suicides, again and again. Robeck shows him what he has found: the letters, the empty datebook, the funeral home's certificate. There are lists of instructions for the new occupants of the house—how to work the furnace; where the bulbs are planted; how long it's been since the chimney was last swept. There is her will, the text of an obituary notice, even an informal outline for a small memorial service, if anyone feels any need to have it. *Please,* she has written, *just a small group of friends, in the living room . . .*

The officer inspects the materials Robeck shows him with interest. "She certainly meant what she said," he muses; "She doesn't want to leave any mess." Then he explains to Robeck that his wife had already been to see them, to discuss with them quite specifically and explicitly her plan, so that no one in the house would be suspected of any ill play, and so that no unnecessary investigation would be required.

"There've been a couple of cases like this in recent years," the officer says. "We've never known exactly what to do with them, when they notify you themselves, in advance. It's not against the law, you know. But usually the person has already got cancer or something, so we just check it with the physician, and let it go at that."

"I don't want her to do it," Robeck says.

"Have you considered psychiatric help?"

"She won't go. I can't force her."

"You could consider a temporary commitment," the officer suggests, and there is a sharper edge to his tone; "there's more than enough evidence here to establish that she's a danger to herself."

After the officer goes, Robeck turns back into the bedroom of the house he and Annis have shared. He opens the doors of the closets and the drawers of the dressers again, and again he realizes that almost everything of hers is gone: her side of the closet contains only dangling hangers, the drawers are empty, the clutter of rougepots and lipsticks and assorted earrings has been swept from the top of the dresser, and even the miscellaneous pictures of the grandchildren stuck in under the edges of the mirror are gone, as if she has already died, and all traces of her existence are being expunged.

He weeps, now. And he calls his sons.

Eighteen

After the valleys she discovers the moors, the high, waste places where the hedge-rows end and the roads do not penetrate and only scattered sheep still graze, where a cold mist from the ocean envelops everyone, everything, almost constantly. Annis walks only a little way the first day, uncertain of the terrain, but she returns again and again, in the fog, alone. She comes to know the landmarks of the moors: small round hills, perhaps fifteen feet across; they are the burial mounds of the ancient peoples who inhabited this area, three thousand years ago. Some of the mounds have caved in, so that they are more like doughnuts than hills; she wonders if they were built that way or whether it is the work of later grave-plundering, but no one she asks can tell her. She begins to visualize an old, frugal, isolated people, living sparse, austere existences in the thick mists of these regions, their tranquility only later disturbed by invasions from the continent, from the Scandinavian islands, from the other parts of England. In her long evenings in the inns, their own few hundred years paltry in comparison with the scope of this long prehistory, she reads what she can of the development of these ancient peoples, their brief and mysterious existences, their disappearance. Perhaps she is one of their issue, she supposes, as are the ruddy English folk she has been recognizing as relatives, and she sees her own life, their lives, all lives, as tiny bits of sand, single little leaves on the gorse bushes of the moors, droplets of the mist that cloaks, recedes, and cloaks the moors again, then again, and again. It is a time of tremendous peace.

It is also time for home.

Nineteen

Long before her eyes are open Annis can feel the bed, its well-familiar contours, the small lumps and hollows that make a bed one's own. She moves just slightly, and finds the pattern into which she and her husband have fit their bodies together over the past half-century. They have conceived their children in this bed, suffered their illnesses in this bed, wept together here in this bed after the death of Luel, but in all the nights and afternoons and mornings in this bed, after the love or weeping or contented conjugal laughter would come the time for sleep, when John would turn on his side toward her, she would turn also on her side, away, and she would fit her smaller body into the angle formed by his. They would lie together motionless, their bodies touching all along their lengths, like one spoon nestled in another, and he would fold his arm gently over her. Sometimes she would feel a tiny, exquisitely gentle shuddering of his body, a kind of contented convulsion, at the moment of sleep; sometimes, she knew, he would feel the sleep coming to her.

But now she sees faces hovering over the bed, and only from time to time can she surface from the depths of her sleep to see them. Roddy. Evan. Both sons appear, leaning over her, their faces concerned; they seem to appear at intervals, though she has no sense of how far apart their visits are, how long they last, or why her sons are here. Sometimes it is a strange face, one she does not recognize, which bends over her in a cautious, professional manner; sometimes she talks with this face, though later she will have little recollection of what it said, or what this face said to her. Her condition is sheer exhaustion from the trip, she knows, exacerbated by age, from the solitude and the long walks in the wet mists of the moors; then too it is the dazed dislocation of altered time zones, so that what is daytime for everyone else is the middle of the night for her, and she speaks to them only through a continuous film of sleep. But then she discovers that the face she has not recognized is a doctor: he leaves capsules for her, rigorously administered by her sons, and it seems to her that they too produce a drowziness through which she cannot quite find herself.

Gradually, though, she begins to recover from her exhaustion, and she sees that she is the center of crisis: the house is full, and there is an air of emergency, urgency, and fear. Rod's small children peek wide-eyed into the bedroom from the door; they are scolded for it by their mother, who hides in the kitchen. The adults take turns sitting by the bed. Evan reads, Rod examines the newspaper, John sits and simply stares ahead. Even Luel's adolescent child sits by the bed, her thin legs knotted up beneath her and her dark hair falling wild across her eyes, but she says nothing. She leaves as suddenly as she arrives, without a word or nod, but she comes again, day after day, and sits beside the bed. For a moment, Annis imagines that it is a summer house, where all the family has come together for those most intimate and joyous times, but then the truth intrudes, and she sees that this is crisis, entirely surrounding her.

She gets out of bed. She examines the pills left on her dresser by the psychiatrist; she studies the contents of her desk. She calls John.

"Why are these people here?" she asks. "I'm only tired from the trip, not ill."

But John does not sit in the chair in her little room; he stands by her desk, his hands planted on it.

"What did you decide?"

"About what?"

"You said you were going on the trip to make up your mind. About whether"— he fishes for a careful circumlocution—"you still intend to carry out your plan."

"Oh, that," she laughs, relieved, "sure, eventually." She tells him what she has been thinking about these past weeks, what it has meant to her to see the roots of her family, her immediate ancestors and the remote, prehistoric ones, of her new free sense of the evanescence and fragility of a single human life, the way one figure yields to the next, and the next, at the centuries-old hearths of the inns.

"I'm not in any hurry," she says. "But it's an extraordinary thing, to feel your life is complete. I think it probably is getting on to be time to die, though it is very pleasant as it goes on."

"You'd still do it, then?" John is still standing, his hands fists.

She remembers something. "You were going to bring home some tablets from your lab."

Robeck stands upright, takes his hand from the desk. He looks at her with a coldness she has almost never seen in him, and he turns to leave the room. At the door he pauses, stops, turns back to her:

"No. Of course not."

Twenty

In the opinion of the psychiatrist, Annis needs not only continued medication, but a change of life-circumstance: her depression is in part reaction to the emptiness of the large family house, in part a delayed grief response to the death of Luel; it is a reaction to future losses too, anticipating a decline in mobility, appearance, health.

"Or you could say it's like a premature decathexis," he conjectures, and he describes the final stages of leave-taking, disinterest, detachment from the world, usually seen only at the end of the long defeat of the terminally ill. "Some people just seem finished with the world."

He recommends that they consider moving. There is an excellent retirement community, he says, not very far away.

John and Roderick and Evan tell Annis.

"It isn't what I want," she laughs. "But I'll be glad to look."

Twenty-One

Rod drives. For the first part of the trip, John sits in the front with Rod, Evan in the back with Annis, but after they stop for coffee they switch Annis into the front: they want her to be able to see. Many miles down the road they see the first groups of stark white buildings spreading across the dry California countryside, low and close together, and as they approach they can distinguish several different types: low, two-story apartment blocks; single-level houses; the several high towers that are the nurse-attended residential units. They drive through the gate of the surrounding wall, past the guard in his glass entry-house, then past vivid green lawns and elaborately tended beds of red semitropical flowers, toward the Information and Sales office. Rod has made an appointment in advance, but the salesman is not the smoothly worded, subtly pressuring sort they had all expected, but an innocently honest, guileless young man, embarrassingly sincere, who has not a touch of the salesman in him, and seems as willing to display the faults of the leisure-world way of life as its advantages. Even so, he recognizes the scene: a slightly skeptical aging couple, piloted through the retirement complex by adult children anxious for a solution of their problem. The adult children stub the toes of their shoes into the grass, and keep themselves from asking questions that might unsettle their parents, while the victims themselves look tremulously about at the vast strange place they are expected to learn to call home.

They begin with the two-story apartment units. These are decorated in garish versions of what the interior decorator clearly believes is the taste of elderly people—heirloom sideboards and corner cupboards and glass-fronted cases for displaying china—with walls papered in deceptively bright designs suitable for people with failing eyesight. The furniture is built to three-quarters scale, so as not to seem too large for the small rooms. Annis notes the grip-rail in the bathtub and beside the toilet, the stoves with large, clear, unmistakable dials.

They tour the single-level houses. Annis notices the complete absence of steps, the capaciousness of the medicine cupboard, the direct intercom system for emergency calls.

"These are called villas," the young man says, and artlessly recites a vast variety of financing plans. This is followed by a cumbersome little speech on the ease of resale, on the way in which financing is designed so that it prepares for extreme disability or even death from the time of purchase, and the way in which one can move from the villas to the nursing-care towers, to the hospital itself.

"You don't need to worry about those things after you come here," he is saying, "it takes care of itself."

"It seems quite sensible," Annis replies.

They tour the sports facilities: a large, well-heated, Olympic-sized pool, most of it shallow, the golf course, the bowling alleys, the game rooms for cards and checkers and chess. Bingo is Tuesday night, duplicate bridge on Thursday, though the young man explains that there are many many informal bridge groups, and the community boasts an astonishing number of masters. Annis is noticing other things—the absence of curbs that might impede people with walkers or wheelchairs, the large number of benches and resting-places on the streets, the very large number of churches, the little jitney buses that transport residents from one portion of the community to another.

"There's a travel club too," the young man says. "This year they've gone to Greece, Morocco, and Japan. Some people seem to travel all the time." They meet the residents everywhere, most of them women with carefully styled hair, wearing leisure wear or pantsuits, but there are men too, tanned and leathery from the sun, driving in from the course in their golf carts, or reading the Sunday papers in the sun. Some of the residents walk with canes or walkers or are pushed in wheelchairs, but they seem few, and most of the people they pass on the streets seem active and well.

"We haven't seen where the older ones are yet," says Annis.

So they tour the nursing-care high-rise, and visit the hospital facilities. Rod had thought Annis ought not see them, since it would certainly discourage her, but she had insisted, and had inspected them with a thoroughness and interest that surprised them all. She had chatted with the on-duty nurses, peered into patient rooms, suggested they try the cafeteria food.

"It seems really quite humane," she says. "If you're going to be old, this must be the place to be."

"A surprising thing happens to a lot of people who thought they were old when they come here," the young man says. "They've been trying to swim in pools that are full of teenagers in bikinis, or play tennis on a court next to an A game. But when they come here they discover that all the people in the pool are as old and slow and full of wrinkles as they are, and all of a sudden they can keep up with the next tennis game after all."

"I suppose it's tremendously rejuvenating," Annis says.

"It is," says the young man fervently. "It is."

"It would certainly be easier than that big old house," Robeck speculates. Annis smiles, and they begin to relax now, the father and the two sons, for they see that Annis is genuinely impressed, and that she discovers merits in the place they had not dreamed of.

"It's only five minutes from the ocean," Rod says. "We'll all come in the summer, and take a place by the water. You and dad can go back and forth if you like, or stay with us."

"You'll be able to write poetry," adds Evan. He turns to the salesman. "Didn't you say there were three poetry-writing groups?"

"Yes, and there's one that does short stories, a script-writing group too. There's every activity you could want." He leaves them with a large number of brochures, a statement of the features of the sale contract regarding disability and death, the terms regarding advanced old age.

"Just give me a call if you need anything," he says, but they are in the car already, Annis in the back, peeling hot shoes from her tired feet, sinking gratefully back on the seats. John sits closely next to her; Evan turns around with his elbows over the back of the front seat. "Eighty percent of them don't have teeth," she chides, but then she is asleep instantly, and Rod grins at them in the rearview mirror.

Twenty-Two

The day begins as if some large family problem were solved: the sons are up early, moving stacks of cardboard cartons from the attic to the basement, inspecting the garden equipment in the garage, thumbing through the Yellow Pages for the names of local real estate agents, whom they might get to sell the house. The grandchildren have free run of the house, and no one scolds them. They dart in to sit a moment on Annis's lap, and are off again. John begins the task he had so much earlier avoided—he begins, as she has already done, to sort through the contents of his dresser, the closet, the cupboards where he keeps his clothes and shoes and golfing hats, and he begins to throw some out, set other things aside to pack and take along. Even Rod's shy wife emerges from the kitchen, to ask Annis if she'd like a cup of tea.

But Annis sets off by herself along the steep path to the sea. The frayed bark of eucalyptus covers the ground, small spiny plants push themselves up through the soil, and the noise of the ocean seems irregular and loud. She thinks of rows of identical villas, one of which is to be prepared for her, of the warm shallow pool and the continuous bridge games and the periodic tours of elderly women through Spain, Portugal, Greece, and the progression from there to the nursing-care units, where help comes at the sound of a buzzer and there is oxygen stored on each floor, and finally the new white impeccably clean hospital facilities, where one could finally come to dying in the expected way. Evan would come, and Rod would fly in at the last, to sit for a while beside the bed of a wasted, incontinent, senile old woman, who would neither perceive the presence of her sons nor succeed in saying goodbye.

Afterward, they would shake hands with the doctor, board their planes back home, and tell the children, "Grandma died."

"Oh," the children would say.

She thinks of their faces now, the giggling children, but she thinks of the older faces too, these expectant, responsible, adult faces, who so much want her to consent, and see the problem safely solved. She sits on the rock where she has so often sat, drains a little sand through her fingers. Can she do this to them, tell them no, she won't go, she will do as she's planned in concluding her life? Can she really say, can she mean, *farewell?* Dying would hurt Rod's pride, of that she is sure, but she thinks it would hurt nothing more. Evan, dear sweet silent Evan, is independent now, and he would understand. Of the children, her dying would have really injured only Luel, needy, unresolved Luel, but Luel herself is dead now, and cannot cry.

Annis picks herself up from the rock, begins to walk slowly back up the beach. Gulls waddle just in front of her along the sand, leaving prints of their three-pronged feet. Small bubbles appear on the surface of the wet sand as new waves slide back; they are made by sand crabs, concealed just below the surface. But what of John? It is here that her trouble is hardest; the children have their own independent lives, but John is tied to her, more so, it seems, every day. Can she simply leave him, and abandon him to the old, old age that is coming, that she herself refuses to endure? But it was John who had originally brought her to this idea, who had first given her a sense of the simplicity and naturalness of life, of death, who with his broad biologist's view had resisted all that talk of mystery, sanctity, the sacredness of life. He would still resist it now, she thought; he is just afraid to die. But she has gained her own new sense of the mystery and sacredness of life, and that is what they do not understand. Ah, John! She has spent herself in many ways for him, for all of them, but this one last, greatest sacrifice—this they cannot ask her to make.

She is not sure whether she feels older or younger now, as she winds her way back up the eucalyptus-covered path. Perhaps, she thinks, age is not really the thing, after all.

Twenty-three

Annis has been asleep since she came back from her walk, though the activities of the family continue uninterrupted; they understand that she is still recovering from her journey, from the excitement, from the sudden prospect of the move. Evan peeks in at her from the bedroom door. She lies heavily on her side, her shoes kicked off, her knees drawn slightly up; there is a blanket barely covering her legs.

He tiptoes in, entranced by the silence of her sleeping. He pulls the blanket gently up around her sleeping shoulders, adjusts the lamp so that it does not shine in her eyes. He stands and looks at her for several moments, visualizing the mother who taught him how to tie his shoes, who scolded him for leaving his schoolbooks on the piano, who smiled at his stories in the school newspaper, who attended nearly every one of the recitals he had given and not remarked on the off-pitch notes. It is the same face still, he sees, with the same deep-set eyes, eyes that would be dark and somehow luminous if she were awake; the same slightly olive skin and wide cheekbones, which have always given her an air of mysteriousness, remoteness, reserve. But the face is older now, much older, and as he seats himself in the chair beside the bed he studies his mother's sleeping face, the lines that group around the corners of the eyes, at the mouth, the soft pale cast of fine-grown hair, the way the cheeks puff ever so slightly below the chin. It is an old face, growing more old, but not unlovely. Dear mother, he thinks, dear, dear mother. He leans over in the chair to kiss her, ever so softly. He is somewhat surprised by himself; he sits back on the chair, and his eyes move around the room. He studies the small-figured wallpaper, the outlines of the chest of drawers, the roseate door-knob that has survived from earlier generations. His gaze falls on the dresser; it is quite bare, except for the small vial of pills and three framed pictures, but beside it is her purse. It is the one she always carries, a plain brown leather purse, large and capacious, soft with use. She has had this purse almost ever since he can remember, he reflects; it never seems to wear out altogether or go out of style, or else she secretly replaces each with an identical one every several years, but in any case his gaze remains rooted to this purse. It is large. It is always with her. And it is almost the the only thing of hers that has not been packed, boxed, labeled for someone else. Almost without realizing it, he finds his hand extended, finds himself reaching for the purse, finds it in his hand now, in his lap as he sits in the chair. He strokes the leather; it is almost as soft as she. A sudden extremely vivid memory comes to him of a playmate being severely punished for taking two nickels from his mother's pocketbook; he, Evan, would never have tried. He looks at his own mother; she is still sleeping. But now he is opening the catch, looking down into the brown interior of the purse: he sees several letters, the envelopes of which are slit open, a packet of tissues, a single lipstick and one comb; the wallet.

He looks at her again; she is still sleeping. He opens the wallet. The credit cards have been removed, and there is only a small amount of money. But there is still a picture of John, and another picture of the family all together, when Luel was still alive, posed on the lawn at some earlier family gathering. Dear mother, he thinks, whose love does not stop. He closes the wallet. He takes out the letters, thinks better of it, puts them back. He closes the catch of the purse, softly, so that it does not awaken her. He sits for a moment in the chair, watching her regular, rhythmic breathing, and then, equally quietly, he opens the purse again. He reaches into it for the letters. They protrude from a small side pocket of the cavernous purse, but as he removes the letters he notices something he had not seen before: at the bottom of the pocket is a small, soft, dark object. He takes it out, sees that it is a coinpurse, apparently full but not heavy. He opens it. His eyes travel instantly to the pharmacist's bottle on the dresser, back to the coinpouch: it is filled with capsules, just like those that are in the bottle.

He sits absolutely rigid for a moment, his hand clasped tightly around the purse. Dear, sweet mother, he thinks, but then he sees: Rod is also pausing at the door. Evan's hand freezes. Rod wanders casually in the door. Evan knows he must close the pouch, stuff it back in the purse, display embarrassment as if he'd been reading the letters, but he does not, and soon Rod is standing over him, looking down into the purse. He lifts Evan's hand and the pouch it is still clutching out of the purse, opens the pouch.

He lets out a single yell that brings everyone running, John, the frightened wife from the kitchen, the still more frightened children, and he pours the pills out onto the dresser.

"Two," he counts, "four, six, eight . . ."

Annis leaps from her sleep, struggling to understand.

"Ten, twelve, fourteen . . ."

"They're mine," Annis whispers, "put them back," but no one hears her now.

"Sixteen, eighteen, twenty . . ." and she watches as they scoop up the capsules, a handful each, and run through the hall to the bathroom. One small capsule rolls to the floor, but a single capsule is no use now, and she follows them desperately into the bathroom: "no," she cries, "they're mine," but she is not as quick or strong as they, and she watches the thirty-seven magical capsules, sweet easy somnolent keys to her prison, drop into the toilet. They bob on the surface of the water, and as she moves closer, horrified, to look, Rod presses the handle of the toilet, the water rushes into the bowl, and the capsules swirl, still on the surface, down and away. Rod and Evan and John talk only among themselves now, agitated and wild.

She retreats back into the bedroom, and she sees Luel's kid slide away upstairs. She can hear Rod on the telephone now; his voice is indistinct, but she knows who he is calling. There is not much time.

Twenty-Four

After that, the men begin to take turns. It happens only informally at first; Roderick asks his brother if he'd stay with Annis while he goes out for a couple of hours to check the correspondence from his office; Evan asks Rod to keep an eye in the afternoon, as he'd like to do some undisturbed reading; both brothers suggest to their father that he sit with Annis, as they'd like to go out to talk together for a while. But they also call Luel's kid from the upstairs room, because they are not quite sure their frail old father could—or would—restrain his wife.

"Just keep an eye on her, will you," they say to the child.

The girl's thin body assumes an automatic, insolent posture, only slightly disguised by the loose shirts she wears. "What for?"

"You know what for." Roderick does not like this girl very much, not just because she so tangibly represents the early indiscretions of his sister Luel, but because she seems to embody so many of Luel's qualities: the remoteness, the aloofness, the utter resistance to authority. In Luel these qualities had been attractive; but there wasn't any Luel now, only this sad, unhappy child, sitting forlornly in her room, responding only with anger, or insolence, or silence to those around her. Sometimes the girl would go off for the afternoon, or the night, walking, or in her car, but she always seemed to return, to wait half-insolently, half-sadly, around the house. Rod cannot understand why she would bother to come here, now that her mother is dead and her connections with them severed; her father had remarried shortly after Luel's death and took no further interest in her family. Rod finds it hard to understand why this child would not stay there, where a new family had been formed around her, or why she would want to watch one old woman's strange obsession cause a perfect family to fall apart.

Rod glares at the girl: "You know what for."

Luel's kid does not answer; she gives her shoulders an almost imperceptible shrug, and moves off down the hall.

When the two sons return, however, they find Annis is gone: the girl has allowed her to go for a walk, even though it is evening and very nearly dark, and even though she is supposed to be watched at every moment.

"She wanted to go for a walk, that's all," the girl says, and her natural insolence is apparent in her voice.

"You were supposed to be watching her," Rod fumes. If she were his own child, instead of the child of his dead sister, Rod would turn her instantly over his knee, as if she were half her age, and spank her.

"I did watch her, that was the trouble. She wanted to be alone." The girl flips her black hair out of her eyes, looks directly at Rod. "How would you like it if you were watched all the time?"

"We don't need help, the way she does."

"She doesn't need *help*. She needs to be left alone."

Rod ignores the girl. "Try the road in town," he growls to his brother. "You stay here in case she comes back," he says to the girl, "and for god's sake, if she comes back don't let her out again. If you do you'll be out too. I'll see if she's gone down to the ocean."

The two men scramble into their coats, clatter out across the gravel in the driveway. But just then they see her coming, an old woman, shrouded in an old dark cloak, moving slowly up the path from the beach.

"Where have you been!" the two men scold, though it is perfectly apparent. "You are not to leave the house alone. And not after dark. And not to go near the ocean." Rod is puffed, agitated, red in the face.

Annis looks at them with genuine surprise. "I didn't mean to worry you," she says, "though it is getting dark. I just wanted a walk. A good walk, by myself." She removes the cloak, spreads it out on the steps of the porch. "Let me tell you what I saw." She is so calm, so mysterious, so enveloping, that as she slowly seats herself on the cloak-covered steps, the two men begin to lose their anger, and slowly sit beside her too. Their sister's child hunches on the step below, at her grand-mother's feet.

"Dearest children," she begins, and she tells them about the broken eucalyptus, the anemones, the rhythm of the waves on the beach. Rod is still a little angry, still puffed, but he allows himself to settle on the steps, almost at his mother's knee. She strokes the head of Luel's child between her hands.

"The older you grow, the more important solitude becomes, and the harder it is to find it. It is hard to find a way to be alone, but that is the most important thing there is." She sits forward on the steps, and her tone alters from that dream-like, distant quality it sometimes has, to the straight sharp matter-of-fact way she often speaks.

"I know it's hard for you to understand why I don't want to move to that villa, and I could give you a bunch of reasons which only maybe would convince you. I could say I didn't want to have only elderly neighbors, or live in a geriatric group. Or that I refused to live somewhere where I couldn't have my grandchildren come to spend a week, with their tricycles and their chewing gum and their nonstop noise. I could say the place is too sheltered, or that I'm politically opposed to walls; I could tell you I don't like bridge or pinochle or poetry guilds or any sort of craftwork at all." She feels Rod tense, but she lays her hand on him to stop, and continues:

"I just don't want it, that's all. I mean, suppose someone offers you a cruise on an ocean liner, and you know exactly what it will be, when the meals will be served, what sorts of clothes the first-class passengers wear, where the shuffleboard courts are, the swimming pools, what time the dancing will end at night. You wouldn't have to go, would you?"

"But it would be fun," says Evan. "You'd meet interesting people, you'd see the sunsets on the ocean, you'd learn interesting new things . . ."

"I've had fun," she answers. "I've met interesting people, learned fascinating things. But I'm ready to be alone now, I just simply don't want any more. I love you all, but I want you to let me go."

There is no answer.

"I want you to let me go," Annis repeats.

There is a long silence again, but Rod's urgent breathing becomes more audible in the dark. "Stop it," he finally explodes. "That's just unthinkable, you can't. You just plain can't. You ought to be in the hospital."

"Besides," Evan adds, "think what it would do to Dad."

Annis is silent a long time, stroking the motionless head of Luel's child. A slight wind stirs the trees; the steady hum of traffic on the main coast road is faintly audible. Rod shifts himself down one step, then up again; he finds the hard stone uncomfortable.

"Didn't your father tell you he was going to do it too?" she asks. "We've lived our lives together, we were going to end them that way."

"No," growls Rod. "Absolutely not."

Now the surveillance increases, and the loose arrangements that had been so informal at first become regimented quickly. Rod spends the morning working on the materials from his office while Evan watches Annis; Evan reads during the afternoon while Rod keeps his eye on her. Rod's wife fills in at lunch and sometimes during supper. John is watching all the time; occasionally he sets out for his office or the lab, but if he arrives at all he does not stay long, and returns quickly home again. Luel's child is not trusted any longer, and when both brothers go out, they hire a sitter in. It is torture to Annis to be watched so continuously, and it quickly begins to be a torture to the watchers too. Roderick and his wife and Evan are impatient to go home, to return to their normal lives, to have the matter settled and under control. But they respond to this tension by redoubling their efforts. They make regular searches of the house, in case there is any little cache of sleeping pills or razor blades they have not yet discovered. They inspect Annis's purse, empty out the pockets of her coat; they buy a child-proof medicine chest, and lock the prescribed pills in it. They remove the knives from the kitchen and let her use them only when Rod's wife is also there. Earlier, there had been talk of retirement communities or perhaps rest homes; now the talk is of hospitalization.

"If you let them put you in there you'll never get out," Luel's child had said to her once. "You'd go crazy."

"I don't think the hospitals are as primitive as that," Annis says gently, but she knows somehow the girl is right; hospitalization, whether for mental or physical distress, is the last thing she wants, when all she wants is peace, tranquility, a surcease of activity, a final stilling of her world.

"That's what they want to do with you, you know," the child insists. "I've heard them talking."

"So have I." Annis says it with her usual composure, but she can feel that composure disturbed—she feels a new urgency, a fear, a claustrophobic, confined feeling, as if the bars of a cage were being nailed up around her one by one.

But Rod sees them talking, and sends Luel's kid to her room. "You shouldn't upset your grandmother," he says. "She needs rest."

The girl turns, flips her long hair insolently at him, slides off down the hall.

"That girl's been here long enough," Rod says to his brother. "She ought to be home with her father."

"I think she feels this *is* her home, as much as she has one any more."

"It's not good for her. It's not good to be around these crazy old people, not for a child like that. I'm going to tell her to go."

Twenty-Five

John Robeck has not managed to come to his office for almost two weeks, and when he finally does arrive, he sees the door of his office open, a large stack of flat, new cardboard cartons propped against it, smartly strapped with a steel band. There are two men inside his office, wearing the blue workshirts of the institute's services staff; he can see them moving about inside. Now one of them appears at the door, takes a small pair of wire clippers from his back pocket, cuts the band that straps the flattened boxes together. The man looks briefly at Robeck; then the other man joins him, and they begin to put the cartons together. It is clear that they have done this often; they are quick and efficient.

Robeck moves into the room. "What's going on?" he asks, in a surprisingly small, old voice.

"Some old geezer's moving over to the emeritus wing," says one of the movers, but he sees instantly that Robeck is the geezer to whom he refers.

"I'm sorry, sir. Are they yours, sir, the books? Would you like them packed in any particular order?"

"No," says Robeck, as he wanders slowly out of the room. Down the hall, he reaches Liller's desk; Liller is not there, and Robeck picks up the phone. He dials the extension of the vice-president he has known for years.

"I'm sorry, sir, he isn't in."

Robeck feels some of his old spleen coming back, he feels the color in his face increase, and a straightness in his spine. "Find him. I want to know why the hell my office's being moved, I haven't agreed to any such thing."

"Just a moment, sir." The voice is young, polite. There is a long pause; he sits in Liller's chair, doodles on the notepad on Liller's desk. He sees the thick stack of the manuscript of his *Defense,* hidden under many piles of other papers; it has not been typed.

The voice returns. "I've checked the records, sir. There was no objection from your office, we've contacted them about it twice."

Robeck draws a vicious doodle on Liller's notepad, gets up, takes his manuscript, and leaves.

Twenty-Six

The continuing conversation between Roderick and Evan, moved from one city to another and then another, as circumstances have required, is fixed now; it takes place in the shabby adolescent beer parlor situated in the nearest corner of the town where John and Annis live. The brothers sit, for the dozenth time since they have both been here, facing each other over an uneven table topped in plastic made to look like genuine wood; they watch the ways the kids drape themselves across the bar's one pinball machine, or flip darts into the target on the wall. Rod loathes this place, but it is close enough to the house to go without his car, and Evan does not care much where they meet. Their conversation would be hard in any place.

But Rod is unusually impatient today. The service in the tavern is almost always slow, if in fact there is anybody on duty at all; it appears to be run largely by the local students, just barely old enough to drink what they sell. Even Luel's kid, they have discovered, sometimes works here.

Rod will not wait to be served; he barks his drink to the man behind the bar.

"Double Manhattan." It is a beer parlor, not the kind of elaborate cocktail lounge in which Rod is at home, but the bartender here is prepared for him. These two strange men, who look so much alike and yet are dressed so differently, who talk so frequently over matters of such apparent urgency, have become regulars in the bar. The bartender upends the bottle of sweet vermouth, which has been drunk bit by bit over the last month by the two men alone, into a glass of whiskey, and places it on the bar.

Rod takes the drink, makes his way to the table at which Evan is already sitting. The room is ill lit, filled with stale smoke and the odor of ashtrays, the rancid flavor of old spilled beer. Rod reflects that perhaps it is the last time they will have to drink here. Things have changed, and they have only a single last question to resolve.

"We can't very well leave him alone in that enormous house."

That is the issue, and they both know what rides on it. They swallow their drinks, and stare at the surface of the table.

"We could hire a housekeeper," says Evan. "Just while Annis is gone."

"We could get him an apartment, or put him in the high-rise at the leisure-world place," says Rod. "They could both move to one of those villas when she gets out."

"She doesn't want to go there."

"Maybe she will, if it's that or the hospital."

There is a long pause, and then Evan finally says what they have both known is coming.

"I don't think we can just ship him off. I think we have to take him in."

Rod does not answer.

"You or me," muses Evan. "We have to take him in."

Rod still does not answer. Then, "You," he says suddenly. "It would be easy. You live by yourself, you could make a little room for him."

"But you've got Alicia to help take care of him and the kids. You could put him in that back apartment, you now, where the maid used to live."

"That's the guest room now."

"There's room enough."

"He'd have to quit work," Rod says, finding another objection.

"He's not working anyway," says Evan, pressuring now, "He just goes over to his office to hang around. Besides, it won't make nearly as much difference in your life as it would in mine, you'd hardly notice him."

"I don't want to do it," says Rod.

"You have to," says Evan. "Or I do. And I don't want to do it either."

Rod fingers a dime, which lies on the surface of the bar table as change from the previous set of drinks. Suddenly he picks it up, flips it, catches it with one hand closed over it against the back of his other hand.

Evan watches the flip; the coin is still covered. "We'll take him two months each," he says, "Until she gets out."

"Who gets him first?" says Rod, holding the coin still covered.

"Tails," says Evan.

Rod uncovers the coin.

"Shit," he says.

But it is done, and at least an arrangement has been made. Rod signals to the bartender for the check, takes out a little pad of paper and begins to make notes. "Let's see, today is Friday. They'll come to get her Monday; we can leave that night." A dark-haired girl who has been waiting sporadically on tables arrives with a little pad, stands figuring the total, but Rod does not look up. He is hurrying now, eager to leave this place he so thoroughly dislikes. "We can get the house listed on Saturday, the rest of the stuff packed on Sunday." The girl who is waiting tables starts to leave, but Rod puts out his hand in a gesture to indicate that he is about to pay, and reaches into the pocket of his coat for his large flat wallet. He does not look at the girl.

Evan sees her: it is Luel's kid, but he says nothing.

"Ten o'clock Monday," Rod says, "that's when the ambulance is coming."

"Why an ambulance?"

"With a sedative."

Evan suddenly understands what Roderick means, and the picture comes to him: his soft, old mother, tied in the coarse white cotton of a straightjacket or immobilized by a hypodermic, taken off to a place from which she would not return.

"I don't think we can do it, Rod," he says.

The girl does not move; Rod is suddenly angry now; he leans forward across the table toward Evan, his hand fastened around the wallet. The girl still does not move.

"It's all arranged," says Rod. "It's what she needs. Maybe they'll cure her."

"I'm not so sure she's ill," Evan says, and he looks again at the girl, Luel's kid.

But Rod does not notice. He picks a bill out of his wallet; the girl still waits.

"Look, Evan," he finally says. "She's a sick old woman. If we don't put her in the hospital she'll kill herself." He places a second bill on top of the check.

Now Evan says nothing.

"Don't you *love* her?" sneers Rod.

"You haven't got the commitment papers," argues Evan. "You can't just put her away."

"And that's where you are wrong," says Rod triumphantly, shoving the check and the small piles of bills toward the girl. "The doctors have signed them. The police have signed them. And I got Dad to sign them this morning." He leans back in his chair, so that the girl can take the money away. He sees her bend over, watches the long, dark hair fall across her face, and realizes who it is.

"It's all arranged," he says to Luel's kid, "whether you like it or not."

They leave through the alley that runs in the direction of the house. It is a warm night in this small town, and behind the beer parlor they walk past slightly urban grime, broken bottles, billboards advertising cheap tequila. At the far end of the parking lot four or five teenagers are sitting on the pavement, smoking, laughing, passing around a bottle of wine. Luel's kid is often among them when these two men, her uncles, pass by on their way back to the house, but tonight she is still inside the bar, removing the Manhattan glasses from the table at which they've sat.

Twenty-Seven

"We'll be leaving Monday night," they tell Annis, and they watch a smile gather, hesitate, then flood across her face.

"Just like that?" she says, disbelieving.

"Just like that," answers Rod. "We've been here long enough."

But they do not tell her that she will be leaving too, and that one of them will take her husband away after she is gone.

"It would only upset her," they say to themselves. "Let's let these last couple of days be good ones."

And, indeed, the last couple of days are good ones. Annis holds her grand-children on her knees; she unearths from one of the cartons a box of old costume jewelry, and gives it to them to play with. They devise skits, where Amy, wrapped in gauzy veils from Annis's youth, is Peter Pan, or little John, enveloped head to toe in grandfather John's ancient hiking knickers, plays Peter and the Wolf. Annis sits for hours with Rod's wife Alicia, hearing all her accounts of the children's growth; but still more she sits with her two sons and her husband, recounting their early years, their disappointments, their dreams. She spends vast amounts of time in the kitchen, fixing the dishes that had always been her family's favorites, her pleasure in them heightened because she knows she is doing these things for the final time. The family will leave. She had once dreamt of summoning them all to her bedside for a last farewell, but she sees now that they could never accept it, and the real farewell is now. But it is good nevertheless, she thinks, and when it comes to Sunday she begins to prepare a last and final meal together. She kneads her hands into the bread she will bake in the evening, feels the potatoes rough and crisp between her hands as she peels them, watches cream swirl slowly into a pie. Every movement she makes is delicious, every dish is examined with affection, every tiny pinch of spice added with love, and even the crazy rancor she has felt toward her husband and sons in these last several weeks is ebbing, now that she knows that the peaceful end at last will come. They will share this final meal, embrace one another, but then they will leave, and she will be free again to com-plete her life in the stillness and tranquility she seeks.

Yet she sees there is someone missing from these final family festivities: Luel's child. Annis moves towards the telephone.

But Rod is already there.

"I want her to be here for this last dinner," Annis says, "before you go."

"We spoke to her at work," Rod says, as he recalls the dark-haired girl bending over the bar table. "She says she can't come." He sees the hurt this brings to Annis; he softens it a little, with another lie. "She says she's sorry, she'll come to see you as soon as she can."

So Annis forgets the girl, and returns to her preparations for the final, farewell meal. She is wholly consumed in the simplest chores, allowing them to summon up a lifetime's memory of other meals cooked for this family, as small roguish toddlers, as sturdy schoolchildren, as painfully maturing adolescents, as full-grown adults. As she peels vegetables into the sink, she sees them now, just as they are, and all that went into making them. She sees the limitations of her little family: Rod's rigidness, for instance, from the time he was a small toddler arranging his toy locomotives in precise and exacting rows across the floor, while Evan and Luel had steered theirs with much greater abandon; she sees Evan's ambivalence and hesitations, from his early childhood, when he had rarely finished drawings because he could never fully decide what to do, until his full adulthood, when he had refused to take any sort of permanent job, but moved from one to another, every several years, in part because the newness of each interested him more than the success that might be gained from staying at one, but in part too because of his central undecidedness, a kind of gentle lack of commitment to the world as a whole. Then there was Luel too, whose impetuous indiscretions had produced this single, solitary child, but whose spirit had been stronger, wilder, more wonderful than any parent could hope for, and who always sought to rise beyond her mild beginnings. Dear children, Annis thinks, as she surveys the cookery in her kitchen, not one of them perfect, all of them loved. Hers had not been a complex or outwardly exciting life, but it had been one of great, secret contentment, a contentment she could feel most strongly now. Of course there had been hard places in this life, Luel's death, first, and other trouble, and now these little harshnesses with Rod and Evan and her husband John in the last few weeks, but somehow that is of no moment any more, not here at the end . . .

But she sees suddenly that in all the wonderful chaos of this final meal, she has forgotten to buy a lemon. One lemon. One small simple thing, for which perhaps a few drops of vinegar would do, but then, she thinks, no substitute will really do, not at the last.

"I'll just pop over to the store and get one," she says, swinging her coat around her.

"Maybe you'd better go with her," Rod says to Evan, as he adjusts his tie in front of the living room mirror. They are all somehow flattered by her delight in making this last dinner perfect; the hard thing has been decided, and the family harmony restored. They have been out to buy a good wine, are dressing for dinner, are conversing with each other in genuine interest. Still the habit of total surveillance is strong, and Evan starts to rise from his seat.

But he stops, looks at Rod. "Oh, let her go if she wants to," Rod says, "she only wants a lemon."

If she were not in a hurry, Annis would take the long route to the store, down along the beach and up again into the town; but as it is she takes the shortcut, through a series of alleys to the little group of stores at the near end of town. It is not yet dusk; a single premature streetlight winks on, but the sun has only begun to spread itself out across the sky. Annis hurries through the alleys, across the parking lot near the shops; at the far end of the lot she sees the little group of aimless teenagers that is always sitting there. Annis does not stop; she is in a hurry now, and cannot see exactly who is there.

But when she is in the store she feels the presence of the child behind her: thin, withdrawn, somehow very shy.

Annis turns to her. "I'm sorry you can't come for the dinner," she says, "they're all leaving tomorrow."

"I know," says the child miserably. "Uncle Rod said I wasn't to come near the house. He says I disturb you."

Annis takes two lemons from the bin, but feels her enthusiasm for the dinner diminished.

"I wanted to see you again before you go," the child persists, and her hair hangs loosely over her face.

Annis gives her a hug, jovial and affectionate. "If you can't come tonight, come tomorrow. Or the next day. I'll be washing dishes for a week."

"But you won't be there," the child protests, "I wanted to see you *before* you go."
"Go?"

"Don't you even know about it?" says the child. "Didn't they tell you?"

Annis finds that she is suddenly feeling weak, nauseous. The girl leads her out
to the cooler air of the parking lot. "My car is here," she says, opening the door
of a rusted Volkswagen. "You can sit in it."

Annis lowers herself limply into the car, and stares at the dials on the dashboard: they are old, small, caked with dust. The girl walks around the car, extracts
a key from the hip pocket of her jeans; she sits in the car, puts the key in the
ignition, but does not turn it on.

"Are you sure?" Annis asks, her eyes fixed dully on the dashboard.

"I heard them talking at the bar."

"I won't go to any hospital," Annis says, suddenly stubborn.

"But they've got commitment papers signed and everything," says the girl. "An
ambulance is coming in the morning."

Annis thinks a long time, slowly, painfully, carefully. "What about John?" she
says at last.

"They're going to take him home with them. Rod first, for two months. Then
Evan, then Rod again."

"Did he agree?"

"John?"

"Yes. To the hospital, did he agree?"

"I don't know," the girl lies, because she cannot bring herself to say *yes*.

Annis turns the two lemons inside their brown paper bag. "They must be
beginning to wonder where I am."

The girl leans forward, turns the key in the ignition. The old motor starts. "Do
you want me to drive you home?"

Annis does not answer, and the child eases the car out of its parking space,
turns out into the street in the direction of the house, crawls slowly up the small
hill. Annis can see the house now, silhouetted against the late-afternoon sky; she
can see the first lights of the porch, where the children are playing, the lights of
the kitchen, where the bowls and pans and mixing spoons are still spread out in
vast, delicious confusion for the meal she has been cooking; she can even see the
lights of the living room where her husband and sons are dressed for dinner now,
reading, or talking, sharing a bottle of wine, savoring the smells of the roast that
is just now fully done in the oven. It is not a lavish scene, but one of great family
contentment, but as the car struggles up toward the house she suddenly sees what
is coming, and what has made this brief, perfect respite possible: the stark starched
regimen of the hospital, the well-trained smiles, the psychotherapy, the medications,
the Sunday-afternoon visits from the children, taking turns, perhaps, if she is no
longer considered a risk to herself, eventual release to a nursing home, perhaps
not, but in any case continuing despair, decay, continuing loneliness without real
solitude, and as they reach the house she can see the figure of her husband silhouetted against the window, looking out. Dear, sad John, she thinks, it will come to
him now too, the unvarying institutional regimen, the bedpans, the feedings, the
lying there alone . . .

"Keep going," she whispers to Luel's kid, and the child puts her foot to the gas; the old car, surprisingly nimble, hurries away, and she sees the door of the house open, a figure look out into the dusk, then go back in. She feels the lemons inside the bag, grips them hard between her hands.

"Just keep going," she says, and the girl drives aimlessly at first, but eventually finds the main road along the coast. The girl settles back, her foot steady now on the gas, and eventually Annis' grip on the lemons loosens a bit.

They drive for two days, not hurriedly, but not slowly either, talking; sometimes they stop for lunch or a cup of coffee in the afternoon, and at night they stop at small, random motels, where they slide in together in the same bed, and Annis sleeps dreamlessly all night. In the daytime, they talk, and though the girl does not say much of herself, she absorbs and cherishes what Annis has to say. But fear travels with them too, that they will be discovered, apprehended, that police bulletins will find them, that they will be taken back, delivered into custody.

By the third day, it is enough, and they reach a small town far up the coast.

"Here," Annis says to the child, as she looks out to the sea. The girl brings the car to a stop in the center of the town, just at the end of the grassy strip next to the beach; she watches the old, soft woman, her grandmother, mother of her own dead mother, climb slowly out of the car.

"Goodbye," says Annis to the girl, but it is more than enough. The girl watches her walk away, still holding the bag with two lemons. The girl makes no objection to her going, but her eyes follow Annis down the street. When she can no longer see Annis, she puts her foot to the gas again, and turns the car in the direction from which they came.

It is midday; the sun is bright in this California town, and Annis picks her way slowly down the street. She reaches a druggist's; without hesitation, without even so much as a glance at the brightness of the sunlight or the waves on the water, she enters, selects from the shelves a large bottle of sleeping tablets, a bottle of aspirin, a piece of rubber sheeting, the sort made for babies' cribs, a box of candles, then a box of rat killer. She decides that the order looks suspicious; she adds to it a dozen paper baby diapers, a plastic baby's cup, a small box of sugar. She pays for the items, steps out onto the street again. Not far away she sees a small, beachfront motel; it is quiet at this time of year, and the beach is uncrowded.

She asks for a room. "Facing the water," she says, "I must have a view."

"Is it just for yourself?" asks the motel owner, eyeing her as he does all of his clients.

"Yes," she says. "I won't be leaving for at least three days." She takes the cash for all three days out of her pocketbook, and puts it on the desk.

"Here," she says, "I'd like to pay it all in advance."

It is a small room, somewhat dingy, decorated in floral chintz of a tasteless sort, but it does have a rather large window, and the window does look out onto the ocean. She sits on the bed, surveying the room around her: flat, dull-yellow walls, a single armchair with a crooked-neck lamp hanging over it. There is a television set staring like one bulging eye into the room; she wheels it into the closet and shuts the door. Now the central item in the room is the bed, a very large bed, but hollowed a little in the middle, where night after night couples have lain together, young couples, old couples, married and unmarried, but always their legs intertwined and their bodies pressed together, while they breathe almost in unison.

"So this is the last room," she says to herself. She takes the items she has brought with her out of the bag: she unfolds the rubber sheet, lifts up the bedcovers and inserts it above the mattress, which though already amply stained, need not be ruined altogether. She puts the aspirin and the sleeping tablets in a night-table drawer, next to the Bible she finds there. She opens the box of rat poison, and discovers that it comes in granular form. She shudders a little, but she will not allow herself to think of the instantaneous tablets that could have been brought from her husband's lab, or the sweet easy capsules that had filled her purse. She pours the granules into the bottom of one of the plastic drinking glasses that the motel supplies, covers them with sugar, and puts the glass in the drawer too. She fills a second glass with water; then she breaks open the two lemons intended for that distant, farewell dinner, and squeezes them into the third of the glasses. It will be the hardest way, she knows, but still better than the other.

Then she looks at the telephone beside the bed. She reaches for it, but thinks better of it. She gets up, takes her nearly empty purse, walks outside. In the middle of the town she finds an anonymous telephone booth; she takes a dime from her purse. But she will need other change too, since she does not want to reverse the charges and thus reveal to an operator the location from which she is calling; she walks back toward the druggist's, where she changes her last two dollars into coins.

She puts the dime into the slot, dials the number of her home.

"One dollar and twenty-five cents," a mechanical voice interrupts, and she feeds the change into the machine. But there is no answer; instead, another mechanical voice tells her the line has been disconnected. She hangs up, and the coins she has inserted into the telephone cascade out again.

She tries her husband's office. "He hasn't been in for a week," Liller tells her. "I don't know where to unpack his books."

At last, she tries Rod's house in the distant city; his wife answers the phone, and after a moment's hesitation calls her father-in-law shrilly to the phone. It is startling to Annis to hear how old and frail John's voice has become, how disconnected his thought, how confused.

"They've brought me here," he says dimly, "until you come back."

"I'm not coming back, John."

Somehow, she had expected the outburst with which he had begun to answer her allusions to death: *No, you can't do that,* he would have said; *No, it's wrong.* But this time it is different. He is silent a long time, as if he were learning the way that has always been characteristic of her, and it is only after a very long pause that he answers. When he does so, his voice is much more firm.

"I understand, now."

She lets the silence of it flood in around her, and she sees this man in perfect, fulfilled clarity—she sees love, and trust, and the trivial pain of suspicion here at the end, erased in the supreme simplicity of his words.

"I love you, John," she says.

"Annis," he says then, but there is pleading now in his voice. "Come back."

Sudden, so sudden is the change from serenity to fear—she visualizes them both, cowering in the rear apartment of Rod's house, shipped out before long to the villa, or the nursing home, or worse. It is all in her power now, what she seeks, and if she slips here, she will not find it again.

"No, John, I cannot," she says, "goodbye." With her finger she pulls down the telephone cradle to break the connection, and replaces the handset noiselessly upon it. She is crying. She opens the door of the telephone booth, steps out into the insolent sunshine, walks silently back toward the motel. She unlocks the door of her room, but does not go in; she tosses the empty pocketbook onto the bed, and walks down toward the beach. She finds a place where there is no one and sits slowly on the sand, at the base of a large, sea-polished rock. The rock forms a little hollow, just the shape of her back, and she leans against it, feeling the triumphant warmth of the sun on her face. She watches the endless repetition of the surf, the little pools that form and vanish among the rocks, the cocky shorebirds that strut among the rocks. She sits there all afternoon among the rocks, while the tide moves in, advances toward her rock, hesitates, then recedes; she sits motionless, deep in contemplation, as the sun drops in the west, sinking through the layers of blood-red cloud, until it is at last extinguished in the sea.

When she moves at last, she finds she is numb. She walks slowly up the beach toward the motel, opens her door. She takes the Do Not Disturb sign that dangles behind the knob and places it on the front of the door; she closes and locks it. The room is still small and ungainly, but she does not notice now; she removes her clothes almost mechanically. She thinks suddenly of the nightgown that had been her mother's and is now in the box for Luel's child; it is the only thing she would now like to have. She finds herself taking a sheet of paper out of the drawer of the desk; it has the name of the motel printed garishly across it.

"If you bury me," she writes, "make it in mother's nightgown." She sits back, looks around the room, looks at the note.

"Nonsense," she thinks to herself. She crumples the note into a ball and throws it across the room toward the wastepaper basket. She begins to get into the bed, but she suddenly realizes they will find the note, even if it is in the wastepaper basket. She retrieves it, sits down at the desk, flattens it out, crosses out what she has written.

"Please remember I'd rather be cremated," she writes, and adds that the nightgown is to go to Luel's daughter. *She doesn't need to wear it,* she thinks to herself. She goes to the bed, turns down the covers, lights two of the candles, one on the night-table at each side of the bed. She wraps the paper baby diapers around herself as best she can, two together, and fastens the adhesive tabs at the sides. Now she slides into the bed, opens the drawer to the bedside table, takes out the glasses she has hidden there. She takes the sleeping pills first, then the aspirin: finally, when she feels the drowsiness coming upon her, she mixes the granules with a little water, and swallows them as quickly as she can. She washes her mouth with the juice of the lemons and settles herself back on the pillows, watching the light of the candles dance into the shadows of the room.

Note

From M. Pabst Battin, *Terminal Procedure,* winner, Utah Arts Council First Prize for Book-length Collection of Short Stories, 1981, not previously published.

HISTORICAL, RELIGIOUS, AND CULTURAL CONCERNS

7

Collecting the Primary Texts

Sources on the Ethics of Suicide

Imagine a collection of texts on the ethics of suicide—all the primary texts that are of philosophical interest, from all of Western and non-Western culture, from all the major religious traditions—from Europe, Asia, the Middle East, Africa, Oceania, and North and South America, including reports from oral cultures where original texts are not available. What might this be like?

The Ethics of Suicide

Is suicide wrong, always wrong, profoundly morally wrong? Or is it almost always wrong but excusable in a few cases? Or is it sometimes morally permissible? Is it not intrinsically wrong at all, though perhaps often imprudent? Is it sick? Is it a matter of mental illness? Is it a private or a social act? Is it something the family, community, or society could ever expect of a person? Or is it solely a personal matter, perhaps a matter of right, based in individual liberties, or even a fundamental human right?

This spectrum of views about the *ethics* of suicide—from the view that suicide is profoundly morally wrong to the view that it is a matter of basic human right, and from the view that it is primarily a private matter to the view that it is largely a social one—lies at the root of contemporary practical controversies over suicide. These practical controversies include at least three specific matters of high current saliency:

- *Physician-assisted suicide in terminal illness,* the focus of intense debate in parts of the world with long life expectancies and high-tech medical systems, particularly the Netherlands, the United States, England, Canada, Switzerland, Belgium, Germany, and Australia
- *Hunger strikes and suicides of social protest,* as in Turkey, Northern Ireland, and wartime Vietnam
- *Suicide bombings* and related forms of self-destruction employed as military, guerilla, or terrorist tactics in ongoing political friction, including kamikaze attacks by wartime Japan; suicide missions used as a strategy by groups from Tamil separatists to al-Qaeda; and suicide bombings in the conflicts in Israel, Palestine, Iraq, and elsewhere

Beneath these specific practical issues lies the question of suicide itself and how it should be regarded from an ethical point of view. A collection of primary sources would be intended to facilitate exploration of such current practical issues by exhibiting the astonishingly diverse range of thinking about suicide throughout human intellectual history, in its full range of cultures and traditions. Such a collection of primary texts would need to refrain from taking sides in these ethical debates; rather, one must hope to expand the character of what have been rather linear recent debates on issues like physician-assisted suicide, suicide in social protest, and suicide bombing by making them, as it were, multidimensional. This is what a rich acquaintance with history and the diversity of cultures brings. For much of the twentieth and on into the twenty-first century, thinking about suicide in the West has been normatively monolithic: suicide has come to be seen by the public and particularly by health professionals as primarily a matter of mental illness, perhaps compounded by biochemical factors and social stressors, the sad result of depression or other often treatable disease—a tragedy to be prevented. With the exception of debate over suicide in terminal illness, the only substantive discussions about suicide in current Western culture have concerned whether access to psychotherapy, or improved suicide-prevention programs, or more effective antidepressant medications should form the principal lines of defense.

Indeed, suicide very often *is* a tragedy, and depression or other mental illness is often in play. However, a full exploration of historical and cross-cultural thought concerning suicide would need to explore the many, many additional ways in which the phenomenon of self-destruction has also been understood—some of them bizarre, some of them profound. It thus seeks to broaden the current rather monolithic view, not replace it, and to provide a much wider context for understanding contemporary issues about self-caused death.

Historical and Cultural Backgrounds

A comprehensive collection of primary texts must cover as fully as possible the immense range of thinking about the ethics of suicide in both the Western and non-Western traditions, as well as in both literate and oral cultures—in short, the full range of human discussion and dispute that leads up to current times. It must be particularly concerned with philosophical reflection on the morality of suicide, but this takes many different forms: some texts are lengthy, discursive, scholarly texts; others involve vivid stories with implicit rather than explicit messages; some are firsthand accounts, others secondary observations; some are exploratory, others didactic or admonitory, and so on. There is a rich diversity in the kinds of materials available as primary texts addressing the ethical issues in suicide, as there is in the eras and cultures from which they come.

The Western record of discussion and dispute about the morality of suicide begins some three millennia ago with a rather personal dialogue between a man and his soul, a dialogue dating from the First Intermediate Period of ancient Egypt. A man in despair is contemplating suicide by fire, but his soul pleads with him not to do so, for if there is no mummification, burial, tomb, or mortuary service and no preservation of the body, the soul will lose his "house."[1] Writing on suicide also begins with the early Hebrews' texts that record (without ethical comment) a handful of suicides, including those of Samson, Saul, and Saul's armor bearer. In a different culture, the ancient Greeks developed somewhat inchoate classifications of acceptable and unacceptable suicides, including those that were subject to burial restrictions (like burying the hand apart) and those that were not. In the following centuries, the Greek and Roman Stoics came to celebrate suicide as the act of the wise man, while the Christian church, from the time of Augustine through the time of Thomas Aquinas, increasingly vigorously condemned suicide as sin. Some Enlightenment writers defended suicide; some Romantic writers glorified it; and some writers during these eras repudiated it, giving a variety of accounts, religious and secular, of what makes it wrong. Debate continued apace until roughly the time of Durkheim and Freu, at the beginning of the twentieth century, when their theories of suicide as socially conditioned and/or pathological, so to speak, broke the ethical debate: they saw suicide as socially or psychologically caused rather than chosen, and hence not culpably morally wrong, sinful, or criminal. While debate still continues, it has until recently been largely obscured by the dominant professional view that suicide is a product of mental illness, committed by people in the grip of depression or otherwise incapable of reasoning clearly, and that therefore there really is no *ethical* issue here.

Thus writing about suicide in the Western tradition, from early Egypt to the present, forms a complex discussion that evolves over time, in many different contexts, with many different authors voicing their views and many different strands of thinking interacting in multiple ways. There are no sudden changes, even in the twentieth century, though pronounced trends and patterns of evolution can be clearly seen in retrospect. In recent years, public discussion, largely confined in the West to the issue of physician-assisted suicide, has been largely a discussion about ethics, yet issues of metaphysics (for example, causation) and matters of epistemology (like the characterization of rationality, the nature of reasons, and projections about afterlife effects) play roles as well. Familiarity with the vast range of primary texts makes it possible to trace the intricacies of this development over time.

At the same time, however, views about self-caused and self-willed death have been evolving in the East, beginning with ancient Hinduism, Buddhism, and Confucianism in India, southeast Asia, early China, and Japan, as well as elsewhere in the non-Western world. These views have been carried forward within different religious and cultural traditions, often modified and exaggerated but nevertheless typically preserving a characteristic unique, fundamental ethical stance. These too must be included in any comprehensive collection of materials.

Also over long spans of history, oral cultures in the Arctic, Africa, in North, Central, and South America, in Oceania, and elsewhere have been evolving, often including practices involving suicide and related forms of self-caused, self-willed death. From the practices of these cultures, it is possible to infer (though such inferences always involve a considerable degree of conjecture) the background normative views in which they rest. These views, and the practices in which they are exhibited, are often strikingly different from those of the literate cultures of the East and West. To be sure, access to records and especially written records is far more problematic in these oral traditions than it is in the literature cultures of the world. For traditional oral cultures, contact with indigenous practices concerning suicide and the background worldviews and belief systems in which they are embedded is to some degree filtered through Western eyes, since the written records from which the views of oral cultures can be distilled have become available only with the incursion of explorers, missionaries, conquistadores, adventurers, and ethnographers, largely themselves from Western cultures. Just the same, the older sources from these cultures are invaluable, since, despite their distortions they depict societies comparatively innocent of Westernized and hence Christianized attitudes about suicide.

Of course, it cannot be assumed that views of all the members of the various eras and cultures about suicide, whether in Western, Eastern, or traditional oral cultures, were or are alike. Cultures are rarely homogenous groups but rather are living collections of people whose views may differ considerably, though they may appear uniform when contrasted with the views of members of other cultures.

The Evolution of Views and Practices over Time

If such a collection of primary texts were to be organized chronologically (though dating is often imprecise and the identities of authors and sources unclear), it would make it possible to trace the development of thought about morality of suicide through a culture over time. For example, one might examine, say, the development of thinking in Judaism, from the Hebrew Bible and its origins in the twelfth to the ninth centuries BC, through Josephus in the first century AD to the rabbinic writers and the Babylonian Talmud of the third to the sixth centuries AD, to the tenth-century Karaite writer Ya'qub al-Qirqisani, the Tosafist writers of the twelfth to the fourteenth centuries, and on to Luria in the sixteenth century and Margoliouth in the eighteenth and nineteenth. Or one might examine the Japanese tradition, beginning with Daidoji Yuzan's portrait of medieval Japan's *Bushido* military and chivalric culture; then Chikamatsu's plays and the developing tradition of love-suicide; then Lord Redesdale's account of *hara-kiri;* and finally the letters from kamikaze pilots written just before their final missions in World War II. Or one might explore the entwined traditions of Hinduism and Buddhism, beginning with the ancient Upanishads of the ninth to seventh centuries BC; the Dharmasastra law codes of the seventh century BC to first century AD; the Questions of King Milinda, dating from around 100 BC to around 200 AD; the Lotus Sutra, composed sometime during the first several centuries AD, Baña, from the late sixth to the early seventh century AD; the anonymous late nineteenth-century Hindu widow describing *sati* or widow-burning; and on to figures of the twentieth and twenty-first centuries, Gandhi and Thich Nhat Hanh. These are long, rich traditions of reflection on this issue.

Chronological organization of reflection on the ethics of suicide would also make it possible to observe that while the various historical traditions initially develop independently, they come to interact and reflect each other over time. For example, reflection on suicide within Judaism begins long before that within Christianity, but in the Talmudic period of the first and second centuries AD and during the Middle Ages, Judaism's view of suicide appears to evolve in part in tandem with that of Christianity—both exhibit an intensifying condemnation and prohibition of suicide, even though the specific details never fully coincide. Islam's view, comparatively uniform over time, is articulated at least two centuries after the Augustinian view that suicide is always wrong had pervaded both Christianity and to some extent Judaism. While Islam's repudiation of suicide in many ways parallels that of Judaism and Christianity, the distinction it draws between suicide and martyrdom—also an issue in Judaism and Christianity—falls in quite a different place. Self-exposure to death and the undertaking of high-risk missions in the defense of the faith are permitted, as in the other monotheist traditions, but the martyr who dies in battle is also celebrated, even if—at least on some accounts—"he wants to sacrifice his soul in order to defeat the enemy and for God's sake."[2] On another continent, the evolution of Hindu spirituality and its fusion with Buddhist views about the illusoriness of life affected thinking about suicide in Confucian China, and in turn contributed to the military and chivalric Bushido culture of medieval Japan that lionized suicide, which in turn influenced Japan's military tactics in World War II. On still other continents, late medieval Catholic attitudes about the sinfulness of suicide were brought to the central and southern parts of the New World by the Spanish conquistadores and the missionaries who traveled with them, while Protestant attitudes—no more tolerant of the sin they saw in suicide than those of the Catholics—were imported into Africa, India, North America, and other places colonized largely by Protestant nations.

Though it would be necessarily imperfect, chronological organization of the principal texts on the ethics of suicide would not only make it possible to compare views among thinkers and traditions and to recognize the huge spectrum of thought about suicide, but also to chart the relative evolution of views about suicide in geographically adjacent cultures—such as Judaism, Christianity, and Islam, or India, China, and Japan—and also in cultures related by colonizing and colonized roles or the spread of religious traditions—like Protestant Europeans in Africa, India, and North America, Catholic Europeans in Central and South America, and Buddhism moving from India into southeast Asia, China, and Japan. It also makes it possible to observe one author's or one culture's distortions of the views of another—for instance Lactantius's exaggerations of the views of Roman Stoics and al-Ghazali's dismissive account of Hindu practices—as well as the extraordinary exaggerations of Christian conquerors and colonizers about the peoples they subdued.

Chronological reflection on suicide is not easily accomplished, however, with respect to texts from oral cultures. Here, because of the usually fragmentary, erratic nature of the sources, the impossibility of determining in a reliable way the duration or scope of the views of the culture described, and the ubiquitous problem of cultural overlay by foreign observers, these selections must be grouped together, entered in the chronological listing by the date of the earliest report. This permits at least a partial view of the range of beliefs and practices within a culture or a group of cultures, though they are filtered through the eyes of outside observers, the only sources available. While the texts of all traditions, both Western and non-Western, require interpretation, and while all texts can pose problems for readers from other cultures, the records of oral cultures require a double inference, both in extrapolating from practices described to the views that may have motivated them, and in subtracting as much as possible the overlay of western, alien ideology (including as well its racism, sexism, and paternalist attitudes about "inferior" or "infantile" cultures) that also shapes such accounts. For this reason, it would be preferable to use the oldest accounts of an oral culture's beliefs and practices, both because it is temporally closer to precontact times and also because the ideological overlay—since it comes from an earlier period of Western history and is thus more evident to contemporary eyes—may be easier to subtract. In any case, whether in continuing oral traditions or in early observers' accounts, there is no "pure" version of these views—and yet they represent some of the most varied, interesting, and challenging of those available.

A second partial exception to the chronological organization to be sought in assembling the primary sources would have to be made in cultures with highly sophisticated oral traditions capable of preserving material with considerable accuracy over long periods of time—early Islam, for example—so that the date of composition of written texts like the Quran and the Hadiths is actually several centuries later than the actual genesis of the material. Further complicating the chronological presentation of sources, many significant texts are no longer extant, including not only individual works like Plutarch's essay *On the Soul* but virtually the entire corpus of a culture, for example the Aztec works destroyed at the time of Western contact.

It would of course not be possible to include all texts from all authors, at all times, in all cultures; this would fill libraries. However, some of the authors to be included would be allies here, themselves providing quite rich surveys of the then-known previous literature. Donne does this for the religious literature; Montaigne does this for the secular, classical literature; and many other authors reflect in comprehensive ways on earlier work in the traditions within which they write.

Conceptual Issues: Similarities and Differences

The broad scope and astonishing variety of such a collection of primary sources would make it tempting to note overlaps, similarities, common assumptions, similar practices, and the like in thinking about suicide from very different time periods and geographic cultures. There are many apparent parallels: for example, Greek and Roman Stoics saw suicide as rational and sensible in certain sorts of circumstances; so did the Bushido tradition in Japan; and so does at least one strain in Buddhism, where taking one's own life is not wrong if it is not done in hate, anger, or fear. Of course, these are loose parallels, and there are many differences among these traditions' views as well. It is important to remain sensitive to background differences in cultural assumptions about metaphysical, epistemological, and religious issues, as well as quite different systems of morality, even while noting striking parallels among texts and practices.

Nevertheless, similar elements and common problems are numerous, even across distant traditions. As already mentioned, for example, for some traditions, like the early Christianity of St. Ignatius and both traditional as well as contemporary Islam, the line between suicide and martyrdom—one prohibited, the other permitted and even celebrated—is very finely drawn, though in subtly different places, even different places at different times. Similarly, the line between the desire to die and suicide is also very finely drawn; this is true for writers from St. Paul to the thirteenth-century mystic Angela of Foligno to the twentieth-century political activist Gandhi. Some writers and cultures think or hint that it is ignoble to die in bed, deteriorating from illness: for the Vikings, the Yoruba, Bushido warriors, and the Iglulik Eskimo, death by violence, including death by suicide, may be the more noble way. Then, too, writers in very different cultures have been concerned with quelling fashions for suicide: Plutarch, for example, describes an ingenious method of stopping the fad among the maidens of Miletus; similarly, Huang Liu-hung, a seventeenth-century provincial Chinese administrator, and Caleb Fleming, a fiercely conservative eighteenth-century English divine, both think exposing the naked body of a suicide in a public place is the most effective deterrent; so too the founder of Methodism, John Wesley, though he did not insist that the body be unclothed. On the other hand, some writers have been accused of fomenting fashions for suicide, for example the playwrights Chikamatsu and Goethe. Roman generals, Bushido warriors, and kamikaze pilots have been alike in seeing military defeat as an occasion for suicide. Cultures in China, Africa, native North America, the Inca empire, Viking-controlled northern Europe, and in precolonial and colonial India have seen suicide and/or voluntary submission to being killed as an appropriate part of funerary customs, especially for wives and retainers of kings and nobles. While such parallels are never exact, they are instructive nevertheless.

There are conceptual similarities and differences among traditions as well. The distinction between killing and letting die, or between self-killing and being killed, or between being killed at one's request and killing oneself, or between self-killing and provoking another into killing oneself, makes an enormous difference in some cultures (Judaism, Christianity, Islam) but little in others (Viking, Akan, Buddhism). Politically motivated suicide may look very different in the East from the way it looks in the West, partly because political systems are so different and partly because assumptions about what a person would accomplish by committing suicide are different. Different authors and cultures have sharply different views about whether concerns about the impact of a suicide on surviving family members or one's society are important. Some think suicide is largely an individual matter, for example, the Roman philosopher Seneca and Paul-Louis Landsberg, who died at Oranienburg in 1943; for others—for example, those in kin-based societies, where the suicide of a young or middle-aged person breaks up social networks but the suicide of an elderly person who has ceased to play such roles does not—suicide is a social issue.

The scope of suicide prohibitions also varies widely, as does the matter of whether exceptions are ever to be made. Then there are group suicides—for example, the mass suicide at Masada described by Josephus, or the ritual self-disembowelment of the 47 Ronins. There are suicides of protest and social protest in many times and places and for many politically diverse reasons: Lucretia, Cato, Thich Quang Doc, and Yukio Mishima; contemporary hunger strikers and suicide bombers may also belong in these categories. In some cultures, especially in Africa, suicide is understood as revenge; in others, it is conceptualized primarily as altruistic, even when some self-killings are clearly egocentric; in some, it is understood as a matter of individual choice, however idiosyncratic the choice of death in that person's specific circumstances may seem to be. Tracing these similarities and parallels would be invited by a comprehensive collection of sources, but at the same time the recognition of huge and often very subtle differences among authors and cultures would also be encouraged.

Definition and Linguistic Issues

To note such similarities and differences raises the issue of definition: exactly what counts as *suicide?* Some definitions are extremely narrow; they count only cases in which a person has knowingly and voluntarily acted in a way that directly causes his or her own death, with the intention that death result; others are much broader, including cases of semi-intentional self-killing, semi-accidental self-killing, self-harm that results in the extinction of cognitive capacities though not the physical body, self-killing in which the person acts knowingly and voluntarily but does not want to die or wants to achieve some other goal, and so on. It can be argued that terminological differences often serve to mark views about the morality of self-killing in various circumstances or for various reasons, and that the wide range of terms used in cases of voluntary, knowing causation of one's own death serves this purpose. "Suicide" is normally differentiated (in English) from "self-sacrifice," "martyrdom," "acquiescence in death," "aid-in-dying," "victim-precipitated homicide," "self-deliverance," and a variety of other terms, but the primary texts, providing the original wording, or as nearly as possible in translation, invite attention to the subtleties of these differences. While definition is important, it would be impossible to confine a collection of sources to any particular definition of suicide, which, after all, would largely reflect the prevailing assumptions in the culture from which it came. Nor should a collection overlook unconventional definitions of suicide. For example, it should include not only Lactantius's insistence that the death of Cato, the Stoic example par excellence of praiseworthy suicide, was actually homicide, as well as Mao Zedong's view that the death of Miss Zhao, a young peasant woman in the China of 1919 who slit her own throat rather than submit to an arranged marriage, was actually murder, but also, equally unconventional,

John Donne's claim that the death of Jesus Christ, the Christian example par excellence of an unjust execution, was actually a suicide.

Linguistic issues also arise in attempts to refer to the performance of the act of suicide. The expression "to commit suicide," (parallel to "to commit a crime") has been common; contemporary suicidologists typically use a variety of less stigmatizing alternatives, including "suicided," "completed suicide," and "died by suicide." Depending on the background view of the ethics of suicide, these variant descriptions disguise much—or little.

Problems of definition also arise as a product of translation from one language to another. Just as English had no unique term for suicide until 1651, when Walter Charleton used it in his *Ephesian and Cimmerian Matrons* ("to vindicate ones self from inevitable Calamity, by Sui-cide is not . . . a Crime"), many other languages refer to this phenomenon in different ways. Greek, Latin, and other European languages did not have an explicit, unique term for suicide, though they had a wide variety of locutions. While English has just one principal term, "suicide," German has four—*Selbstmord, Selbsttötung, Suizid,* and *Freitod,* the first three of which have varyingly negative or neutral connotations but the last of which has generally positive ones; this means that German speakers can talk about suicide in a range of ways English speakers cannot. Wider exploration would no doubt reveal differences among other languages as well.

Issues of definition are also important in examining the practices of traditional cultures. The only available early reports of practices in oral cultures, especially those made by clerics, conquistadores, and others not trained in ethnography, may distort the meanings of native words considerably. For example, in the translations of the Seneca myth called the *Code of Handsome Lake*, Edward Cornplanter speaks of "sin" and of the "Great Spirit"; these are probably imported concepts and mistranslations influenced by European sources, even if there is no adequate correct translation in English. On the other hand, some traditional practices that are not apparently conceptualized as suicide might meet contemporary Western definitions, insofar as they involve the knowing, voluntary taking of an action intended to bring about one's own death: for example, the practice of the Ga people of western Africa of holding individuals accountable for dying at times or in ways that are impermissible suggests that these deaths are understood as a matter of voluntary choice. Then again, some practices that are apparently conceptualized as suicide and, given the group's beliefs, would meet common Western definitional criteria are nevertheless strikingly at odds with Western categories: for instance, the Mohave belief that stillborn infants are suicides, beings who (knowingly) surveyed the world into which they were about to enter but (voluntarily, deliberately) decided against it.

Negative Cases

An adequate collection of primary sources would also have to try to recognize—though to do so exhaustively would prove impossible—the significance of *negative* cases: the writings or accounts of individuals who did not consider suicide (like the thirteenth-century mystic Angela of Foligno); or who considered suicide but did not do it (like Job); of authors who did not discuss it (like John Stuart Mill); of texts where it is hinted at, if at all, only by implication (Sophocles' *Oedipus at Colonus*); of cultures (e.g., the Tiv of central Africa) where it was apparently not practiced; and religious traditions where it was not mentioned at all (e.g. Shinto). This is a tricky matter, but important, if the full range of thought about suicide is to be displayed. What is not thought, not done, not said about this issue can play an immense role in reflection and action about life and death as well.

The Bases of Analysis

Among the many issues raised by the full range of views on suicide is the question of the bases of analysis. The collection envisioned here focuses on the *ethical* issues in suicide; but there are substantial differences in what it is that is to be assessed. Is it the act itself that is the focus of normative assessment? Is it the intention under which it is done? Is it the pattern of behavior or cultural tradition within which it occurs? Is it the outcome of the act, its effects on other individuals or social groups, and if so, how broad is the scope of these effects?

Issues concerning the bases of analysis also challenge traditional classifications used in the assessment of the ethical issues in suicide. Of particular importance in such a collection is the fact that no attempt has been made to differentiate what Durkheim understood as "sociologically caused" or institutional suicide from the sorts of suicide usually understood under the label "suicide" in Western, professional contexts—roughly, between suicide expected in certain circumstances as a normal part of the practices of a culture, and suicide that is conceptualized as the individual's own idiosyncratic act, whether reasoned or the product of mental illness or psychopathology. The background sources will clearly reveal that the line between "institutional" and "individual" suicide is not nearly so sharp as is often assumed, and that even in the anomic modern industrial cultures of which Durkheim spoke, individuals respond to quite subtle societal expectations. The West has seen only a few clear examples of what it recognizes as institutional suicide: the expectation that the Prussian army officer unable to pay his gambling debts kill himself, for example, or that the captain go down with his ship. Yet the expectation of, say, early Christianity that martyrdom is to be sought, or of Romantic culture (evident in Goethe's *The Sorrows of Young Werther*) that suicide is to be preferred to a life of ordinary everydayness, may not seem institutional at all until examined against the broader backdrop of contrasting eras and cultures.

Nor should such a collection overlook the difficulties of differentiating between suicide and euthanasic suicide, suicide and protest suicide, suicide and tactical suicide, or sorting out suicide by causes or motives like despair or revenge. That is the work to be done by examining the selections themselves.

Furthermore, even if such a collection were to focus primarily on the ethics of suicide, it would be impossible to treat the phenomenon as entirely isolated. The act of suicide is necessarily connected with background views about the meaning of death, the value of life, the relationship between the individual and the community, the nature of suffering, the significance of punishment, the existence of an afterlife, the nature of the self, and many other deep philosophical questions. The issue of suicide challenges all of these: as Camus wrote, "there is but one truly philosophical question, and that is the issue of suicide," but it is also against the background of all these philosophical questions that the issues about suicide are played out. Full understanding of the significance of any of the primary texts would, of course, require full exploration of all these issues in an author's or culture's work; the issue of the ethics of suicide can be said in some ways to be the entry point and challenge point to these issues. Just one thing is clear: a comprehensive collection of sources cannot *start* with the assumption that all suicide is pathological, or that it can be attributed either to pathological mental states or mental illness, or that it is a matter of biochemical abnormality, or that it is always wrong, or that there are no real ethical issues about suicide. These views are to be discovered in the texts themselves.

Nor could such a collection conclude with the uniform assumption that suicide is the causal product of mental illness, the normatively monolithic assumption seemingly so prevalent in contemporary times. In bringing the discussions of the world's widely varying traditions up to the present, it might conclude with three or four selections that raise fully contemporary questions. For example, it could offer Sylvia Plath's essentially autobiographical account of her own multiple suicide attempts and what would turn out to be her own actual suicide; this is an account that, as clearly as any, exhibits the contemporary health professional's view of suicide as pathological at the same time that it exhibits her own singular reasoning. This is not to say that earlier texts do not also exhibit views of suicide as pathological—for example, Hippocrates' account of suicide in premenstrual dysphoric disorder, Sophocles' portrait of the mad ravings of Ajax and his subsequent remorse, and Burton's portrait of the anatomy of melancholy all do so as well; but Plath's is depicted as a fully contemporary suicide. Thich Nhat Hanh, in contrast, describing the suicide of the monk Thich Giac Thanh, which, like that of Thich Quang Duc and other Buddhist monks and nuns protesting the Diem regime during the Vietnam War, involved deliberate self-immolation, portrays it in the opposite way—as a suicide of principle, a difficult act but one undertaken in a fully reflective, thoughtful, aware way, one with deep roots in the Buddhist tradition, and one in which psychopathology plays no role. Mao's account of Miss Zhao also describes resistance to an abusive society, but resistance that takes the wrong form: Miss Zhao should have stayed alive to join the revolutionary effort. A selection from contemporary Western bioethics might sketch some of the very extensive argumentation played out in the ferment over physician-assisted suicide. Here the tension between autonomous choice and the hopelessness of terminal illness as well as risks of abuse play a real role. Finally, a selection from the Islamic *jihad* tradition could pose the issue of tactical suicide in a contemporary light; it too would illuminate the earlier distinction between suicide and martyrdom so carefully drawn in Islam since its beginning and would raise the issue of whether this distinction has been distorted for political ends. To be sure, this will be a continuing history, as cultural conceptions of suicide and related issues like self-sacrifice, heroism, social protest, self-deliverance, martyrdom, and so on in each of these contexts evolve, but in an increasingly global world in which once-independent traditions interact more and more fully and in the process shape and reshape each other, it may be useful to be able to view these issues' deeper roots. It is to this end that a collection of primary sources would be devoted.

Notes

1. "A Dispute Over Suicide," from *Ancient Near Eastern Texts Relating to the Old Testament*. James B. Pritchard, ed., John A. Wilson, trans. (Princeton, N.J.: Princeton University Press, 2nd ed., 1969), 405–407.

2. Christoph Reuter, *My Life Is a Weapon. A Modern History of Suicide Bombing*. Helena Ragg-Kirkby, trans. (Princeton, N.J.: Princeton University Press, 2004), 123, quoting Dr. Abdulaziz al-Rantisi, second in command of Hamas's political wing, in a statement made in 2001.

8

July 4, 1826

Explaining the Same-Day Deaths of John Adams and Thomas Jefferson (and What Could This Mean for Bioethics?)

John Adams and Thomas Jefferson, respectively the second and third presidents of the new United States of America and long-term colleagues, competitors, and correspondents, both died on the same day, July 4, 1826. Both were old men—Adams was 90, and Jefferson was 83—and both were ill, though Adams had been in comparatively robust health until just a few months earlier and Jefferson had been ill for an extended period. They had been rivals, indeed enemies, for some time, and Jefferson had defeated Adams in the presidential election of 1800, but they had repaired their differences and had pursued an active correspondence with each other in the years before their deaths. On that final day, the fiftieth anniversary of the signing of the Declaration of Independence, Adams died at his home in Quincy, Massachusetts, and Jefferson died at his home in Monticello, Virginia, the two separated by hundreds of miles and by many days of overland travel time.

Although the fact that Adams and Jefferson died the same day is taught to practically every schoolchild, asking why is not. What could explain this and what would the implications be for reflection in bioethics about the end of life? There are at least six principal avenues to explore, but *all* of them raise further issues.

Potential Explanations

1. Coincidence

That the two deaths occurred on the same day could be a coincidence, as it is often assumed. But if so, it is a coincidence of considerable magnitude, since it involves three distinct components:

Same day (same day of the year; same year)
Same significant date (July 4, Independence Day)
Same historic anniversary (50 years)

That any individual dies on a given day of the year has, on average, a probability of about 1 in 365, though in nineteenth-century Massachusetts deaths typically peaked during the winter and then spiked again during the summer. The statistical probability that two individuals die in the same year is a function of age and health status as well as the size of the background population; Jefferson was seven years younger than Adams but his overall health worse. The probability that the two would die on the same significant date is more difficult to quantify, and there are other significant dates in the American calendar—Christmas, Easter (Lincoln would be assassinated on Good Friday), Thanksgiving—but Independence Day would have been the date of greatest importance to figures in political life, indeed, former presidents. And the fact that the death dates for both Adams and Jefferson fell on a historic anniversary—the fiftieth anniversary, not the forty-ninth or fifty-first—may seem to stretch beyond the point of sheer plausibility the claim that this was mere coincidence. But when appeals to coincidence are insufficient, we must look for explanations in common circumstance or common cause, or for causation from one case to the other.

2. Divine Intervention

As the news of the two deaths reached the public (depending on where people lived, first of one, then the other), the same-day demise was widely interpreted as a matter of divine intervention. John Quincy Adams, John Adams's son and by then himself president, wrote in his diary the night he heard the news that the fact that his father and Jefferson had died on the same day and that it was the Fourth of July could not be seen as mere coincidence but was a "visible and palpable" manifestation of "Divine favor."[1] In Baltimore, Samuel Smith delivered a eulogy that attributed the timing of Adams's and Jefferson's deaths to an "All-seeing Providence, as a mark of approbation of their well spent lives . . ."[2] In Boston, Daniel Webster delivered a two-hour eulogy in Faneuil Hall, insisting that the fact that the deaths had occurred on the nation's fiftieth birthday was "proof" from on high "that our country, and its benefactors, are objects of His care."[3] The view that divine intervention was involved was widely held at the time.

3. "Hanging On"

Perhaps the two old men were hanging on, so to speak, waiting for the same important anniversary; when they reached it, they just gave up on the same day and died. There are several possible variations of the "hanging on" explanation: that each was independently hanging on, trying to reach the significant anniversary; that each was waiting to die but hung on because the anniversary was near; or that they were in effect competing with each other to remain alive until the important day but would each give up if they made it. Indeed, Adams's next-to-last words are said to have been "Thomas Jefferson survives" though the last word may have been indistinct.[4] Jefferson, on the evening of the 3rd, the evening before his death, and then again after midnight, asked "Is it the Fourth?"[5] Clearly the anniversary would have had a great deal of meaning for each of them. Each had been invited to participate in the fiftieth anniversary celebrations, for which there was a great deal of public anticipation. Adams's son, John Quincy, would be officiating as president. And Jefferson had written his famous defense of self-government, that "the mass of mankind has not been born with saddles on their backs, nor a favored few booted and spurred . . . ,"[6] though it was only a short letter and even so he would not able to deliver it.

Some writers of that time interpreted the deaths in this way. In a eulogy delivered in New York City about two weeks after the deaths, C. C. Cambreleng said of Jefferson that "The body had wasted away—but the energies of a powerful mind, struggling with expiring nature, kept the vital spark alive till the meridian sun shone on our fiftieth Anniversary—then content to die—the illustrious Jefferson gave to the world his last declaration."[7]

Each variant of the "hanging on" explanation assumes that whatever the motivation for hanging on may have been, both men "gave up" on the same day and died. Some more recent studies have sought to document the phenomenon of "hanging on," presumably followed by giving up, in connection with birthdays, religious holidays, or other important events. A 1972 study found that for three groups of well-known men, the most famous were least likely to die in the period before their birth month—indeed, they were five times less likely to die in the month before their birthdays than the average person.[8] Another study looked at patterns of death for Jewish men around the time of Passover, a religious family celebration in which the male head of the household plays a major role: it found a 24% decrease in the week before a weekend Passover and a 24% corresponding increase in the week afterward, a pattern interpreted as showing that Jewish men "delayed" their deaths until after this event of personal significance.[9] Yet another study found that mortality from natural causes in elderly Chinese women dropped by more than a third in the week before the Harvest Moon Festival and increased in the week after it by 35%.[10]

These studies are interpreted within what is known as the biopsychosocial model of health and illness to show that the "will to live" is an important factor in remaining alive—"that our minds are powerful in determining life and death, health and well-being."[11] These results obtained for three classes of natural deaths: stroke, heart attacks, and cancers; deaths due to infections were not affected.[12] (According to one analysis of the historical evidence of reported symptoms by a contemporary physician, Adams probably died of congestive heart failure, Jefferson of unidentified causes among a multitude of medical problems, including prostatic enlargement.[13]) However, observations of patterns of delay and date-timing of deaths, whether in heart disease, cancer, or other conditions, nevertheless do not explain precisely how this effect occurs, if indeed it does; a 2004 analysis of Ohio cancer deaths between 1989 and 2000, responding to these and similar studies, found no evidence that patients are able to postpone their deaths to survive Christmas, Thanksgiving, or their own birthdays.[14]

4. Being Allowed or Caused to Die by Others:
Intervention by Physician or Family

Perhaps, instead, other people were involved. One possible explanation suggests that there could have been a silent conspiracy among physicians, family members, and other caregivers to help their patient "make it" to the 4th, an effort discontinued when that goal was reached. A more active account asks whether the respective physicians of Adams and Jefferson, Amos Holbrook and Robley Dunglison, could have played a role in their patients' deaths, either inadvertently or deliberately— not out of malice, but perhaps seeking to relieve the sufferings of the dying, and choosing the historic anniversary as the appropriate occasion? Adams had written to Benjamin Rush in 1810 that "You Physicians are growing so familiar with Hem- lock, and Arsenick, and Mercury Sublimate, and Laudanum, and Brandy and every Thing that used to frighten me, that I know not what you will do with us."[15] Could Adams and/or Jefferson have been administered substances—perhaps laudanum, an alcoholic tincture of opium—in an attempt to control pain, with an extra-heavy dose on that historic day? Adams's granddaughter Susan Boylston Clark, who was living in the Adams household at the time, reported that the doctor gave her grand- father a "medicine" the day before he died, saying both that "I should not be surprised, if he did not live twenty-four hours" but also that "If the medicine which I shall give him operate favourably, he *may* live a week or two." [her italics][16] Dr. Holbrook himself told Adams's son, John Quincy, then president, that his father had "suffered much" the night before he died[17]; this would make the administration of a heavy dose of opium even more plausible. "Double-effect" intervention by physicians resulting in death, though not intentionally, would be in keeping with present-day attitudes about the permissibility of the overuse of morphine or other opioids for the control of pain "foreseeing though not intending" that they may cause death; direct intervention by physicians or others to bring an easier—or perhaps more symbolic—death might also be in keeping with some practices in contemporary medicine, either where euthanasia is underground or where it is legal. Could physicians or family members have done essentially the same thing?

In a letter to his friend Dr. Brockenborough, John Randolph of Roanoke, who had been on an ocean voyage and datelined the letter The Hague, Tuesday, August 8, 1826, wrote, "And so old Mr. Adams is dead; on the 4th of July, too, just half a century after our Declaration of Independence; and leaving his son on the throne. This is Euthenasia [*sic*], indeed. They have killed Mr. Jefferson, too, on the same day, but I don't believe it."[18]

However, there is no direct evidence for either a "double-effect" or direct euthanasia claim. We do not know what drug Adams was given. Whether Jefferson was given any new medication before his death is not known; indeed, Jefferson is known to have refused the laudanum he had been taking the night before he died.[19]

5. Allowing Oneself to Die

In 1813, at age 77—some thirteen years before he actually died—Adams wrote a letter to the physician Benjamin Rush (a mutual friend of both Adams and Jefferson), a letter ostensibly penned by his horse Hobby. Perhaps I should do him a favor, Adams imagines Hobby as saying: perhaps I should stumble (and thus cause his death). Could this provide evidence that Adams hoped his death would be brought about or that circumstances would be set up that would allow him to die? Hobby is foreseeing his master's future burden of years:

> Add such another 12 [years] and you make him 89: withered, faded, wrinkled, tottering, trembling, stumbling, sighing, groaning, weeping! Oh! I have some scruples of Conscience, whether I ought to preserve him: whether it would not be Charity to stumble, and relieve him from such a futurity. . . .
>   Remember too it is a Horse that asks the question, and that Horse is
>
>   Hobby.[20]

Adams's concerns, translated into Hobby's words, might be interpreted in a variety of ways: that Adams wished to die, that he perceived himself as a burden, that he feared the illness and decrepitude that old age would bring, that he was depressed. But they also hint at one mechanism of "allowing to die": exposing oneself to the risk of death that might come about through a carefully disguised "accident"—for example, one brought about knowingly and deliberately, indeed loyally, by Adams's trusted horse-friend.

Jefferson had also had concerns about the debilities of aging. In a letter dated June 1, 1822, four years before they died, Jefferson wrote to Adams describing the evidently senile Charles Thomson, who was then about 93:

> It is at most but the life of a cabbage, surely not worth a wish. When all our faculties have left, or are leaving us, one by one, sight, hearing, memory, every avenue of pleasing sensation is closed, and athumy, debility and mal-aise left in their places, when the friends of our youth are all gone, and a generation is risen around us whom we know not, is death an evil?

>   When one by one our ties are torn,
>   And friend from friend is snatched forlorn
>   When man is left alone to mourn,
>   Oh! then how sweet it is to die!
>   When trembling limbs refuse their weight,
>   And films slow gathering dim the sight,
>   When clouds obscure the mental light
>   Tis nature's kindest boon to die![21]

Could Jefferson's wish to die have been an active one? In a eulogy delivered in Richmond a week after the deaths, John Tyler said of Jefferson, "One other theme dwelt on his lips until they were motionless-It was the Fourth of July-He often expressed the wish to die on the day."[22] Could Jefferson's refusal to take his medications in his last hours be interpreted as a more direct effort to allow his own death to occur, or even to bring it about? Of course, it cannot be supposed that the medications were actually efficacious in keeping him alive; nevertheless, the refusal of further medication might seem to be evidence of what contemporary bioethicists would describe as "withholding or withdrawing treatment" or "allowing to die."

However, the historical record provides no more direct evidence for this explanation, nor any indication of Jefferson's intention in refusing medication.

In mid-June 1822, about ten days after Jefferson had written to Adams with the poem just quoted, Adams replied. Adams was also clearly burdened by ill health at that time:

> I answer your question, Is Death an Evil? It is not an Evil. It is a blessing to the individual, and to the world. Yet we ought not to wish for it till life becomes insupportable; we must wait the pleasure and convenience of this great teacher. Winter is as terrible to me, as to you. I am almost reduced in it, to the life of a Bear or a torpid swallow. I cannot read, but my delight is to hear others read . . .[23]

What remains unclear is whether Adams's view that "one ought not to wish for [death] till life becomes insupportable" would or would not countenance allowing oneself to die, whether by refusing medication or in any other way: ought one not wish for it at all, or not wish for it until truly bad circumstances prevail?

6. Causing Oneself to Die

Could the two old men have hastened their own deaths, or deliberately brought them about? They might each have seemed to have some reason for suicide: Adams was familiar with tragic, apparently self-caused death in his family. His son Charles had been driven to an early death, ending his life in an alcoholic stupor in 1800, and his grandson, George Washington Adams, may have committed suicide in 1829 by jumping off a ship in Long Island Sound while on his way to visit his parents in Washington; whether he jumped or fell remains a mystery, though he was quite troubled and apparently very agitated the night he disappeared. John Adams's daughter Abigail had died an extremely difficult death of breast cancer in 1813, having already had a breast removed without anesthesia, and his wife Abigail had died in 1818. Meanwhile, Jefferson, who had also lost a child during his presidency, was afflicted by many troubles toward the end of his life in addition to his failing health: his political world was collapsing, enrollments were poor at the institution he had been heavily involved in founding, the University of Virginia, he had huge debts, and a public raffle had had to be instituted to try to save Monticello.

Of course, causing oneself to die need not carry the pejorative label *suicide;* it can be seen, rather, as a matter of self-deliverance in preference to the sufferings and indignities of protracted dying. Adams, a deeply religious man, would probably not have conceived of ending his life in a comparatively deliberate way as "suicide," something that was universally denounced by the clergy of the era. Jefferson's religiosity was far more idiosyncratic. Still, it is not clear in either case that their religious views would entail that they could not have played an active role in the ends of their own lives.

Indeed, some writers have intimated that these men did play active roles in their own deaths. Among the eulogists of the time, Caleb Cushing hints at this in saying that these lines could truly have been written of each:

Nothing in his life
Became him like the leaving it. He died
As one that had been studied in his death.[24]

The contemporary biographer Joseph Ellis calls Adams's expiring on the Fourth "the last and most symbolic act of his life,"[25] particularly because he was willing to die on the 4th, not the 2nd (Adams had initially viewed July 2 as the date of real importance in the birth of the United States, since it was on that date that he had persuaded the Congress to adopt the Declaration of Independence; the document was merely signed on the 4th). Ellis also describes Adams, who was sitting in his favorite chair in his upstairs study on the morning of the day he would die, the 4th, as perhaps trying to "resist the swells of satisfaction he might be expected to feel on that special day"[26]—though this hardly explains how he could go from a condition of such alertness and good feeling to death within a few hours. Adams was dead by 6:20 that evening. And Fawn Brodie writes, "If ever two men in history chose and controlled the moment of their dying, they were John Adams and Thomas Jefferson."[27]

Such comments appear to be sheer speculation. But perhaps there is an argument for the intimation that Adams and/or Jefferson hastened their own deaths. Adams was apparently familiar with lethal drugs: in 1811, he wrote to Benjamin Rush in connection with Rush's anti-alcohol campaign that "The Table of Cyder and Health and Poison and Death I have given to Dr. Tuft [Dr. Cotton Tufts], who will propagate it. It is a concise but very comprehensive Result of long Experience, attentive observation and deep and close Thought."[28] Just two years later, in 1813, Jefferson wrote to Dr. Samuel Brown about the matter of lethiferous drugs:

> The most elegant thing of that kind is a preparation of the Jamestown weed ["Jimson weed"], Datura Stramonium, invented by the French in the time of Robespierre. Every man of firmness carried it constantly in his pocket to anticipate the guillotine. It brings on the sleep of death as quietly as fatigue does the ordinary sleep, without the least struggle or motion. Condorcet, who had recourse to it, was found lifeless on his bed a few minutes after his landlady had left him there, and even the slipper which she had observed half suspended on his foot, was not shaken off. It seems far preferable to the Venesection of the Romans, the Hemlock of the Greeks, and the Opium of the Turks. I have never been able to learn what the preparation is, other than a strong concentration of its lethiferous principle. Could such a medicament be restrained to self-administration, it ought not to be kept secret. There are ills in life as desperate as intolerable, to which it would be the rational relief, *e.g.,* the inveterate cancer . . .[29]

However, there is no evidence that either Adams or Jefferson considered, tried to, or did take such a drug on July 4, 1826.

The Inadequacy of Explanations

Unfortunately, each of these six explanations for the same-day deaths of Adams and Jefferson is inadequate on its face: the coincidence is too great; divine intervention requires background theological assumptions beyond the scope of rational explanation; "hanging on" and "giving up" require pathophysiological assumptions not well understood; and the various forms of direct-causation explanations, including inadvertent or deliberate allowing to die, physician or family-performed euthanasia, and suicide, all suffer from lack of compelling evidence. It isn't necessary that the explanation of the cause of death be the same for both Adams and Jefferson; yet whatever each explanation involves, we still need an explanation for the remarkable synchrony of their deaths.

Furthermore, the issue of synchrony—whatever the individual explanations for their deaths—also leaves us with the further question of coordination. Did Adams and Jefferson think alike but act independently? Could they have had some joint understanding, reached perhaps in 1813—when each had been corresponding with a physician, Adams with Benjamin Rush about a horse's deliberate stumble and Jefferson with Samuel Brown about lethal drugs—that they then recalled later on? Did their physicians or families think alike but act independently, or perhaps in concert? Could their families and caregivers have lied about the precise dates of their deaths, seeking to lend their demises a greater grandeur? Or was there a more orchestrated plan here, known only to these two men, or to their physicians and families, that accounts for the extraordinary "coincidence" or "grand design" of their deaths? Could it have been the mode, so to speak, to die on the Fourth if at all possible, by whatever means? After all, not just Adams and Jefferson, but *three* of the first five presidents of the young United States died on the 4th of July. In 1831, just five years after the deaths of Adams and Jefferson, James Monroe, the fifth president, did so as well.

If it was the mode, something that Adams and Jefferson or their caregivers somehow deliberately brought about, however, there is no remaining evidence of any such plan.

What Does the Way They Died Mean to Us?
The Contemporary Politics of Dying

Given the insufficient historical evidence available, we can't know the truth about why Adams and Jefferson died on the same day—the same date, the same year, the same hugely important anniversary. But we can reflect on whether it would make a difference to us if one or another of these explanations turned to be true. After all, the six possibilities these explanations raise are central to the very questions about death and dying that are so controversial today, almost two hundred years after the deaths of Adams and Jefferson, as disputes over withdrawing and withholding treatment, allowing to die, the overuse of morphine, terminal sedation, physician-assisted suicide, and euthanasia play huge roles in friction over modern medicine.

Two quite different postures are in competition in these disputes. One insists that the patient play a comparatively passive role in accepting death when it comes—whether it is explained as the product of divine intervention, sheer coincidence, or failure to hang on. The other casts the patient in a potentially active role, as the intender or designer or cause of his own death, whether he deliberately gives up or actively brings about death. Where we stand with respect to these two basic postures may influence how we explain the deaths of Adams and Jefferson.

On the one hand, if we assume that Adams and Jefferson so to speak simply let death come to them, and it just happened to occur on that extraordinary day, we need a more persuasive account of coincidence or perhaps divine intervention, or other comparatively passive mechanisms of dying. Did they hang on, but then give up, on that day—and if so, is this a matter of passive acceptance or active self-termination? If passive acceptance of death is what these heroic figures of our history did, is that all we should allow? If we see their death as a matter of intentional "hanging on" and intentional "giving up," we need an adequate, causal, biological account of how hanging on and then ceasing to do so can result in death: what is the *exact* pathophysiological mechanism of death that occurs when a person ceases to 'hang on"? Much of the end-of-life literature, popular culture, and even medical discussion assumes that this is possible—doctors say this is a common phenomenon, and the biopsychosocial literature assembles information about correlations between death rates and symbolic occasions—but *evidence* for such a process is not provided anywhere, nor any plausible explanation of how such a process might work. Can people simply will themselves to die at a certain time, and if so, exactly how does such a choice shut life-sustaining bodily processes off? This is not just a problem in accounting for the deaths of Adams and Jefferson, but for accounts of dying people everywhere, both in the past and today.

Or, on the other hand, could some more active process have been at work? Did physicians or family caregivers play a causal role in the deaths of Adams and Jefferson, deliberately allowing or helping them to die? Did Adams and Jefferson themselves not only will themselves to die on that day but do something to make it occur? Did they refuse treatment with that intention? Suppose they took a drug like Condorcet used: would we count that as suicide or self-deliverance, and if so, should that have bearing on the currently volatile issue of physician-assisted suicide? If we think they could have done this, even discreetly and without clear evidence in the historical record, why shouldn't we allow ourselves to die in the same way?

Thus what we say about Adams and Jefferson, in the absence of compelling historical evidence, may in the end reflect what we want to say about ourselves. In our current legal and political climate, in which the original intent of the Founding Fathers is treated with extraordinary gravity, what we believe about the deaths of Adams and Jefferson (and Monroe) may play a very large role in our views about the what we call "the right to die" and what deaths we make legal or illegal for ourselves. Further historical evidence, were it to become available, could play a major role in deciding current controversies. If evidence of direct causation were found, whether in the form of physician or family-administered euthanasia, or self-undertaken or physician-assisted suicide, this might sway more conservative thinkers who are most opposed to liberalization of the right to die and legalization of physician-assisted suicide but who on the other hand are most concerned to honor the Founders' views; if on the other hand it could be definitively established that Adams's and Jefferson's same-day deaths were coincidence, nothing more, it might challenge many of the forms of negotiated deaths that are ubiquitous in modern medicine now.

Notes

I thank Herbert Sloan, Dominic Albo, Celeste Walker, Sam Karlin, Brooke Hopkins, Beverly Hawkins, Mary-Jane Forbyn, Vince Cheng, Jay Jacobson, Peter von Sievers, Eric Hutton, and many others for discussion of this topic.

1. Allan Nevins, ed., *The Diary of John Quincy Adams, 1794–1845* (New York: Scribner, 1951), 360, cited in David McCullough, *John Adams* (New York: Simon & Schuster, 2001), 647.

2. Baltimore, Maryland, July 20, 1826, in *A Selection of Eulogies, Pronounced in the Several States, In Honor of Those Illustrious Patriots and Statesmen, John Adams and Thomas Jefferson* (Hartford, Conn: D. F. Robinson & Co. and Norton & Russell, 1826), 88–9.

3. Boston, Faneuil Hall, August 2, 1826, in *Selection of Eulogies,* 156.

4. Susan Boylston Adams Clark to Abigail Louisa Smith Adams Johnson, July 9, 1826, A. B. Johnson Papers, Massachusetts Historical Society, cited in McCullough, *John Adams,* 646; Andrew Burstein, in *America's Jubilee: How in 1826 a Generation Remembered Fifty Years of Independence* (New York: Alfred A. Knopf, 2001), 266–274, examines the evidence for this claim and finds it wanting; it is established only that Adams spoke the name "Thomas Jefferson" but what followed apparently was inarticulate.

5. Burstein, *America's Jubilee,* 263.

6. Jefferson to Roger C. Weightman, June 24, 1826, Monticello, Va., in Willson Whitman, *Jefferson's Letters* (Eau Claire, Wisc.: E. M. Hale, 1930), 373–4. This was Jefferson's last letter.

7. C. C. Cambreleng: pronounced in the city of New-York, July 17, 1826, in *Selection of Eulogies,* 66.

8. D. P. Philips, "Deathday and birthday: An unexpected connection," in *Statistics: A guide to the unknown,* ed. J. M. Tanur (San Francisco: Holden-Day, 1972), 52–65, cited in Oakley Ray, "How the Mind Hurts and Heals the Body," *American Psychologist* 59 (January 2004): 37.

9. D. P. Philips and E. W. King, "Death takes a holiday: Mortality surrounding major social occasions." *Lancet* 2 (1988): 728–32, cited in Ray, "How the Mind Hurts," 37.

10. D. P. Philips and D. G. Smith, "Postponement of death until symbolically meaningful occasions," *Journal of the American Medical Association* 263 (1990): 1947–51, cited in Ray, "How the Mind Hurts," 37.

11. Ray, "How the Mind Hurts," 37.

12. Ibid., 37.

13. Bumgarner, John R., MD, *The Health of the Presidents: The 41 United States Presidents Through 1993 from a Physician's Point of View* (Jefferson, NC and London: McFarland & Co., 1994), 14, 24–5.

14. Donn C. Young and Erin M. Hade, "Holidays, Birthdays, and Postponement of Cancer Death," *Journal of the American Medical Association* 292 (2004): 3012–16.

15. John Adams to Benjamin Rush, August 6, 1810, Quincy, Mass., in Alexander Biddle, *Old Family Letters* (Philadelphia: Lippincott, 1892), 23.

16. Susanna Boylston Adams Clark to Abigail Louisa Smith Adams Johnson, July 9, 1826, Quincy, Mass. Courtesy, Massachusetts Historical Society.

17. Burstein, *America's Jubilee,* p. 266.

18. Hugh A. Garland, *The Life of John Randolph of Roanoke.* New-York: D. Appleton & Company; Philadelphia: Geo. S. Appleton, 1850. Vol. 2, p. 273.

19. Sarah N. Randolph, *The Domestic Life of Thomas Jefferson* (Charlottesville: University Press of Virginia, 1978), 428, cited in McCullough, *John Adams,* 646.

20. John Adams to Benjamin Rush, January 4, 1813, Quincy, Mass., in Biddle, *Old Family Letters,* 333–4.

21. Jefferson to Adams, Monticello, June 1, 1822, in *The Adams-Jefferson Letters,* ed. Lester J. Cappon (Chapel Hill: University of North Carolina Press, 1988), 578.

22. John Tyler: pronounced at Richmond, Virginia, July 11, 1826, in *Selection of Eulogies,* 16.

23. Adams to Jefferson, Montezillo, June 11, 1822, in *Selection of Eulogies,* 579.

24. Caleb Cushing: pronounced at Newburyport, Massachusetts, July 15, 1826, in *Selection of Eulogies,* 22–3.

25. Joseph J. Ellis, *Passionate Sage: The Character and Legacy of John Adams* (New York: Norton, 1993), 234.

26. Ibid., 215.

27. Fawn M. Brodie, *Thomas Jefferson: An Intimate History* (New York: Norton, 1974), 468.

28. John Adams to Benjamin Rush, Quincy, Mass., July 31, 1811, in Biddle, *Old Family Letters,* 342.

29. Jefferson to Dr. Samuel Brown, Monticello, July 14, 1813, in *The Writings of Thomas Jefferson: Definitive Edition,* ed. Albert Ellery Bergh (Washington, D.C.: The Thomas Jefferson Memorial Association, 1907), 13:310–1.

9

High-Risk Religion

Informed Consent in Faith Healing, Serpent Handling, and Refusing Medical Treatment

In some of the more colorful groups on the American religious spectrum, the religious faith of believers involves a willingness to take substantial physical risks—risks to health, physical functioning, and even the risk of death. In several of these groups, the risks a believer takes are indirect, as in refusing blood transfusions or medical treatment; in others, the risks are direct and immediate, as in drinking strychnine or handling poisonous snakes. We may think of these practices as extraordinary tests of religious commitment. We may take willingness to risk death as a demonstration of the extraordinary value religious goals can have for believers. In fact, willingness to risk death for religious reasons is often extolled as the highest test of faith. But this willingness also raises a set of disturbing moral issues concerning the ways in which religious groups bring it about that their adherents are willing to take such risks. In what follows, I want to take a closer look at the influence of religious groups on their adherents' choices, focusing on high-risk decision making that can result in death. In addressing these issues, I do not wish to suggest that a religious believer's willingness to risk death may not be sincere and devout; rather, I want only to cast a morally inquiring eye on the way in which religious institutions engender these sincere, devout beliefs.

Risk Budgets and Styles

To pose the problem more precisely, we can conceptualize it as it might be addressed in the field of professional ethics. Drawing on issues concerning the formation and manipulation of choice, especially in medicine, we can approach this problem under the general rubric of *informed consent.* This conceptualization permits us to begin with the first prong of an analytic pincer, involving the application of norms from professional ethics to practices within organized religion.

In everyday life, risks that a person voluntarily and knowingly takes can be described as the result of a prudential calculation, however rudimentary that calculation may be in practice, in which he or she elects a course of action hoping it will produce a gain or avoid a loss, though at the same time recognizing that it may either concurrently or alternatively result in a (further) loss. This prudential calculation involves a survey of the range of possible outcomes of the action proposed, an assessment of the likelihood of the various possible outcomes (the decision is made *under risk* if the probabilities are known, *under uncertainty* if they are not), and an assessment of the relative desirability or undesirability of each of the possible outcomes. Typically, avoidance risk taking weighs two or more projected negative outcomes against each other; gain-oriented, positive risk taking may weigh various positive outcomes against each other, or a positive outcome against both the cost of failing to achieve it and the cost of failing to take the risk. Whatever the specific context of the risk decision, the decision maker properly makes the calculation by multiplying the value of each possible outcome times the probability that it will occur, if known, or the best approximation to it, and then choosing the course of action promising the highest expected utility. That this calculation may be made in a completely intuitive, nonquantitative way does not obscure its nature: conscious decision making under risk or under uncertainty always involves acting so as to produce some preferred outcome despite recognition that this action may instead produce a different, undesired result.

Each individual, Charles Fried has pointed out, has a distinctive *risk budget*— the degree and severity of risk he or she is willing to accept in order to avoid certain losses or to achieve certain gains.[1] The risk budget is a function, of course, of the possible courses of action the individual foresees, the probabilities he or she assigns to the various possible outcomes, and the utilities he or she attaches to each of these, influenced by any characteristic errors the person may make in performing the prudential calculation that indicates what course of action promises the greatest expected utility. But while the risk budgets of ordinary individuals in a culture appear to be fairly uniform with respect to the background risks of everyday life (for example, in drinking the water in a given locality or in using electricity in one's home), there is considerable divergence in the willingness of individuals to accept specific higher foreground risks—for instance, in financial dealings or in high-risk sports like hang gliding or mountain climbing. This is just to say that some members of a culture take risks that other members of the culture won't.

Furthermore, each individual has a distinctive *risk style:* the degree of deliberation or abandon he or she exercises in making a prudential calculation under risk or uncertainty. Some people assess perceived risks with meticulous, painstaking care, regardless of whether the risks are mild or severe and the amount of information they have about the probabilities of various possible outcomes; others take both big and little risks in a comparatively cavalier way. Different individuals also process relevant information in very different ways. For instance, some are naturally optimistic, focusing primarily on the benefits to be gained; others are comparatively pessimistic, attending to possible losses—even when their estimates of the probabilities of the outcomes are the same. In processing information, some individuals may be more prone to characteristic errors of reasoning in risk assessment than others. Like risk budgets, the risk styles of persons within a culture are relatively uniform with respect to background risks, but may vary considerably among individuals with respect to certain more conspicuous risks. Some people make their choices about risks in ways that other people would regard as foolish.

The problem presented by the practices of certain religious groups arises with an observation about risk budgets and styles. The members of a culture ordinarily exhibit broad commonalities in both risk budgets and styles with respect to background risks; they also typically exhibit a range of idiosyncratic, individual risk budgets and styles with respect to certain conspicuous, higher-risk decisions. However, the risk budgets and styles of the members of certain religious groups display striking uniformities not so much with respect to background risks, but with respect to major, conspicuous, foreground risks—direct risks to health, physical functioning, and even risks to life. Furthermore, the kinds of risk characteristically taken by members of these groups often fall well outside the risk budgets and, in addition, violate the risk styles of most other members of society—even outside the quite broad range of individual variation in risk budget and style that members of the culture ordinarily display in their decisions. Put another way, the members of certain religious groups take risks other people do not and decide to do so in ways that other people would not, but they nevertheless do so in remarkably uniform ways. Nor are these trivial risks; some are potentially fatal ones.

These characteristic risk-taking patterns, each distinctive of a particular group, may seem to be just another element in the colorful spectrum of American religious diversity. But this diversity cloaks substantial moral issues about the ways in which religious groups influence and shape individual decision making among their members. It is not merely that these people take risks other people do not and decide to do so in ways other people would not; it is the very uniformity of these group-specific risk budgets and styles and the degree to which they fall outside the ordinary range of variation that invites scrutiny of the mechanisms by which they are produced. What we will find, I think, are systematic, doctrine-controlled violations of the principle of autonomy—that is, of that moral principle familiar in professional and ordinary ethics that requires both protection of an individual's capacity to choose and respect for the substance of that choice.

If there are violations of the principle of autonomy, they can be identified by locating the precise point at which they occur in the paradigmatic decision-making process, evident in varying forms in the four religious groups to be examined here. These are groups whose adherents regularly make choices that indirectly or directly expose them to risks of death. Are these choices *informed?* Do they involve *consent,* genuine consent that is voluntary and uncoerced? In answering these questions, raised in approaching the problem from the standpoint of professional ethics, it will become clear that some of the ways in which religious groups shape and control high-risk decision making are morally indefensible. However, this is not true of all the ways in which high-risk decision making is influenced—even among the four groups isolated for discussion here—and it will be necessary to develop a general criterion for distinguishing morally indefensible practices controlling religious decisionmaking from those that may be morally defensible. This criterion will serve in concert with the topology of doctrinal claims developed in the previous chapter [of my book, *Ethics in the Sanctuary*] to fix more precisely the range within which we can discern and address *ethical* issues generated within organized religion.

Three of the groups we shall examine participate in practices that impose varying degrees of indirect risk of death by refusal of medical treatment or some component of it—Christian Science, Jehovah's Witnesses, and the Faith Assembly. The practices of a fourth group impose, in addition, a direct threat of death—the various serpent-handling, strychnine-drinking pentecostal groups within the Holiness churches. Two of these, the Faith Assembly and the Holiness churches, are generally regarded as cults or fringe groups; the other two, Christian Science and the Jehovah's Witnesses, occupy intermediate positions between the fringe and the mainstream of American religious groups. That these are all generally Christian denominations, though differing considerably in their teachings, should not suggest that similar moral issues do not arise in other world religions, but only that the issues of high-risk decision making in religious commitment are particularly prominent in certain strands of the Christian tradition.

Risk Taking in Four American Religious Groups

CHRISTIAN SCIENCE

The First Church of Christ, Scientist, takes the refusal of conventional medical treatment in favor of Christian Science healing as central among its practices and as indicative of faith.[2] According to Christian Science belief, what we (mistakenly) call "disease" is produced by a "radically limited and distorted view of the true spiritual nature and capacities of men and women"[3]; illness results from "human alienation from God,"[4] produced by fundamental misunderstandings. Disease is symptomatic not of physical disorder but of underlying spiritual inadequacy and a failure to understand one's true spiritual nature. When a faithful member of the church falls ill, he or she consults a Christian Science practitioner to seek treatment which consists "entirely of heartfelt yet disciplined prayer."[5] The practitioner, who is often consulted by telephone (sometimes long distance) and need not make a bedside visit, has no medical training in either diagnosis or treatment. The practitioner does not physically touch or examine the patient. Rather, the practitioner assists the ill person in prayer, the objective of which is to relieve physical symptoms by promoting the correct and reverent understanding of the true nature of disease—that in reality there is no such thing. Hence, prayer is believed to be incompatible with conventional medical treatment, since medical treatment presupposes the misleading assumption that there is such a thing as disease, that it is of physical origin, and that it can be treated by physical means. Properly, one cannot speak of *cure*, for there is no disease to be cured; rather, the relief of symptoms is a "demonstration" of the correctness of the principles upon which Christian Science is founded. Christian Scientists do generally use the services of dentists and oculists and sometimes have physicians perform what they call "mechanical" procedures not involving medication, such as setting broken bones, but other than this, no conventional medical procedures, either diagnostic or therapeutic, are used.[6] For services rendered in praying for and with the individual who is ill, the Christian Science practitioner receives a fee roughly comparable to the fees conventional physicians charge. This fee is reimbursable by many insurance companies (including some Blue Cross/Blue Shield plans) and by some state and federal Medicare and Medicaid programs.[7] There are about five thousand Christian Science practitioners who practice healing through prayer on a full-time basis.[8]

Frequently, the choice between Christian Science healing and conventional medical treatment does not constitute a subjectively recognized *risk* for the devout Scientist, since belief in the efficacy of Christian Science healing may be very strong. In such cases, the individual may be confident that Christian Science healing will provide relief from the condition that troubles him. Nevertheless, the choice to accept treatment from a Christian Science practitioner rather than an M.D., or not to accept treatment at all, resembles in structure any other prudential calculation under risk: various possible outcomes—cure, continuing illness, incapacitation, and death—are foreseen under specific valuations and under more or less quantifiable expectations about the likelihood of their occurrence. Christian Scientists are, of course, aware of the availability of conventional medicine; medical treatment is a possible choice, but one that, on prudential grounds, the believing Christian Scientist does not make. The believing Scientist not only thinks he or she is acting in accord with the dictates or expectations of the faith, but also that he or she will maximize the likelihood of achieving the outcome with the greatest expected utility—namely, a successful cure—by preferring Christian Science healing to conventional medicine. It is in this choice that the risk taking lies, though for the believing Christian Scientist, of course, it is seen as a good risk.

JEHOVAH'S WITNESSES

Jehovah's Witnesses refuse a single component of medical treatment, the transfusion of blood or blood derivatives into their bodies. They do so on the basis of a variety of scriptural passages, especially Genesis 9:4 ("Only, you shall not eat flesh with its life, that is, its blood"), Leviticus 17:12 ("Therefore I have said to the people of Israel: No person among you shall eat blood, nor shall any alien who resides among you eat blood"), Deuteronomy 12:23–25 ("Only be sure that you do not eat the blood; for the blood is the life"), and Acts 15:28–29 ("For it has seemed good to the Holy Spirit and to us to impose on you no further burden than these essentials: that you abstain from what has been sacrificed to idols and from blood and from what has been strangled and from fornication"); they believe that the scriptural prohibition of eating or drinking blood includes any form of taking the blood of another into one's own body, including by transfusion.[9] Although they will accept the infusion of nonblood solutions to expand blood volume, faithful Witnesses consent to surgery—even major surgery—only under the understanding that it be performed without additional blood.[10] They will not accept blood in emergency situations or accidents, and relatives are asked to refuse consent on behalf of those who are unconscious. Nor will they accept blood or blood derivatives in treatment for diseases of the blood, such as anemia or leukemia. In a series of cases, the courts have generally upheld the right of competent, adult Jehovah's Witnesses to refuse blood transfusions, even where the risk of death is high, provided that the patient has no obligations to dependents that cannot otherwise be met.[11] However, the courts have generally not permitted pregnant women to refuse transfusions, nor parents to refuse transfusions for their minor children.

For Jehovah's Witnesses, the situations in which these choices arise are comparatively rare, though when such situations do arise they may be extremely serious or life-threatening. Frequently, too, such decisions must be made in conditions of extreme urgency, as for accident victims, where exsanguination is an immediate, life-threatening risk. Despite the urgency, however, such choices also conform to the risk-taking paradigm: the two principal possible outcomes—survival with transfusion, versus death without transfusion—are foreseen under evaluations assigning great weight to obedience to church belief and the highest value to an expected salvific afterlife, versus a great but comparatively lesser value to continuing physical existence. As in all risk taking, that option believed to promise greater utility under the assigned valuation is the one that the prudent, rational Witness will choose.

THE FAITH ASSEMBLY

The Faith Assembly, a small fundamentalist group centered in northeastern Indiana, at its height prohibited its members from consulting doctors or from using any medical treatment at all, including vaccination and other preventive treatment, assistance in childbirth, emergency treatment, prostheses, eyeglasses, or hearing aids. This group was founded in the mid-1960s by Hobart Freeman, a former Southern Baptist minister who had been dismissed from the faculty at a fundamentalist theological seminary for failing to conform to its beliefs. Freeman started the church in his basement, moved it to a rural barn (the "Glory Barn") and after a dispute with the owner, moved the church again to its present center near Goshen, Indiana. Freeman taught the members of the fledgling church to shun doctors and to rely on prayer and faith for healing—a teaching that stiffened into a rigorous antimedical policy enforced by the threat of expulsion from the group. Freeman also claimed that he would never die.

In the spring of 1983, two reporters from the *Fort Wayne News-Sentinel* investigated evidence of fifty-two deaths attributed to the group's prohibition of medical treatment.[12] The dead included twenty-eight babies whose mothers refused prenatal care, seven children with untreated illnesses and injuries, ten adults with untreated illnesses, and seven mothers who died of untreated complications of childbirth. The reporters also identified a living 5-year-old child with a basketball-sized tumor of the abdomen whom they expected to become the fifty-third death. But they also found evidence that compliance with the group's policy of refusing medical treatment was by no means universally voluntary. They documented the existence of an underground network by which mothers were taking their children to physicians in neighboring cities to seek medical treatment without fear of exposure, punishment, or excommunication for themselves or the children. They also described in detail the case of Sally Burkitt, a twenty-seven-year-old woman who hemorrhaged following the unassisted delivery of her child: medical attention was denied her and she bled to death fifty-six hours after delivery—despite her explicit, repeated pleas for a doctor. ("We'll get the best doctor there is," her husband had promised, but what he meant was Jesus.)[13] By late 1985, at least ninety deaths had been attributed to the practices of the group; by 1988 the figure had reached one hundred. Hobart Freeman had been indicted in connection with the death of a 15-year-old girl, but in December 1984 he himself had died—with advanced heart disease, gangrene in one foot, pneumonia, and possible diabetes, having refused all treatment. By 1988, eleven parents had been convicted in the deaths of their children, and without Freeman, the group had begun to relax its prohibition of medical care.

THE HOLINESS CHURCHES

Serpent handling is a practice found in many cultures, including those of certain southwest American Indian groups, but is particularly widespread in the Appalachian regions of the southeastern United States. It was apparently introduced in 1906 in Grasshopper Valley, Tennessee, by a man named George Went Hensley, who carried a rattlesnake in his hands down from a ridge where he had been bitten. Hensley evangelized throughout Appalachia; his legacy includes many of the small, independent Holiness churches found in the region. While not all Holiness churches practice serpent handling and while it is illegal under state law in Kentucky, Virginia, and Tennessee and under municipal ordinances in North Carolina, the practice is nevertheless found in rural areas in much of Appalachia.

Serpent handlers base their practices on a literal interpretation of Mark 16:17–18: "And these signs will accompany those who believe: by using my name they will cast out demons; they will speak in new tongues; they will pick up snakes in their hands, and if they drink any deadly thing, it will not hurt them; they will lay their hands on the sick, and they will recover."

At the Scrabble Creek Church of All Nations (about thirty-seven miles from Charleston, West Virginia), prayer meetings are held in a small, one-room building with benches or pews and an open area at the front. The meeting is attended by members of all ages, including infants and children, and sometimes by visitors as well. Meetings may last four to six hours, two or three times a week, and consist of hymn singing, preaching, foot washing, healing, and personal testifying of increasing emotional intensity. Participants dance, sing, shriek, shout, crouch, or lie on the floor and may exhibit glossolalia and motor automatisms, including spasms, jerks, and seizures. At the climax of these meetings, live poisonous snakes (usually rattlers or copperheads from nearby mountains) are produced from a box or wicker basket and passed among those who wish to handle them. Some participants simply touch or hold the snakes; others coil the snakes around their arms, heads, or throats.[14] The purpose, participants say, is to "receive the Holy Ghost" or to "confirm the word of God" in Mark 16. Bites do occur, but although one source claims that George Hensley said of his forty-six years with the Dolley Pond Church that he had been bitten four hundred times until he was "speckled all over like a guinea hen,"[15] bites are not particularly frequent. Many members also refuse medical treatment if bitten, claiming that the bite provides a further test of God's will.

Many serpent handlers claim that they are "afraid of snakes like anybody else,"[16] but that they lose this fear when they are "anointed" to handle snakes and enter an ecstatic condition. Said Sister Eunice Ball of Newport, Tennessee, "When the anointing's on me, I'm not afraid of the serpents. Other times I'd run. I've taken up as many as six serpents at one time—five copperheads and a large rattler. I've not ever been bitten. There's something there that you know without a doubt that it won't harm you. My hands don't get stiff. I can move my hands, but the feeling's still there."[17] Serpent handlers variously believe that they will not be bitten or that if bitten they will not die, that recovery from snakebite is a miracle wrought by God, and that each snakebite death that does occur is a sign that the Lord "really had to show the scoffers how dangerous it is to obey His commandments."[18] Detractors' claims that the snakes have been de-venomed, drugged, or otherwise deliberately rendered harmless are clearly false, and naturalistic explanations such as that grasping snakes by their midsections produces cataplectic reactions in the snakes or that human body heat or motion disturbs their reflexes also seem inadequate.[19] Between 1910 and 1977, the total number of deaths attributed to religious serpent handling was about forty.[20] Fatalities are also reported from drinking strychnine (sometimes called a "salvation cocktail"), especially in serpent-handling groups in West Virginia.

Religious Risk and Freedom of Religion

Of course, showing that risk-taking conduct occurs in various forms and degrees of potentially fatal risk among different religious groups is not to reach a normative conclusion. It cannot simply be assumed that risk taking is wrong, however extreme the consequences for the person taking the risk. Quite the contrary, it is plausible to defend risk-taking conduct in religion under the general principle of autonomy, regarding religious choice as one kind of choice an individual is entitled to make by virtue of his or her right of self-determination. Furthermore, since religious belief may be at the heart of an individual's identity and since action according to these beliefs may be central to the individual's maintaining this identity in the world, religious choice—even where it involves serious, potentially disabling or fatal risks—may seem particularly worthy of protection and respect. Of course, some religiously committed individuals may not perceive their behavior as involving risk, nor, for that matter, as involving any choice or decision at all. In fact, it may be those most firmly committed who see themselves as having no options, in that they feel bound to do whatever God or the specific religious group requires. Some may even believe that they cannot do otherwise not only in a normative sense but in a metaphysical sense as well: ultimately, they believe, God determines both what shall happen and how they shall act. Still others may recognize a single antecedent choice—for instance, the choice "for Jesus" or "for God"—but hold otherwise theodeterminist views. Nevertheless, many believers recognize the distinction between subjective and objective risk, and even if they feel their personal commitments oblige them to make certain choices rather than others, acknowledge that in many religiously relevant situations it would be possible to perform any one of several alternative actions, each of which would yield differently valued outcomes and incur different degrees of risk. The principle of autonomy defends all varieties of high-risk choice in religion where choice is voluntarily and knowingly made—that is, where the criteria of informed consent are met—even when the outcome may be death.

A principal objection to the view that autonomous risk-taking conduct in religion should be respected, the only objection with legal standing, appeals to the harm principle by citing the social costs of such behavior. Under this principle, risk-taking religious conduct may be morally condemned, as well as restricted or prohibited under law, where it imposes harm or substantial risk of harm to others. For instance, emotional and financial costs for immediate family members or the dependents may be severe if the risk that person takes turns out badly. Whether a parent dies because he or she has undergone surgery without blood, or was fatally bitten in a serpent-handling prayer meeting, or died after refusing medical treatment for a curable illness, the consequences for a dependent child are the same. Some legal cases appear to restrict religious risk taking on the ground of obligations to dependents, as in the Jehovah's Witnesses cases, but this remains a much-disputed issue.

Religious risk taking may also be restricted if the risk involves not only the individual who voluntarily assumes it but bystanders and dependents as well. For instance, in *Swann v. Pack,* a 1975 case, the Tennessee Supreme Court outlawed serpent handling on the ground that it constitutes a public nuisance. In this case, a prayer meeting of the Holiness Church of God in Jesus Name was described by the prosecution as involving the "handling of snakes in a crowded church sanctuary with virtually no safeguards, with children roaming around unattended, and with the handlers so enraptured and entranced that they were in a virtual state of hysteria,"[21] although the defense presented further evidence to show that the snake handling was performed on a stage in front of the audience and that the area was roped off with guards stationed at intervals to prevent any snakes from escaping. Although laws explicitly prohibiting serpent handling have been passed in only a handful of states, observers suggest that in many other states such practices would most likely be construed as constituting a public nuisance.

The costs society must absorb for those who are injured, incapacitated, or killed in religious risk taking may, of course, be considerable. However, a general analysis that focuses on the social consequences of religious practices must surely cut the other way: a great deal of the behavior encouraged by religious groups is strongly risk reductive, especially where nonviolent, continent ways of life are required, and results in social savings rather than costs. Methodists and Mormons do not drink; Seventh-day Adventists avoid food additives, stimulants, and meat; Quakers do not go to war. Catholics, like those in most Christian groups, are forbidden to commit suicide. The Amish generally shun modern conveniences, such as motor vehicles and electric power appliances and tools, and thus risk fewer accidents. Most Christian-based groups discourage pre- and extramarital sexual activity and violent lifestyles, thus reducing the risk of injury, pregnancy, and sexually transmitted disease. Where these prohibitions are effective, they lower the risks of health and life considerably, and the social savings that result clearly vastly outweigh the social costs of increased risk taking by those who refuse medical treatment and the handful of snake handlers in rural Appalachia. Of course, an appeal to the harm principle introduces the extremely interesting further question of whether a religious group ought to encourage or require its members to consider the potential impact of their own risks on others before taking them, and just how the impact ought to weigh in their choices. The more fundamental issue, however, directly concerns the ways in which members of religious groups come to take such major risks in the first place.

In this examination of the ways in which four specimen groups—Christian Science, Jehovah's Witnesses, the Faith Assembly, and the Holiness churches— elicit risk-taking behavior, it has been assumed that their practices do, in fact, increase risks of ill health, disability, or death. Comprehensive, reliable figures for the actual rates of risk or the frequency of negative outcomes are not available for any of these groups, however, and for some of them information that might provide evidence of increased risk is either not collected or very closely guarded. Of course, there are some scattered data on which to base this assumption. As we have seen, by 1988 one hundred deaths had been attributed to the practices of the Faith Assembly in its two decades of existence. A joint study by the Indiana State Department of Health and the Center for Disease Control in Atlanta calculated that in Elkhart and Koscuisko counties, Indiana, where many Faith Assembly members live, mothers in the sect were one hundred times as likely to die from complications of pregnancy as other women in Indiana and that babies up to one year old were three times more likely to die.[22] About forty deaths had been reported by 1977 among snake-handling groups. The coroner of King County, Washington, did a retrospective analysis of deaths in the years 1949–51; he found eleven apparently preventable deaths among Christian Science children and calculated that 6 percent of all Christian Science deaths were preventable. This study, though simplistic in its methodology, also reported that among Christian Scientists, the death rate from cancer was double the national average. In King County, the average longevity of Christian Scientists was very slightly lower than the average longevity of the non-Scientist population.[23]

Case-by-case data on deaths of children in religious groups that reject conventional medical treatment are available from CHILD, Inc., in its extensive newsletter.[24] This group, founded by Rita and Doug Swan, former Christian Scientists whose young son died of meningitis after receiving only Christian Science healing, lobbies actively to have religious exemptions from requirements for medical care for children removed from state law. However, case data cannot provide reliable estimates of the increase (or perhaps decrease) of risk in these religious behaviors. Rigorous statistical analyses of morbidity and mortality patterns associated with treatment refusal or direct risk are not, in general, available for any of the groups considered here.

No complete figures are available, for instance, on the number of Jehovah's Witnesses who have died as a result of refusing blood transfusions, though certain individual cases can be documented from court or medical records. On the contrary, Jehovah's Witnesses often claim that surgery without blood or with only nonblood volume expanders may offer equal or better results than surgery with blood transfusions, partly because of the risks of disease transmission in transfusion and partly because of the greater surgical caution and skill employed by the surgeon who must operate without using blood.[25] Nevertheless, it is believed that many Witnesses have been denied surgical treatment by surgeons unwilling to assume the risks of operating without blood. For instance, although accurate figures are not available, it was rumored some years ago that one of the busiest trauma hospitals in Dade County, Florida, had a blanket policy of refusing to treat Witnesses.[26] As surgical techniques improve for operating without blood and as recognition for Witnesses' firmly established legal right to refuse blood becomes more widespread, however, the risks for Witnesses are declining, though they still remain higher than for persons receiving competently performed surgery with blood where needed. For a variety of reasons, the use of transfusion is no longer virtually automatic in major surgery even where religious belief is not an issue; some conjecture that this can be attributed to better surgical and laser techniques as well as to volume expanders developed partly in response to the dilemmas that surgery on Jehovah's Witnesses had presented.

Similarly, until very recently there has been no controlled study of the mortality of Christian Scientists compared with persons accepting conventional medical care. A 1989 report in the *Journal of the American Medical Association* comparing mortality data for the graduating classes from 1934 to 1983 at Principia College in Elsah, Illinois, a small liberal arts college for Christian Scientists, with a control population of graduating classes from the College of Liberal Arts and Sciences at the University of Kansas in Lawrence found that the death rate for Christian Science alumni was significantly higher—especially for women.[27] That their religious practices increase the risk of ill health or death would, of course, be disputed by many Christian Scientists—who sincerely believe that theirs is a tradition of consistent, effective healing—and perhaps by the Faith Assembly and Holiness churches as well. Nevertheless, there is no persuasive evidence to the contrary, and there is good reason to think that the risks are in fact substantially elevated in all these groups: they forgo blood transfusions, they avoid medical treatment known to be effective, and they handle poisonous snakes.

Altering Risk Behavior

That the members of these four religious groups exhibit distinctive commonalities in risk budget and style that fall well outside the risk budgets and styles of most other persons in society is evident enough, but these commonalities do not all arise in the same way. If we examine the practices and policies of the four groups more closely, four quite different mechanisms are in evidence by which these commonalities are produced. Each involves autonomy-compromising interference with the paradigmatic decision-making structure at a different point. It is the varying nature of the interferences that renders the practices of each group subject to a different point of moral critique and that makes it possible to distinguish between those interferences that are morally defensible and those that are not. In the actual world of religious practice, of course, none of the mechanisms ascribed to each of these groups occurs in isolation, and each group has some of the features of the others— as do many other religious groups as well. Nevertheless, these mechanisms—artificially isolated here—are clearly most prominent in and distinctive of these groups.

COERCION

One way a religious group (or any group) can alter the risk-taking behavior of its members is by coercion. Within the Faith Assembly, although some members voluntarily accepted its policy of refusing medical treatment, others—according to the accounts of the two Fort Wayne reporters—did so only under threat of other sanctions. These included public humiliation, repudiation by spouses, friends, and other members of the group, and expulsion from the group altogether. Coercion operates by introducing a new outcome variable into the calculation that the risk taker makes. Not only must the risk taker weigh the probabilities and costs or benefits of possible negative or positive outcomes, but also the very large cost that will be imposed if he or she refuses to take the risk. Coercion thus suppresses the possibility of the initial choice. The force of the coercive measure is a function of the perceived costs to be imposed and the likelihood that the measure will actually be imposed, weighed against the costs and benefits of the risk itself. However, such sanctions are typically viewed as virtually certain to be imposed—especially those that involve not only institutional discipline but humiliation and rejection within the group. A number of religious groups, especially among the cults and new religions, are said to use coercion in securing compliance with fasting, socialization, work regimens, expressions of loyalty and group commitment, and the contribution of one's financial and other resources to the group: the Oakland Family of the Unification Church, or Moonies, and the International Society for Krishna Consciousness, or Hare Krishna, are often cited in this regard. The People's Temple at Jonestown provided no doubt the most horrifying example. Within the Faith Assembly, the sanctions were comparatively mild, but still strong enough to produce compliance in many cases where the risks apparently would not have been voluntarily sustained.

ALTERING RISK STYLES

A second way a religious group can alter the risk-taking conduct of its members is by altering their risk styles. For instance, a group may work to make its members consider certain choices more carefully than they ordinarily might, often to the individual's ultimate advantage. This may be the effect of much of the pastoral marriage counseling that many mainstream and other religious groups provide, since counseling usually encourages the individual not to leave a marriage impetuously or in temporary anger, but only after sustained reflection, thought, and prayer. However, some religiously induced changes in risk style appear to work in the other direction, toward less considered, less cautious styles of taking risks; it is these that present deeper moral issues.

Among serpent-handling groups, for instance, individual choices to touch or hold a snake appear not to be coerced; there is no sanction, either official or informal, during the prayer meeting or afterward for declining to handle snakes. Nor are snakes thrust upon people; those who choose to handle them must come forward to do so. Many members of Holiness churches where serpents are handled attend prayer meetings on a regular basis but never touch snakes. In fact, the teachings and traditions of this group explicitly encourage members to handle snakes only when they feel called or moved—"anointed"—to do so, and urge them not to do so otherwise. Persons are not blamed or chastised for failing to become anointed or for not handling snakes. Thus, serpent handling in the Holiness churches appears to be free of the kind of coercion characteristic of the Faith Assembly's refusal of medical treatment.

However, serpent-handling meetings involve active participation by many of the members. Services consist not only in singing and preaching, but in moving about the room, touching, shouting, and shrieking; this very high level of activity is sustained over several hours. These factors tend to produce an extremely heightened level of emotionality, which in turn invites the trembling, tactile hallucinations, glossolalia, and physical convulsions that members believe are the identifying signs of being anointed to handle snakes. But, according to the teachings and practices of the group, it is in precisely this (abnormal) condition that an individual's choice to handle serpents on this specific occasion must be made. One cannot decide in advance to handle snakes; one must wait to be "called." Reverend Robert Grooms describes his first anointing, which occurred at the Holiness Church of God in Jesus Name, Carson Springs, Tennessee, in 1970, in the following way: "It was like a bucket of water pouring over me. I was tingling all over. I was so anointed with the power that I was just shouting. . . . It's sort of like feeling the heat from a light bulb. It's tremendous. It came over me in such a fantastic way. I felt it through my whole body. I just went plumb out in under the power. But I knew exactly what it was for. God was telling me to take up the serpent."[28] This is the condition that the prosecution in *Swann v. Pack* called "so enraptured and entranced" that worshippers can be described as in a "virtual state of hysteria." It is in this agitated condition, then, that the risk of sudden death is undertaken.

While it is easy to point out the moral deficiencies of coercive alterations of risk budgets or styles, alterations brought about by producing heightened emotionality may be somewhat harder to assess. Under the principle of autonomy, recognized by both ordinary morality and professional ethics, self-harming choices ought not to be honored where emotion is heightened, at least not if it is so heightened as to impair the capacity for autonomous choice. Instead, paternalistic intervention may be necessary to protect autonomy where the individual's decision-making capacity is impaired. Nevertheless, we do in practice respect many sorts of risk-taking decisions made in emotionally heightened conditions, for instance, those made in love, in patriotic fervor, in moments of altruistic self-sacrifice, in daredevil sports adventures, in emergency rescues, and so on. Thus, we have rather ambivalent antecedent standards concerning impairment in risk-taking choices. It is not properly the actual risk involved in serpent handling that should arouse moral suspicion (especially since the risk of death from snakebite may not be greater than in certain dangerous sports, such as hang gliding), but rather the way in which the group engenders a highly charged emotional climate and then requires that risk-taking choices be made in this impaired condition.

Of course, the antecedent choice to attend a serpent-handling prayer meeting is not made under the same emotionally charged conditions, and thus is not subject to the same ethical reservations. However, participants claim that they do not know in advance whether they will in fact be anointed to handle snakes at a particular meeting; they do not decide in advance to handle snakes, but rather they simply decide to attend the meeting. Of course, to decide to attend the meeting is to decide to expose oneself to the risk of deciding to take the risk, but it is not a decision made while confronting the snakes or in the volatile surroundings of the prayer meeting. The specific decision to handle snakes is not made during earlier, calmer, or presumably more rational moments—namely, those moments in which a serpent handler might say "I'm afraid of snakes like anybody else"—but only at the meeting under the extraordinary conditions that occur there.

ALTERING RISK BUDGETS

Even when the risk taker's prudential calculation is neither skewed by the imposition of coercively large costs for failing to take the risk nor made in an emotionally heightened condition, there are still two further ways this calculation can be distorted. Like any other group, a religious group can influence the individual's estimate of the probability of the various outcomes he or she foresees, or it can change the evaluations assigned by the individual to these outcomes, or both. In both cases, the effect of the influence is not to coerce choice or to impair its quality by altering risk style, but to alter the individual's risk budget.

ALTERING ASSESSMENTS OF PROBABILITIES

A person reasonably conversant with the circumstances of the world knows certain facts: that malnourishment impairs health, that rattlesnakes are poisonous, that acute appendicitis can be fatal, and so on. These commonplaces are as familiar to the religious person as to the nonreligious; they are part of the common stock of background information shared within a culture. Hence, the religious risk taker— at least when the risks are understood to be common, physical ones—will have a fair amount of background knowledge about the risks he or she takes. A snake handler knows that rattlesnake bites can be fatal; that is what makes snake handling important and why it serves as a test of faith.[29] Similarly, Faith Assembly members know that hemorrhage in childbirth can be fatal; that is why it is a test of commitment to the church's beliefs to refuse treatment and why Sally Burkitt pleaded for a doctor instead. Of course, in many cases religious risk takers will not know the precise degree of risk involved—as most of us do not know the precise risk from hemorrhage in childbirth or from untreated rattlesnake bites—but we all share a general conception of the relative dangers of these threats. It is against this background conception of general estimates of danger that religious risk taking occurs.

Yet it is possible to change an individual's estimate of the likelihood that various possible outcomes will occur. Given an array of evaluated possible outcomes, this may involve making specific positively valued outcomes seem more likely, or making specific negatively valued ones seem less likely, or both, so that a recalculation of the risk would result in a different choice.

Take, for instance, the case of the Christian Scientist with acute appendicitis who seeks relief. Like other members of contemporary society, he or she will have some background understanding of the likelihood that untreated appendicitis could result in death. Although this is by no means a scientifically rigorous conception, the person can say, for instance, that the likelihood of death is greater in untreated appendicitis than in, for example, untreated influenza. However, the teachings of the individual's church persuade him or her that although this background information is accepted by nonbelievers and correctly describes the probabilities confronting them, the probabilities are quite different for persons who understand the nonphysical nature of illness, the power of Christian Science healing, and the true nature of prayer. The believer holds that achieving a correct understanding of illness as resulting from defective mental attitudes will free him or her from illness—even when the risks would otherwise be very high—and that the way to achieve this correct understanding is in prayer. Thus, the Christian Scientist will hold, the risk of death from acute appendicitis treated only with Christian Science prayer is, in fact, much lower than the shared cultural conception would insist—in fact, that it is actually lower not only than the risk from untreated appendicitis but lower than the risk in appendicitis treated with conventional medicine. Prayer, in this view, is the most effective treatment of all. This shared perception of risk explains why Christian Scientists exhibit similar, though unusual, risk budgets in medical choices of this sort; but it also invites us to ask how this shared perception of risk is attained.

How does the believing Christian Scientist reach this still lower estimate of the probability of death? Let us look at the kind of evidence with which the believer is supplied and upon which he or she bases prudential calculations of risk.

Support for claims of the efficacy of Christian Science healing, following the pattern of assertions made in *Science and Health with Key to the Scriptures* and other writings of Mary Baker Eddy, is provided largely by the testimonials of those who recount the ways in which they have been healed from disease or injury. These testimonials are typically quite detailed and fervently sincere in tone; they are direct, firsthand accounts of what is often an extremely powerful, faith-confirming experience. For example, a woman living in the Mojave Desert area of California writes: "On a warm afternoon last May while coming into our house through the laundry room (which is part of the garage), I felt a sharp pain in my right foot. Looking down, I saw what appeared to be a rattlesnake, disappearing under the washing machine."[30] She goes on to recount her fear, the assistance of the Christian Science practitioner in praying for her recovery, the development and eventual subsiding of a discolored, numb swelling on her foot, and the confirming effects this experience had upon her faith.

This testimonial is typical of the handful published in each issue of the *Christian Science Journal,* a monthly periodical widely circulated among Christian Scientists and, like the weekly *Christian Science Sentinel,* a primary source of information about the church. The *Journal* asserts that "the statements made in these testimonies with regard to healings have been carefully verified,"[31] and that it retains on file the originals of testimonials together with the three written verifications or vouchers required for publication. Since 1900, some 53,900 testimonials of healing have been published in the periodicals of the church; they are said to be "the most important body of evidence concerning Christian Science healing."[32]

According to a First Church of Christ, Scientist, authority defending healing in a recent issue of the *New England Journal of Medicine,* a careful examination of testimonials published in Christian Science periodicals between 1971 and 1981 shows "647 testimonies concerning illnesses that had been medically diagnosed, in some cases both before and after a healing . . . [including] leukemia and other neoplasias, both malignant and benign; diptheria; gallstones; pernicious anemia; club feet; spinal meningitis; and bone fracture, among numerous others."[33] This figure includes 137 pediatric cases. Healing in such cases might seem to constitute an impressive record. But the record is wholly anecdotal in form, appealing simply to isolated cases without reference either to general patterns or trends or to comparisons based on control groups. The effect of this kind of information—independently of whether the claims are actually true—is to exacerbate one of the most common, frequent errors in decision-making under risk.

Many kinds of error are possible in risk-taking choice. Objective errors include misidentification of the range of possible outcomes and assignment of faulty probabilities to possible outcomes (often as the product of subjective factors such as unwarranted optimism or pessimism), misidentification of the values one assigns to possible outcomes, self-deception, and so on. But there is a common, documentable error characteristic of rational choice, frequently discussed with reference to informed consent in medical situations. This is the tendency to overrely on case information and to underrely on base-rate information.[34] Ordinary patients in ordinary medical contexts do this: they tend to base decisions on anecdotal accounts, supplied by physicians, friends, personal experience, or other sources, and to downplay or ignore information about the rates of incidence of specific conditions, side effects, self-limiting conditions, spontaneous recovery, and so on. But while ordinary medical patients do this rather naturally, Christian Scientists in situations of medical risk are in effect encouraged to do so, since they are supplied with information that makes miscalculation inevitable. What are *not* available from the Christian Science church or from its publications are data that might counteract this tendency or that could contribute to establishing reliable base-rate information: How often, given a specific medical condition, does Christian Science healing appear to be effective? This is a much easier question to answer than "How often is Christian Science healing actually effective?"—but even for the easier question about apparent results no data are available.

Clearly, 647 documented cases over a ten-year period is sparse evidence, in view of the number of Scientists and the frequency within the general population of the diseases involved. There might, of course, be many undiagnosed, undocumented cases or a lower incidence of the conditions among the Christian Science population, but these conjectures do little to provide the Christian Scientist with a reliable sense of the frequency with which Christian Science healing, once attempted, is effective. Testimonials of failures are, of course, not published in the church's periodicals. Furthermore, the lack of negative information is compounded by false positives—cases in which Christian Science healing is credited with the cure of a condition that was self-limiting or would have resolved spontaneously anyway—as when the cold that vanishes after troubling a person for two weeks is taken as proof that Christian Science really works.[35] Even the account by the woman bitten by the rattlesnake under her washing machine should be seen in light of the fact that rattlesnake bites, especially at distant sites on a limb (the woman was bitten on the foot), are comparatively seldom fatal; but this information was not provided. Yet it is only with adequate base-rate information, making it possible to calculate overall frequencies of success and failure in non-self-limiting conditions with given forms of treatment, that a person can rationally compare conventional medical treatment with Christian Science healing of the same condition, and make a choice in an informed way.[36]

To assert that Christian Science healing cannot be chosen on a rational basis is, of course, not to assume that Christian Science healing is in fact less effective than conventional medical therapy (a point possibly conceded by some critics of the group, given substantial rates of iatrogenic illness in conventional treatment and the fact that a very large proportion—variously estimated at 75 or 80 percent—of the "illnesses" initially seen by physicians are either self-limiting or psychogenic in origin), but only to point out that the basis on which a Christian Scientist makes a choice in seeking relief from symptoms is not rationally defensible. Christian Science healing might, in fact, be more effective than conventional medicine, but even the Christian Scientist would have no way of knowing this. Yet the church does claim to supply persuasive, empirical *evidence* for the efficacy of healing; this is part of the point of *Science and Health with Key to the Scriptures* and part of the point of providing testimonials at all.

Nicholas Rescher takes the crucial distinction in risk assessment to be that between *realistic* and *unrealistic* appraisal.[37] But despite the fact that the individual Christian Scientist's choice to rely on Christian Science healing is not rationally defensible, it cannot be said to be unrealistic in a general sense. This is because the individual Scientist has not exaggerated, underestimated, misinterpreted, or otherwise misapprehended or distorted the available evidence. Given the evidence he or she has, the tools provided for assessing it, and the surrounding claim of a trusted institution that the evidence is compelling, he or she makes a subjectively realistic assessment; the fault is not the Scientist's, given that he or she is both a believer and a member of the church. In fact, the Christian Scientist characteristically believes that such a choice is a good, sound decision based on a large body of compelling evidence—evidence that, though ignored by non-Scientists, is rationally persuasive. As one Scientist wrote;

> My own family has relied on Christian Science for generations. I have never considered prayer a gamble. Please understand: I'm not speaking of some crude kind of "faith healing" that implores God to heal and says it was His will if nothing happens. I'm speaking of responsible spiritual healing practiced now over a century by many perfectly normal citizens and caring parents.
>
> I'm concerned about not being taken seriously—that nobody in the media . . . is really taking into account that these healings have been happening over many

years. Not just in my family, not just my friends. I'm speaking of the massive, long-term experience in a whole denomination.[38]

If this believer's assessment of risk is objectively unrealistic, any moral complaint must be directed not primarily against the believer, nor against church teachers and officials, since after all they too share the same set of assumptions as members of the church. Rather, blame should be directed primarily against the institutional perpetration of the claim that the evidence is valid, and the complaint should point out how the encouragement of belief in the efficacy of healing rather than objective confirmation of it compromises the possibility of autonomous choice. Of course, there is fault on both sides: the medical establishment has been as uninterested in examining alleged Christian Science healings (being generally content to assert that they must either be spontaneous recoveries—perhaps associated with the placebo effect—or have been inaccurately diagnosed in the first place) as Christian Science has been to provide well-documented evidence, in particular evidence scrutinized under contrary hypotheses.

But there is a further complexity to the risks Christian Scientists take in choosing healing over conventional medical treatment. Not all healing is successful; some people remain incapacitated, some are sent to Christian Science sanitariums or nursing homes, and some die. Christian Science teaching explains this at least in part as the result of a failure on the part of the patient to understand fully his or her own nature as a spiritual being or to pray adequately for release from incorrect attitudes; the devout Scientist believes that the risk of death from disease correctly understood and adequately prayed for is nil. But what the Scientist, devout or otherwise, is not encouraged to assess in making risk-taking choices is how likely it is that he or she will correctly understand and adequately pray for release from the condition. This crucially relevant factor in a prudential risk calculation under these religious assumptions is simply not brought into question or discussed, nor is any evidence bearing on it, anecdotal or otherwise, provided. How often does the explanation of a patient's failure to recover appeal to the claim that the patient failed to pray appropriately or had the wrong attitude? This information, too, is of great relevance in risk-taking choices, yet is nowhere forthcoming.

Furthermore (although there is some lack of agreement on this issue)[39] Christian Science generally holds that healing through prayer is incompatible with conventional medical treatment, since prayer consists in achieving an understanding of the nature of disease that contradicts the causal, physicalist assumptions of medicine. Stories abound of people being denied continuation of the services of a Christian Science practitioner if they also enter the care of a physician. Patients who enter Christian Science sanitariums receive care only from nurses who are members of the church and from church practitioners; the nurses are prohibited from doing anything "material" to evaluate or relieve disease and suffering.[40] Thus, although conventional physicians are quick to recognize the psychotherapeutic value of ordinary prayer by the patient, whatever advantages might accrue to the ordinary patient from a combination of medical treatment and religiously supported hope are not available to the Christian Scientist. Rather, the Scientist is forced to make a choice between therapies without knowing whether the chance of survival with both kinds of therapy is better or worse than with only one or the other. Christian Science periodicals do not print testimonials from persons who see doctors as well as healers, any more than they do from persons who see doctors alone.

The institutional practice of altering persons' risk budgets by providing only anecdotal information unaccompanied by base-rate data, as Christian Science does, and by ignoring the incidence of failed cases and of any special conditions that must obtain for the supposed course of action to be effective, fails to satisfy the third basic initial criterion for autonomous choice: not only must it be voluntary and rationally unimpaired, it must be adequately informed. It is true that anecdotal information of the kind provided in Christian Science periodicals can be extremely effective in stirring faith and may be of great significance in a person's life. It may well produce a sizable placebo effect. And it is possible that Christian Science healing is actually efficacious, even in cases of non-self-limiting, serious illness. But insofar as merely anecdotal information is put forward as the evidence for claims of efficacy in healing and as a basis for refusing conventional medical treatment, it is clearly an inadequate basis upon which to encourage people to take such substantial risks. Neither their reliance on religious healing nor their refusal of conventional medical treatment meets the conditions for "informed consent." Hence, if we are to assess the practices of this church in the same way we would assess those of medicine or other secular professions that encourage people to take life-threatening risks without granting them the right to give informed consent, we would be tempted to say that they involve manipulation, callousness, or deceit.

The analysis given here of evidentiary claims concerning the efficacy of non-medical healing applies not only to Christian Science, but to any religious group that appeals to alternative varieties of healing, whether the healing involves denominational practitioners, faith healers, or the assumed direct influence of a divine being. The Faith Assembly, for instance, regards Jesus as the sole physician, but, at least if the scant evidence available concerning this group is correct, relies on much the same persuasive structures (where it does not directly coerce) as does Christian Science to produce acceptance of its claim. So do individual faith healers of various sorts, groups such as the Church of the First Born and the Faith Tabernacle Congregation, and many of the contemporary "televangelist" preachers. One might also want to inquire into the way in which beliefs about the efficacy of healing are furthered at such institutions as the Roman Catholic shrine at Lourdes, as well as into the practices of groups which accept faith healing but do not reject conventional medical treatment, such as the Assemblies of God and certain charismatic subgroups of Catholicism and Anglicanism. Thus, while Christian Science may provide the most conspicuous example of a certain sort of religious intervention in high-risk decision making, it will have many features in common with other groups, and ethical censure, if it is appropriate at all, ought hardly be reserved for this group alone.

ALTERING EVALUATIONS OF OUTCOMES

In addition to altering assessments of probabilities, risk budgets can be altered by changing the evaluations that the risk taker assigns to various possible outcomes.

Since the prudential calculation the risk taker makes is the product of assessments of the probabilities of the various outcomes times the value he or she assigns to them, changing evaluations will alter risk behavior as effectively as altering estimates of probabilities.

The Jehovah's Witnesses, who refuse blood transfusions although they accept other components of medical treatment, accept a risk—death—that is as serious as that taken by serpent handlers, Christian Scientists, and members of the Faith Assembly. However, the prudential calculation that the Jehovah's Witness makes has quite different ingredients. Whereas the Christian Scientist seeks a cure for his or her illness (although the Scientist does not call it a "cure" nor recognize the condition as an "illness") and makes a decision whether to accept conventional medical treatment or to rely on Christian Science healing based on a calculation concerning the efficacy of the two forms of treatment, however ill-informed, the Jehovah's Witness, in contrast, does not seek a cure at all. To be sure, the Witness hopes to get well, and hopes not to die. But the primary commitment is to honor a prohibition that he or she believes to be divinely mandated, *whatever* the costs in health or life, in order to ensure eventual salvation. Of course, the Jehovah's Witness will be party to the culturally shared background information concerning the likelihood of death in whatever medical condition he or she is suffering, whether it is acute appendicitis or intestinal hemorrhage, but the church makes no attempt to alter the individual's assessment of these probabilities. What the church does instead is supply him or her with a reevaluation of outcome states.

The Jehovah's Witness suffering an intestinal hemorrhage, for instance, will have at least a general awareness (sometimes intensified by an unsympathetic surgeon) that the chance of surviving with both surgery and blood transfusion are good, but that the chances of surviving with surgery alone, without blood, are markedly reduced, though they are not so low as the chances of surviving without any treatment at all. The church does not disguise these facts, nor does it encourage the Witness to base his or her choice on anecdotal information in the absence of base-rate data. But there is something new in the picture here, not much evident in the Christian Scientist's choice between medicine and healing as the better risk for staying alive: the Jehovah's Witness sees the choice as one for maximizing the chances of eternal life rather than temporal existence. Clearly, the Witness does not want to die; otherwise, he or she would not consent to surgery at all. But the believing Witness wants something else still more, obeying the divine command because he or she believes that failure to do so might end all hope of salvation. Thus, although the believer's prudential calculation is in structure just like the calculations made by the serpent handler, the Christian Scientist, and the member of the Faith Assembly, its scope includes a wider set of possible outcomes. This range of outcomes believed possible is expanded by the teachings of the church, which supplies not only the claim that there is such a condition as salvation, but a set of conditions for attaining it; it also identifies in its doctrines a particular act, accepting blood, that would preclude reaching this state.

To expand the range of possible outcomes a person foresees in this way has two associated consequences: it forces that person to reassess the disvalue he or she has assigned to the possible loss or adverse consequences previously expected, and it forces the person to reassess the value of the previously expected probable benefit or gain. Reassessment typically takes the form of diminution of the extreme values assigned to the previous best and worst outcomes, though they remain possibilities within the schema, and distinctively religious outcomes are substituted that now assume the most extreme values. These altered value rankings are so strongly bipolar and so extreme that one, salvation, acquires complete priority over the other, damnation, and over all intermediate outcome states as well. Life and death become trifles in the face of these new outcomes so that they come to play a subsidiary role, if any, in risk-taking choices.

It is this double substitution in the value rankings of outcomes that is characteristic of religious recommitment and conversion, and it is the adoption and maintenance of these value rankings that is central to much religious education and to convert seeking. (It is also this feature of reevaluation that distinguishes this type of risk-budget alteration from simple coercion, discussed earlier. There, additional sanctions were added to the individual's perceived range of outcomes, but this did not produce reevaluation of the initial possible outcomes foreseen.) A reevaluation of outcomes of this sort would have evident effects on the risk-taking calculation: virtually any risk that might secure salvation would be worth it, whether it cost one's life or anything else, provided only that failure in the risk would not preclude future chances of achieving salvation after all. Similarly, one could venture *no* risk of damnation, no matter how attractive the intermediate gain.

To be sure, this starkly bipolar conception of an afterlife is too rigid and primitive for the many more liberal, contemporary forms of religious faith; heaven and hell in a hereafter are not the outcomes envisioned by every religious consciousness. Many religious groups (or at least the more liberal elements within them), especially among mainstream Protestants and some Catholics, have been discarding traditional notions of the afterlife. But this does not diminish the capacity of the more liberal religious groups to alter their members' evaluations of outcome states in risk-taking situations. For some modern groups, "heaven" and "hell" are taken to apply to conditions of this world, and there is no life after death; heaven and hell label states of human consciousness, but are equally strongly to be sought or avoided. These states are not to be confused with pleasure and pain or happiness and unhappiness. Borrowing Catholic terminology, they might best be called "beatitude" and "sin," though this conception is by no means confined to Catholicism. They are distinctively *religious* conditions, though they may on occasion coincide with positive and negative hedonic states.

The more contemporary interpretations of traditional afterlife notions exhibit a second way in which religious groups can alter evaluations of outcomes in risk-taking calculations; they can divert the individual's assignment of maximal value from secular states of happiness, pleasure, or utility, generally defined, to the distinctively religious condition of this-world beatitude. This change might seem to be merely terminological, if an individual is simply to switch risk-taking strategies from maximizing utility in the secular sense to achieving this-world beatitude: it is still the state the individual most strongly prefers. But while secular states of pleasure or happiness are by and large identifiable both by the agent and, though less reliably, by external observers, it is the religious group, drawing on the theological tradition behind it, that stipulates what counts as beatitude. It is also the religious group that defines the conditions for identifying it. Thus, the religious group both promotes achieving the state and urges the believer to be willing to risk all to gain it, and yet at the same time identifies what that state is and provides instructions ("discipline") concerning how to attain it. For some strains of Catholicism, for instance, this-world beatitude seems to be identified with "the beauty of suffering": what one should want most is to be like Christ and to feel the full measure of Christ's sacrifice. In other strains of the same tradition, it is identified with humility, with mystic transport, or with complete self-sacrificing charity. In still other traditions, particularly those influenced by Eastern religions, the maximally valued state (often called "enlightenment") is stipulated as egolessness, detachment, or perhaps complete obedience to a "master." The range of this-world conditions that are identified as maximally valued possible outcomes may vary widely from group to group, but in each case it is the religious group that identifies the condition and assigns both its preeminent status in the believer's value schema and its capacity to reevaluate or eclipse ordinary value rankings. It is in this way that a religious group alters the risk budgets and hence the risk behavior of its members, first by stipulating what sorts of outcomes they should be willing to risk serious harm or death to attain and then by urging them to take the risk.

Looking back at the three forms of intervention in high-risk decision making previously described, it is easy to see where moral analysis gains a foothold. The Faith Assembly methods involved clear-cut coercion, at least on some occasions. The Holiness churches avoid coercion but foster a kind of circumstantial manipulation resulting in impairment of decision-making capacities. Inasmuch as Christian Science practices involve providing only partial, misleading information wholly inadequate for the sort of choice to be made, they involve manipulation, callousness, or deception. Coercion, manipulation, deliberate impairment, callousness, and deception are familiar themes in moral analysis. But risk encouragement by a reevaluation of outcomes, as occurs among the Jehovah's Witnesses, may prove a difficult matter to assess by ordinary moral analysis. There are two principal reasons for this difficulty. First, since encouraging risk taking in this way does not seem to involve coercion, deception, or impairment of the individual's reasoning processes—at least not to the same conspicuous degree as in the three other groups examined here—it does not appear to violate the conditions of autonomous choice. Second, the reevaluation of values is a familiar, accepted strategy for behavioral change and is characteristic of many other enterprises: education, psychotherapy, moral training, discipline, criminal justice, and so on. In each of these areas, reevaluation proceeds by persuading the individual that the old goals, aims, fears, objectives, and so on, were unsophisticated, immoral, or foolish, and by encouraging him or her to accept new, better, healthier ones. The new goals then assume preeminent status; as the older ones are completely eclipsed or recede into triviality, the reevaluation is achieved.

Although reevaluation may make use of a variety of specific techniques, moral objections to deliberate alteration of an individual's valuation of outcomes, where it does not involve coercion, deception, or impairment of reasoning processes, typically attach not to the fact or methods of reevaluation but to the altered valuation itself. Regardless of its methods, we object when an institution—a school, for example—attempts to turn a humanitarian into a bigot, but are much less likely to object when a similar institution using similar methods seeks to reverse the process. By and large, we take the reevaluation to be a salutary one when it assigns greater importance to rationally defensible value rankings such as happiness over unhappiness, pleasure over pain, beauty over ugliness, health over illness, compassion over cruelty, and so forth, both for the agent and for those affected by the agent's actions. However, in a religious context like that of the Jehovah's Witnesses, the reevaluation can move outside the range of rationally defensible value rankings to assign preeminent status to distinctively religious conditions.

It is this that makes it difficult to evaluate some forms of risk taking in religion and to assess the means by which some religious groups elicit such behavior. The altering of risk budgets by reevaluation of outcomes that characterizes Jehovah's Witness practice should, presumably, be evaluated by assessing the actual moral value of those outcomes that are assigned the highest rank in the individual's new evaluative scheme. Of course, it is not possible to supply morally objective, non-faith-based assessments of these outcomes, nor for that matter objective, non-faith-based evidence for the reality or attainability of such outcomes. The Jehovah's Witness may be quite willing to risk death by refusing blood transfusions in order to attain salvation, but he or she has only faith-based "evidence" that there is such a thing as salvation or that keeping the commandment to avoid blood will be instrumental in attaining it. Similarly, the traditional Catholic who seeks beatitude in suffering has only faith-based evidence, supplied by the doctrines or teachings of the church, to assure him or her of the intrinsic superiority of this condition over pleasure, happiness, or other secular states. Nonbelievers will be skeptical of both claims and hence quite ready to say that these (erroneously) expected outcomes do not warrant the risks made in their names. Consequently, the skeptics will further argue, the institutional church that promotes risk taking to achieve these outcomes has no warrant for controlling the behavior of its adherents in this way. It may be one thing to hold or even teach such beliefs; it is quite another, the skeptics will add, to encourage or require persons to make high-risk personal decisions based on these beliefs, especially when it may cost them their lives. Where religious risk taking is elicited by a reevaluation of outcome states in a way that deviates from rationally defensible rankings of outcomes, there is no way to defend such practices but little way to denounce them either, since they are to be evaluated on the basis of religious outcome values that cannot be assumed either true or false. Thus risk encouragement by reevaluation cannot be attacked in the direct way that risk encouragement can be attacked when it proceeds by coercion, impairment, or deception, but it cannot be granted a clean bill of ethical health either.

It is now possible to see why it is often difficult, in the religious situations covered here, to distinguish between decisions under risk and those under uncertainty. In many or most of these decision situations, the individual has very little, if any, knowledge of the actual probability of the outcomes he or she can foresee; objectively, decision is made under uncertainty. But in most cases a believer's religious group supplies both a general conception of the likelihood of various outcomes and a conception of what the range of possible outcomes is, though these conceptions are likely to be conveyed by trading on hopes, conveying promises, supplying assurances, discounting counterevidence, and so on. Significantly, the religious group typically supplies the believer with a conception that the probabilities are very strongly favorable ("Since Jesus loves you, mere serpents cannot harm you"), though he or she has little or no objective evidence that this is so. Thus the individual *believes* he or she knows the probability of possible outcomes; subjectively speaking, the choice appears to be a decision under risk, though to an external view, it is a decision made under uncertainty of the most complete sort.

The Doctrinal Status of Risk Taking

To show that risk-taking religious conduct occurs in various forms and with various amounts of risk in various religious groups is not yet to reach a normative conclusion. It cannot simply be assumed that the making of decisions in which one risks death is wrong, nor can it be assumed that there is something wrong with the mechanisms that religious groups employ to influence people in making these decisions—however extreme the risks, however manipulative the manner of encouraging them, and however severe the consequences for both the risk taker and for others. These are the features that an examination of religious practices using professional ethics exposes; yet to identify features is not to establish that they are morally intolerable, since such conduct is governed not only by moral considerations, but also by the doctrines, teachings, and authoritative pronouncements of the specific religious groups.

In examining the issue of confidentiality in confession in the previous chapter [of *Ethics in the Sanctuary*], a typology was developed to distinguish various levels of doctrinal assertions with respect to the ethical dilemmas involved. The typology recognizes four distinct levels or orders of doctrinal assertions: zero-order or base-level doctrines, the fundamental imperatives of a group (often, though not always, stated in scriptural texts); first-order doctrines or teachings, which stipulate ways of putting basic imperatives into practice but which characteristically generate new moral problems in doing so; second-order doctrines or teachings, which establish a position that attempts to resolve the ethical problems presented by first-order doctrines; and third-order doctrines or teachings, which function as excuses for residual moral problems. This four-level typology provides a basis for distinguishing the more fundamental religious imperatives of a group from dictates that, though they may have achieved similar doctrinal status, exhibit later historical or theoretical development within a tradition and are best viewed as "answers" to and "excuses" for the moral problems posed by the fundamental imperatives and the ways they are put into practice. Because of their derivative status, whatever doctrinal position they may enjoy, they are to be treated as initially more vulnerable to ethical review than the basic imperatives of the tradition within which they arise.

In surveying the huge variety of risk-taking practices evident among various Christian and Christian-influenced groups, this typology serves to differentiate between those risk-taking dictates that are more vulnerable and those that are less vulnerable to ethical criticism. Of course, since the risk-taking practices described here do not form a coherent, unified, single tradition but occur in a spectrum of denominations and sects with differing histories, application of this typology will not be completely tidy or uniform. Nevertheless, it is possible to identify doctrines, directives, teachings, and other authoritative pronouncements at all four levels.

This identification is most difficult at the zero-order, base level, since most Christian groups do not point to a single, explicit statement of a risk-taking command in their scriptural texts in the same way that they point, for instance, to scriptural commandments to confess. Although suggestive biblical passages do exist, they do not yield a clear, fundamental imperative. Nevertheless, even in the absence of explicit biblical texts that clearly mandate the taking of risks, it is fair to characterize Christianity, with its history of heroism, persecution, and voluntary martyrdom, as a religion of personal commitment and sacrifice: it is a religion in which one must be fully committed and "risk one's all" for God. (This feature of Christianity is particularly evident when compared to Hinduism, Buddhism, and other Eastern religious traditions.) Of course, Christianity also offers comforts, including assurances of divine benevolence and of eventual personal salvation, but these comforts are available only to those who are willing to risk themselves for the faith. Christianity, at least in its earlier forms, is not simply a religion of gradual, confident, relatively automatic self-development and unfolding, but a religion in which one's future is always at stake: one is dared, so to speak, to put one's faith in God, even when doing so will invite hardship, sacrifice, penalty, or death.

If this central challenge to risk oneself in religious commitment constitutes the fundamental, albeit penumbral imperative underlying religious risk taking—that is, the making of high-risk decisions by opting to take the risk—the emergence of first-order doctrines stipulating *how* the risk is to be taken can be expected. Here there are two divergent developments that become increasingly distinct in later, post-Reformation periods of Christian history. In some groups, teachings emerge that interpret risk as a matter of faith or belief and do not promote physical risk to health or life at all. It is coming to *believe* certain things that, in these traditions, constitutes the risk one must take for God. Risk lies in the "leap of faith," not in the danger of bodily harm. The tendency to treat the risks of religious commitment as wholly mental, emotional, or spiritual is characteristic of the Protestant tradition and of some recent contemplative, Eastern-influenced Christian groups as well. Catholicism, with its traditional emphasis on fasting, mortifications of the flesh, celibacy, pilgrimage, crusade, and martyrdom, has not always interpreted the risks of religious commitment in a wholly mentalized way. Contemporary mainstream Catholicism—except perhaps for its monastic communities, political activist groups, penitential communities, and organizations such as Opus Dei—may now much more closely resemble Protestant practice. At the other extreme, the groups considered here understand the risks that religious commitment poses as primarily physical, though the distinction is not sharp and psychological risks may be intertwined with them. No doubt, many of the members of groups that construe risk as largely mental would say that they are prepared to risk their lives and physical selves should the occasion demand it; but they do not belong to groups that have adopted high-risk behavior *as a practice* of the group. It is this latter feature that is central to the groups considered here. Thus the crucial distinction at this first level of doctrinal development concerns institutionalized risk-taking practices, which determine how the fundamental imperative is to be honored, and specifically whether these practices are institutionalized primarily as mental or as physical risks.

These schematic claims may seem to raise again the "relativism" issue: How can zero-level imperatives be identified reliably? Even if the historical account given here of the general relationship between the fundamental Christian imperative to risk one's all and derivative, upper-order practices interpreting these as mental or physical risks seems intuitively accurate, the groups discussed in this chapter will not seem to fit this model very well. However, there is a reason for this: these groups are not representative of the full scope of practices associated with the fundamental imperative, but only a small part of it. To display the full spectrum of risk-taking practices characteristic of Christianity, we would need to include groups ranging from mainline Protestantism, where risk is typically understood to be largely mental, if any risk is undertaken at all, to those groups whose practices involve such complete submission to physical harm that it barely seems meaningful to speak of "risk." Such groups might include some that are no longer extant, such as the second- and third-century North African Donatists, who deliberately courted martyrdom at the hands of the Romans, or the Donatist subgroup called the Circumcellions, who in addition practiced religiously motivated suicide. Groups engaging in high-risk penitential practices might also be included, like the Spanish-American group found in the high plateaus of the Sangre de Cristo mountains in northern New Mexico and southern Colorado, the Brothers of Jesus of Nazareth, better known as the Penitentes. The Penitentes' practices involve reenactment of Jesus' passion and crucifixion; they are performed by flagellating oneself, enduring severe scourging with cactus whips, and dragging huge wooden crosses up a hill. Although the practice of using nails to fix the penitent to the cross was last observed in 1908,[41] these penances still sometimes result in fatalities. However, these more extreme groups are not the focus here. In this chapter, unlike the previous one, a range of groups chosen to represent the broadest variety of possibilities for expression of a fundamental imperative well distributed across a spectrum is not addressed. Focus, rather, is on a few groups that exhibit similarities and differences within a much tighter range. Even within these limits, it is still possible to differentiate upper-order, developed practices within a group from its basic zero-level doctrines.

For example, in the serpent-handling groups it is Mark 16 that serves as a zero-level imperative—a basic, nonnegotiable, fundamental commandment, functioning in approximately the same way that Matthew 18 did in the Collinsville Church of Christ's disciplining of Marian Guinn. Similarly, the serpent-handling groups observe a highly specific imperative, one that if honored at all in other groups would be viewed as derivative from a more general mandate. But while the serpent-handling groups take Mark 16 as basic, this passage stipulates nothing about how serpents are to be handled. It does not say how, where, when, or with whom serpents are to be handled, or even whether serpent handling is to be initiated at all, rather than performed only in response to confrontation with a snake. The Holiness churches have developed practices that settle these questions: serpents are to be handled on a specific occasion—the prayer meeting; in a specific location—the church; in the presence of other individuals—the congregation; and in ways that pose very substantial risks—picking them up, coiling them around one's arms, trunk, or neck, and doing so without protective equipment or surgical devenomization of the snakes. The how, where, when, and with whom questions that Mark 16 does not answer are made determinate in these practices; they are first-order practices, developed to put the basic imperative into practice. Of course, the biblical imperative to handle serpents could have been put into practice in various forms. For instance, it could have been taken to require handling snakes alone, in the woods, without music, singing, praying, or other background noise. It could have been taken not to encourage handling snakes, but only to require not avoiding them when they are encountered. The minister of a West Virginia Full Gospel church that does not practice serpent handling explained that he interpreted the phrase "they shall take up serpents," as it occurs in the King James translation of the Bible—the one most serpent handlers would be familiar with—as instructing people to "remove" snakes where they find them.[42] To put the biblical commandment concerning serpents into practice by handling serpents *at religious services* is already a developed, upper-order practice and hence one open to ethical critique. Of course, this developed, first-order practice of handling serpents at religious services poses obvious moral problems, among them those of voluntariness and of danger to participants and observers. To "answer" these moral problems, second-order doctrines and practices emerge: those recognizing the distinctive condition of anointment and holding that it is prerequisite to handling snakes; those discouraging criticism of church members who do not handle snakes, those precluding offering snakes to visitors or to children, and so on. These are all ways of minimizing the physical and emotional damage the practice itself can create; but these doctrines, too, are open to ethical review.

Similarly, for Jehovah's Witnesses, the zero-level imperatives the group observes can be identified by inspecting the texts it regards as fundamental: Genesis 9:4 and similar passages prohibiting the drinking of blood. The group's developed practices are those that involve interpreting these biblical passages as applying to blood transfusions (after all, transfusions are not explicitly mentioned in the Bible) and the structures of religious education and reinforcement that promote this interpretive teaching. Here, obviously, it may be difficult to distinguish the development of a practice from the development of an interpretation; but as in all groups, the development of a practice occurs simultaneously with the emergence of a doctrinal interpretation. The distinctive nature of the Jehovah's Witness interpretation and practice based on Genesis 9:4 and other texts can be more clearly seen by contrasting it with that of Judaism, where the same texts prohibiting the eating or drinking of blood are differently interpreted as dietary laws and have developed together with an extensive code of kosher slaughtering, food preparation, and food serving.

Within the practices examined here, some risks eventuate badly: some persons who take these physical risks suffer serious damage to their health; some die. The typological model employed here predicts the emergence of a further level of doctrinal, quasi-doctrinal, or authoritative claim, identified as third-order doctrine, that provides "excuses" for the residual moral problems the practices in question generate. For instance, when a Christian Scientist practicing his or her beliefs by relying on healing refuses conventional medical treatment and dies, some account consistent with both the basic doctrinal imperative and with the first- and second-order teachings is needed to explain or justify the negative outcome. Similarly, since serpent handlers act to honor the assertion in Mark 16 that "they will pick up snakes in their hands, and if they drink any deadly thing, it will not hurt them," the group's continued acceptance of the basic religious imperative depends in part on providing a doctrinally acceptable account of how snakebites and snakebite fatalities can occur—that is, an excuse for the negative outcome resulting from the risks a person takes in relying on the scriptural assurance that no harm will come from handling snakes.

These third-order teachings or excuses for failed risks are usually easy to identify, though they are not always encoded in official doctrine. When a Christian Scientist who refuses medical treatment and relies on prayer worsens or dies, the most frequent explanation, as observed earlier, is that he or she failed to pray adequately and hence failed to achieve the proper understanding of the nature of disease. Similarly, the Faith Assembly member who dies after refusing treatment is said to have lacked faith in Jesus' power to heal—an accusation so prevalent in this group that Hobart Freeman extended it even to those who use automobile seat belts. The serpent handler who is bitten is sometimes said to have failed to be sure he or she was genuinely anointed before taking up the snakes. For instance, in an informative cautionary tale circulated among serpent handlers, the story is told of a woman who *planned* to display her powers to handle snakes at a prayer meeting the following Sunday. She kept a snake in a jar for this very purpose. When she took out the snake at the announced time she was bitten and died—clearly, so the tale holds, because she had failed to wait for the appropriate anointing by God. A variant form of excuse appeals to higher purposes. For instance, not long before receiving a bite on the toe, Reverend Clyde Ricker of Hot Springs, North Carolina, offered this account: "I'd say that if I get bit, and I swell up, that's not a sign that I denied the faith, or that I wasn't anointed . . . God was just using me to prove to somebody that the serpents have teeth, and to show what snakes can do to you."[43]

Not only is it easy to identify these third-order teachings or excuses for the negative outcomes that a group's risk-taking practices have brought about, but it is easy to see a common feature of many of them. They explain the negative outcome as a result of a failure on the part of the individual harmed. This is true in the Faith Assembly, the Holiness churches, and Christian Science. Even Clyde Ricker's prescient attempt to explain the bite on his toe as "God using me to prove that serpents have teeth" is preceded by an attempt to defuse the usual institutional explanations—that he denied the faith or was not anointed. Thus, in examining the excuses various groups encode in their doctrines, we can begin by considering whether excuses that lay the blame for unsuccessful risk taking at the feet of the risk taker are themselves morally defensible, or whether a defensible excuse must be of some other form.

In contrast, the Jehovah's Witnesses appear to offer no excuse when a Witness refuses transfusion and dies. Notice, however, that under the reevaluation that is characteristic of Jehovah's Witness practice, there is nothing to excuse. The faithful Witness who dies because he or she refuses blood—according to the teachings of the group—nevertheless achieves salvation, even if it means the loss of life. Achieving salvation is, under the reevaluation, the maximally valued outcome the choice could yield, whereas losing one's life under the reevaluation assumes much lesser importance. Consequently, for the devout, the death need not be excused.

The Moral Evaluation of Risk Taking in Religion

In looking at the practices of our four specimen groups, it has been tempting to draw the immediate conclusion that these practices cannot be morally defended—and, furthermore, that they should be denounced on moral grounds. We have already established that the developed practices and teachings of religious groups, as distinct from the fundamental imperatives, are vulnerable to ethical critique, and when we now look at these practices, we see that they involve clear abuses of identifiable, uncontroversial moral principle. In examining issues in confidentiality [in the previous chapter of *Ethics in the Sanctuary*], we found practices that variously involved lying, nonconsenting disclosure, manipulation, and the permitting of serious, preventable harms. In looking at issues in risk taking in this chapter, we find coercion, impairment of rational capacities, manipulation, callousness, and deception. No doubt we could look further and find more. But to identify these apparent moral abuses is not to establish that they are abuses in religious contexts; we have only seen them this way because we instinctively appeal to principles familiar in secular life. Yet even though we have established that certain religious doctrines and practices are open to ethical evaluation, we cannot simply assume that the principles presupposed by this catalogue of apparent abuses are applicable here.

Of the moral principles these apparent abuses seem to violate, that of autonomy is central. This principle is highlighted by the strategy of using the apparatus of professional ethics to examine issues of religious risk taking—in particular the concept of informed consent. The principle of autonomy, received in both its Kantian form and in the utilitarian version defended by John Stuart Mill, is not itself contested in either ordinary or professional ethics, though there certainly are continuing, vigorous debates about how it should be interpreted, about the degree to which individuals are capable of genuine autonomy, and about when, if ever, the principle may be overridden. This principle has been central in contemporary professional ethics. Here, too, disagreement virtually exclusively concerns the conditions under which paternalistic or harm-based exceptions to the principle are legitimate; there are no real challenges to the principle of autonomy itself.

Throughout our examination of the practices of various religious groups, both in confession and in high-risk decision making, we have seen repeated violations of autonomy. Though they are often explicated within professional ethics in more elaborate ways, the conditions for autonomous choice involve three criteria: (1) the decision must be uncoerced, (2) it must be rationally unimpaired, and (3) it must be adequately informed.

As we have seen, these are precisely the conditions that the practices of these groups violate. The Faith Assembly, at least on some occasions, coerces its members into refusing medical treatment. The Holiness serpent-handling groups encourage making potentially fatal decisions about handling snakes under extreme emotional impairment, calling that condition an anointment for taking the risk. Christian Science provides selective, anecdotal information only, without base or failure rates, in a way that is inevitably deceptive in influencing high-risk choice. Nor is it apparent that these interferences in autonomous choice can be excused on the ground of limiting risks to third parties or for compelling paternalist reasons. Consequently, since these practices are vulnerable to ethical critique and the infractions of the principle of autonomy are so clear, it would seem that moral conclusions could readily be drawn.

But I do not think this is so. Since our apparatus for evaluating religious practice is not yet complete, the principle of autonomy cannot be directly employed. Upper-level doctrines and practices are *candidates* for critique; but we have yet to establish on what basis the critique can be made. To condemn practices for violating conditions of autonomous choice involves an unwarranted leap in ethical evaluation, even though these criteria are well established in both professional and ordinary ethics. It is a leap we can make—and then only in limited ways—only after our initial typology is supplemented with the appropriate critical principle.

The principle to which we shall appeal, the fiduciary principle, is a distinct moral principle not reducible either to that of autonomy or to those of nonmaleficence and beneficence. Most explicitly articulated in law, it is vaguely recognized in various forms in all of the secular professions. The fiduciary principle serves to identify the obligations of the professional vis-à-vis the client in professional contexts and, except for a few distinctive interpersonal relationships, it is usually thought to be limited to professional contexts.

To employ a principle adopted from professional ethics to examine organized religion is not to presuppose that religious functionaries are all professionals in the fullest sense. Clergy of the mainstream denominations have traditionally been regarded in this way, though cult leaders, evangelists, faith healers, gurus, and the like have not. But while the fiduciary principle has been developed in professional contexts, its scope is broader and provides a crucial distinction in assessing religious practice.

The fiduciary principle, which applies to all aspects of professional-client interaction, regulates practice by stipulating that it must be possible for the client to *trust* the professional in the course of the interaction, even though the professional's own interests may conflict with those of the client. Put another way, the fiduciary principle prohibits the professional from taking advantage of the client—that is, violating the client's rights or harming his or her interests—in the course of the professional relationship, though of course the professional's superior status, power, and knowledge would make it easy to do so. For example, the lawyer has fiduciary duties to the client; this means that the lawyer must use his or her professional skills to advance the client's interests or, at least, not to harm them. Similarly, the trustee, as fiduciary to the beneficiary of a trust fund, must refrain from usurping the beneficiary's interests in the fund, just as the director of a corporation must refrain from promoting his or her own interests at the expense of the corporation. The fiduciary principle may seem similar to the more general principle of non-maleficence, but it has a specific application to the professional-client relationship and to the characteristic imbalance of power this relationship exhibits. It is broader in scope than the comparatively narrow principle of autonomy; it requires the professional not only to respect the client's autonomous choices and to protect the client's capacity to make them, but also to ensure (and this does not rule out paternalistic intervention) that the client's interests are served. Thus, the principle is a complex one, with conditions often in tension between autonomist and paternalist demands, and not reducible to the simpler principles often cited in professional and ordinary moral discourse. To say, as Charles Fried does, that the fiduciary "owes a duty of strict and unreserved loyalty to his client"[44] is correct, and makes it clear that the professional's primary obligation is to the client, rather than to the professional's own interests, to the institution, or to others who might be involved, but leaves open the question of how the sometimes conflicting requirements of this complex principle are to be satisfied.

Inasmuch as the fiduciary principle has autonomist components, the three conditions for the protection of autonomous choice identified above—noncoercion, freedom from rational impairment, and adequate informedness—can all be derived from it, though in some circumstances they may be in tension with paternalist components of the principle. In professional areas such as medicine and law, these three conditions protect the client from the professional in very specific ways. The client, it is assumed, consults the professional in order to advance his or her aims and interests; the protection needed is protection from possible dishonesty, manipulation, or greed on the part of the professional. For instance, when the patient consults the doctor for help in curing an illness, he or she occupies an unequal, vulnerable position in the relationship (the patient, after all, is both sick and un-trained in medicine) and must rely on the physician's obligations as fiduciary to keep from being made worse off—specifically from being made worse off with respect to health. The legal client consults an attorney for help in protecting his or her rights and similarly relies on the attorney's fiduciary obligation to a client. Since the attorney is far more skilled in the law than the client, the attorney could easily jeopardize those rights. Professionals are also often in a position to jeopardize other interests of the client (both doctors and lawyers, for instance, can easily threaten a patient's or client's emotional, social, or financial well-being), but it is with respect to the specific interest or set of interests about which the client has consulted the professional that the fiduciary principle most directly applies.

Like other professionals, the religious professional, whether minister, priest, rabbi, pastor, evangelist, faith healer, or guru, is in a position to make individuals within the group either better or worse off. He or she can affect their emotional, social, financial, or other peripheral interests. The religious professional can also affect either positively or negatively the specific aim or interest for which they seek help in the first place; it is this fact that initially supports the appeal to the fiduciary principle made here. What the fiduciary principle requires is that the priest or the preacher not treat those who come as prey, even in the most subtle ways, or use them either for self-interested ends or other institutional goals, but instead remain worthy of trust.

To construe the relation between the religious professional and member of the religious group in this way invites us to identify precisely what it is that the religious believer comes to the religious professional for, that is, what interests he or she hopes to serve in approaching the religious professional. Although this may be very difficult to do for a specific case, we can venture certain general observations. Consider, for instance, the reasons why the Christian Scientist or a member of the Faith Assembly has contact with the leaders of his or her group, as contrasted with the reasons why, for example, a member of a serpent-handling group might do so. The Christian Scientist calls a practitioner when he or she is ill and does so for help in restoring health. Similarly, the member of the Faith Assembly rejects medicine and relies on Jesus in order to get well, but he or she also acts to retain membership and avoid humiliation by the group. The serpent handler, on the other hand, attends a prayer meeting and handles serpents in order to satisfy the injunction he or she believes Mark 16 states; there is less evidence here of some particular external objective. Then again, the Jehovah's Witness appears to refuse blood in order to satisfy the biblical commandment, much as the serpent handler does, but does so in order not to jeopardize his or her chances of salvation.

Of course, identifying reasons why people engage in religion is a murky business at best; a full psychological explanation of such behaviors is far more complex than can be treated here. Nevertheless, it is evident that strikingly different degrees of rational prudence, in the pursuit of self-interest, are exhibited by the members of various groups. The Christian Scientist seeks to get well, just as any ordinary patient seeing any ordinary doctor does; in doing so, the Scientist acts to promote one of his or her interests—health. The Scientist does not call the condition "illness" nor recognize its symptoms as those of "disease," nor does he or she understand the end-state sought to be a "cure," but rather a "demonstration" of the truth of the principles of Christian Science. Indeed, the Scientist rejects the entire causal metaphysics of medicine. Nevertheless, he or she accepts, and the church promotes, a variety of external similarities, many dating from the earliest period of the church,[45] which reinforce the claim that what the believer seeks is what any ordinary patient does: help in regaining health. For instance, the Christian Scientist calls the practitioner only when he or she has discomforting symptoms (whether or not viewed as symptoms of disease). The practitioner can be found by looking in the Yellow Pages; an appointment is made; the practitioner's services are paid for at rates roughly comparable to those of a physician; and, in some states (Massachusetts, for instance) Blue Cross will pay the bill. To put it another way, Christian Science functions as an alternative health-care system, though it denies medicine's metaphysics and makes no use of medical techniques; we can easily identify the professional institution to which Christian Science promotes itself as an alternative.

Not all risk-taking practices function as alternatives to secular professional institutions. The serpent handler, for example, does not so clearly seek to advance his or her interests by risking health or life but instead acts simply to obey an injunction he or she believes is what the Lord demands. There do not seem to be external similarities promoted by the group that would reinforce the claim that in handling snakes the believer attempts to further the same aims and interests that clients of other professionals do. Serpent handling is not an *alternative* anything; it is simply a practice of the group.

Noting these differences should allow us to see why the fiduciary principle, while vaguely asserted in the secular professions, is not discussed much there, and why—in contrast—it is of particular interest in the religious sphere. The fiduciary principle prohibits the professional from violating moral principles in such a way as to undermine those aims or interests for which a client seeks protection or advancement in using the professional's services. In medicine and law, as in other secular professions, this covers the entire range of cases: patients and legal clients use the services of doctors and lawyers in order to protect and advance their own aims or interests, or those of organizations and causes with which they identify, and generally not for any other reason. They come to lawyers and doctors to protect their rights, broadly construed, or to get well. Since virtually all of the activities in which the professional engages with the client are initiated in response to such purposes on the part of the client, there is nothing distinctive in these areas of professional practice that the fiduciary principle might isolate and identify as protected under this principle. Of course, some clients do not voluntarily consult professionals, but are delivered to them, such as the unconscious emergency patient or the impoverished defendant in the criminal justice system, but even in these circumstances the fiduciary principle applies by extension. On some occasions a client might consult a professional for purposes that do not appear to serve his or her self-interests, as, for example, when a person consults a doctor to donate a kidney to someone else, but even here the patient does so with the aim of protecting his or her interests as well as those of the recipient, and does not ask the doctor to remove the kidney without regard for his or her own health. Even if the fiduciary principle is not particularly conspicuous in the secular professions, largely because it covers virtually all available cases, it will nevertheless play a central role in sorting out those cases in religion to which ordinary moral norms apply and those to which they do not.

The fiduciary principle functions in critiquing religious practice by identifying under what conditions upper-level practices and doctrines may be reviewed with the moral principles available in professional and ordinary ethics—such principles as autonomy, nonmaleficence, and beneficence; while the working typology developed earlier makes it possible to distinguish between fundamental, zero-level imperatives and upper-level, developed doctrines and practices, it does not specify whether all of the latter are actually open to critique. The fiduciary principle functions as a second general principle, supplementing the earlier typology, and further limits the application of moral norms to religious practices. The fiduciary principle does not in itself aid in sorting out conflicts and tensions between the demands of autonomy, nonmaleficence, and beneficence, either in general or in specific cases like those of Faith Assembly members or Marian Guinn; this is work for the applied professional ethicist concerned with organized religion, the "ecclesioethicist," to do. But the principle does tell us when the ecclesioethicist can get to work, by telling us under what conditions the basic moral principles can be applied to upper-level doctrines and practices. In religious contexts, the fiduciary principle asserts that *the developed practices, doctrines, methods, and teachings employed by religious professionals or their religious organizations must meet (secular) ethical criteria wherever the individual participates in these practices to advance his or her self-interests.* The fact that the religious professional is *religious* does not exempt him or her from treating clients in ways that are morally binding in the secular professions, as well as in ordinary morality, wherever the client approaches the religious professional for the same sorts of self-interest-serving purposes as he or she would approach a secular professional—even if the client is also a believer and adherent of the group. For example, if the Christian Scientist seeks help from a Christian Scientist practitioner *in order to get well,* then he or she is entitled to the same freedom from coercion, from impairment, and to the same adequate information to which an ordinary medical patient would be entitled in seeking to get well. In a word, the religious believer, like the medical patient, is entitled to the protections of informed consent; one's status as a believer does not abrogate this right. However, if a believer approaches a Christian Science practitioner not to get well, but in order to deepen his or her faith—as many devout Christian Scientists clearly do—then it is not so clear that these constraints apply. Many Christian Scientists conceive of healing not as an alternative medical system at all, but as a process of prayer that is part of the effort to achieve a certain spiritual condition—of which a side effect, though not the central purpose, may be the restoration of health.[46]

It may seem that the religious organization, or the religious professional within it, can have no such fiduciary obligation, inasmuch as neither the professional nor the organization has control over the reasons for which an individual approaches them. Of course, this is not so, for the way in which a religious organization, including its officials, is approached is very much a function of the way in which it announces or advertises itself. After all, announcing or advertising an organization is an interactive process between the organization and the individuals who approach it. The process is not much remarked upon in the secular professions since most secular professions announce themselves in uniform ways, but it is a process of tremendous variability in religion. Christian Science, for instance, announces and promotes itself as an alternative healing system by the very fact that it distributes testimonials that recount favorable recoveries using Christian Science healing (even though these testimonials are described primarily as serving to give thanks to God) and by asking Blue Cross to cover the services it renders. In response to the way in which Christian Science announces and promotes itself, prospective users of the church approach it in kind, seeking to receive these services in order to further their aims and interests in getting well. At the same time, that prospective users of Christian Science healing, both members and prospective converts, seek to further their aims and interests in getting well leads the church and its officials to promote the church's services in this way. Similarly, for example, the Church of Scientology promotes itself as providing help in achieving psychological stability and growth; in this sense, it attempts to function as an alternative psychotherapeutic profession. As in Christian Science, Scientology's public stance is interactive with the aims and purposes for which prospective users of its services approach the church: it announces itself as able to provide psychological help and personality development, and people who seek these things turn to it.

In the secular professions, when we talk about why a client seeks a professional, we are saying as much about the professional and the background organization as we are about the client. Thus, to phrase the fiduciary principle in terms of what the client seeks is also to identify specific professional and institutional postures. In religion, since the fiduciary principle underwrites the application of standard ethical principles—autonomy, nonmaleficence, beneficence, and justice—when adherents approach with self-interested aims, it thus also underwrites the application of these principles when the religious group and its officials announce themselves as available to help persons pursue their interests.

Of course, it may be that virtually all religious invitation contains some appeal to self-interest. Insofar as a group makes such an invitation, however, under the interpretation of the fiduciary principle advanced here, it is obligated to protect and promote the aims and self-interests to which the invitation is directed. The church that announces itself as able to satisfy certain interests of persons who are attracted to the church in this way opens itself to *secular* moral critique of the practices and doctrines it employs in satisfying those interests. Not all of the upper-order practices in a religious group will be susceptible to ethical critique under the fiduciary principle; but many of those that have been traditionally protected by the notion of religious immunity will be clear targets for ethical examination and can be assessed using the secular moral criteria developed in ordinary and professional ethics. (Curiously, the distinction between upper-level practices that are vulnerable to ethical critique and those that are not is reflected, though somewhat crudely, in the growing area of clergy malpractice insurance; malpractice insurance is available in approximately those areas in which clergy do what other professionals do, especially counseling, but not for practices much less directly related to the satisfaction of individual self-interests, such as the performance of rites, the maintenance of beliefs, or the upholding of orthodoxy.) The distinction is not always clear; most groups give off mixed signals and are approached for mixed reasons. Nevertheless, the theoretical importance of this distinction is considerable.

This chapter began with a discussion of the practices of four religious groups in encouraging their adherents to take risks. In that discussion, appeal was made to both general moral principles, such as autonomy, nonmaleficence, beneficence, and justice, and to their application in requirements such as informed consent. But while it was established earlier that upper-level practices such as these, which encourage risk, are candidates for moral critique, we did not see why critique is appropriate in these specific cases. Use of the fiduciary principle provides an answer. At least in the cases of the Christian Science, Jehovah's Witnesses, and the Holiness churches, there is good reason to think that individuals consult religious professionals to promote their own interests and that these groups promote characteristic practices under a corresponding appeal to self-interest of the members of the group. Christian Scientists choose prayer over medicine in order to get well; the church promotes prayer as a means of healing. The Jehovah's Witness refuse blood to avoid precluding salvation; this church and its officials promote the practice of refusing blood at least in part with this rationale. If it turns out that the serpent handler does not after all act only to obey the biblical commandment but simply seeks the heightened sensory or emotional experience provided by the dangerous thrill of handling snakes, then this, too, belongs under ordinary ethical scrutiny. After all, heightened sensory or emotional experience is available in ways that are less life-threatening.

The distinction drawn by the fiduciary principle also explains why it seems natural to examine confidentiality in religious confession with the secular apparatus of professional morality: confession is often seen chiefly as a mechanism that allows people to pursue self-interests in relieving guilt or enhancing their spiritual status and ultimate rewards. Confession is not primarily conceived as of something done for the sake of the religious group or for God but for one's own sake—to rectify one's conscience, repent of sin, and hence to advance one's prospects of salvation. If this is so, then the principles employed in secular discussions of confidentiality are also applicable here.

Applications of the fiduciary principle in organized religion are not likely to be easy in practice. The principle refers to the reasons for which people use religious services, as induced by the religious organization and vice versa, and these reasons may be multifarious and obscure. Nor can we assume that the reasons for which people consult religious professionals are anywhere nearly as uniform as the reasons for which they consult doctors or lawyers. Individuals go to church or see their ministers for an enormous variety of reasons, including relieving anxiety, coping with fear, preserving a marriage, restoring health, increasing security, dealing with grief, curbing aggressive or suicidal impulses, maintaining social standing, and so on. A very large part of what leads the religious believer to a religious professional involves the protection and advancement of interests like these; a very large part of the comforts that religious groups offer are directed toward the satisfaction of these interests. Self-interested religious behavior may be very difficult to distinguish from self-interested nonreligious behavior. However cumbersome applications of the principle might be in practice and, consequently, however poor a basis it might make for policy formation, it is an appropriate basis for distinguishing those religious activities and practices that are proper targets for ethical critique from those that are comparatively immune.

It is also a proper basis for scrutinizing the way that religious groups advertise themselves and their services, both in securing continuing commitment from their members and in attracting new ones. The televangelist groups and their leaders are particularly revealing targets for scrutiny. Oral Roberts, for example, makes a direct appeal to the financial interests of prospective contributors by promising immediate material reward. Roberts sends multicolored prayer sheets to his "prayer partners" to be mailed back (together with a contribution) with a list of needs for which he can pray: "The RED area is for your SPIRITUAL healing; the WHITE area is for your PHYSICAL healing; the GREEN area is for your FINANCIAL healing. Check the needs you have and RUSH them back to me."[47] Roberts is by no means the only media preacher who announces his brand of religion as likely to enhance a believer's interests in material comfort and financial success; but because they invite persons to approach them for the same sorts of reasons for which one might approach a secular financial counselor or investment firm, they are open to the same sort of ethical critique. In general, religious operatives promising satisfaction of their audience's financial interests provide a ripe field for further inquiry.

However, not all individuals approach religious professionals or organizations to promote their own self-interests. Consider, for instance, the person who describes why he or she sees a minister or goes to church as wanting to "strengthen my faith." This seemingly central religious purpose bears close scrutiny, for it must be asked why the believer wants to strengthen this faith. If, for instance, it is evident that the believer seeks assistance in strengthening faith to "be sure to go to heaven," the motive sounds very much like the kind of self-interest that other forms of rational prudence display. Once it is assumed or believed that there is a heaven, then it is not so much a matter of *religion* to want to get there; it is a matter of rational prudence, particularly considering that the only available alternative under this belief system is hell. Consequently, even the apparently purely religious purpose of strengthening one's faith in consulting a religious professional or participating in religious practices falls under the fiduciary principle just articulated. Hence, the professional's methods of providing these services and the established church practices that support them are subject to the same working moral criteria as other areas of professional ethics, at least if we assume that the religious professional is in any way capable of either advancing or undermining the interests a person seeks to advance.

This conclusion does not mean, however, that the same local principles or rules of professional ethics apply in religion as they do in medicine or law, for while the fiduciary principle may provide a basic moral standard for all areas of professional practice—including organized religion—it may be that specific applications of the principles derived from it, as well as local rules such as confidentiality and truth telling, differ from one area of professional practice to another. Thus, for example, principles governing the protection of autonomy in decisionmaking under risk may differ from psychiatry to medicine to sports coaching to religion, but they must all satisfy the general fiduciary requirement that the professional be loyal to and not take advantage of the client.

Although having one's faith strengthened in order to get to heaven may not be a distinctively religious purpose for consulting a religious professional, some purposes are. A person who initially expresses a desire for help in strengthening faith might explain that he or she seeks this help because God is supremely worthy of worship and therefore he or she wishes to worship God more fully—regardless of the impact this fuller worship might have on himself or herself. This kind of purpose in seeking assistance from a religious professional does not involve seeking to advance one's own interests, thereby putting them in a position vulnerable to the professional's influence. Consequently, it is not a purpose to which the usual strictures of professional morality under the fiduciary principle apply. For instance, some Christian Scientists, as perhaps some Faith Assembly members, Jehovah's Witnesses, and Holiness church members, may observe their church's teaching not to enhance their health or to secure salvation, but simply because—as they believe—it is the word of God. As yet, we have no basis for applying secular moral criteria in cases like these—regardless of the nature of these practices and doctrines that have developed or the group's methods in promoting this behavior. (This is not, of course, to say that they are justified.) However, these cases may be very few, and such people as rare as saints. If most religious behavior is actually the pursuit of self-interest under a special set of metaphysical assumptions, then the "professionals" who are the purveyors and caretakers of these assumptions in the form of religious doctrine, teachings, and practices are obligated—as in any fiduciary relationship—to protect these persons in that pursuit.

Notes

Chapter 2 in Margaret P. Battin, *Ethics in the Sanctuary: Examining the Practices of Organized Religion,* Yale University Press, 1990, pp. 74–128. © 1990 Yale University. Reprinted by permission.

1. Charles Fried, *An Anatomy of Values: Problems of Personal and Social Choice* (Cambridge: Harvard University Press, 1970), 167.
2. See Thomas C. Johnsen, "Christian Scientists and the Medical Profession: A Historical Perspective," *Medical Heritage* (Jan/Feb. 1986): 70–8, for a loyal account of the historical background; also see Robert Peel, *Spiritual Healing in a Scientific Age* (San Francisco: Harper & Row, 1987), for a loyal attempt to address scientific issues.
3. Arnold S. Relman, M.D., "Christian Science and the Care of Children," *New England Journal of Medicine* 309(26): 1639 (Dec. 29, 1983).
4. Nathan A. Talbot, "The Position of the Christian Science Church," *New England Journal of Medicine* 309(26): 1631–44 (Dec. 29, 1983). See especially p. 1642.
5. Talbot, "The Position of the Christian Science Church," 1642.
6. On the distinction between mechanical procedures and other medical treatment, see Arthur E. Nudelman, "The Maintenance of Christian Science in Scientific Society," in *Marginal Medicine,* ed. Roy Wallis and Peter Morley (New York: Free Press, 1976), 42–60; also see William E. Laur, M.D., "Christian Science Visited," *Southern Medical Journal* 73(1): 71–74 (Jan. 1980). See especially p. 73.
7. Rita Swan, "Faith Healing, Christian Science, and the Medical Care of Children," *New England Journal of Medicine* 309(26): 1640 (Dec. 29, 1983).
8. Constant H. Jacquet, Jr., ed., *Yearbook of American and Canadian Churches* (Nashville, Tenn.: Abingdon Press, 1988), 42.
9. See the pamphlet supplied by the Watchtower Bible and Tract Society of Pennsylvania, "Jehovah's Witnesses and the Question of Blood" (1977).
10. Some Witnesses will also accept closed-loop extracorporeal recirculation of their own blood during surgery and in hemodialysis.
11. See, e.g., J. Skelly Wright's decision in "Application of President and Directors of Georgetown College," 311 F.2d 1000 (D.C. Cir.), certiorari denied, 377 U.S. 978 (1964).
12. Jim Quinn and Bill Zlatos, series of stories beginning May 2, 1983, in the *Fort Wayne News-Sentinel,* Indiana; see, also, Ron French, ibid., Aug. 25, 1987, and June 8, 1989.
13. Quinn and Zlatos, story in *Fort Wayne News-Sentinel,* May 5, 1983, 1.
14. Robert W. Pelton and Karen W. Carden, *Snake Handlers: God-Fearers? or, Fanatics?* (Nashville, Tenn.: Thomas Nelson, 1974), provides a useful pictorial essay on these practices.

15. *Swann v. Pack* 527 S.W.2d at 105. This case notes that Hensley died of a diamondback rattlesnake bite during a prayer meeting in 1955.

16. Nathan L. Gerrard, "The Serpent-Handling Religions of West Virginia," *Trans-Action* 5(7): 23 (May 1968).

17. Pelton and Carden, *Snake Handlers,* p. 12 of Appendix.

18. Gerrard, "The Serpent-Handling Religions of West Virginia," 23.

19. Weston La Barre, *They Shall Take Up Serpents: Psychology of the Southern Snake-Handling Cult* (Minneapolis: University of Minnesota Press, 1962), 19–20.

20. Findlay E. Russell, *Snake Venom Poisoning* (Philadelphia: J. B. Lippincott, 1980), 527.

21. *Swann v. Pack* 527 S.W.2d at 100.

22. *Fort Wayne News-Sentinel,* June 2, 1984, 6A.

23. Gale E. Wilson, "Christian Science and Longevity," *Journal of Forensic Sciences* 1 (Jan.–Oct. 1956): 43–60.

24. CHILD is an acronym for Children's Health Care Is a Legal Duty, Inc. The organization's address is Box 2604, Sioux City, Iowa 51106.

25. See J. Lowell Dixon and M. Gene Smalley, "Jehovah's Witnesses: The Surgical/Ethical Challenge," *Journal of the American Medical Association* 246(21): 2471–72 (Nov. 27, 1981).

26. Dixon and Smalley, "Jehovah's Witnesses," 2472.

27. William Franklin Simpson, "Comparative Longevity in a College Cohort of Christian Scientists," *Journal of the American Medical Association* 262(12): 1657–58 (Sept. 22/29, 1989). An extended critical analysis of the statistical methods of this study, by Prof. David Nartonis, is available from the church.

28. Pelton and Carden, *Snake Handlers,* 29–30.

29. Members of the Holiness churches insist that serpent handling is not to be understood as a "test of faith" in the sense that reciting a creed might be, but that it is a "confirmation" of God's word. Glossolalia, serpent handling, strychnine drinking, and similar practices are the "signs following" belief in God but are not evidence for it. See Pelton and Carden, *Snake Handlers.*

30. Merrily Allen Ozengher, *Christian Science Journal* 101(9) (Sept. 1983).

31. Footnote appearing at the beginning of the "On Christian Science Healing" section of testimonials in each issue of the *Christian Science Journal.*

32. Talbot, "Position of the Christian Science Church," 1642; see also, *A Century of Christian Science Healing* (Boston: The Christian Science Publishing Society, 1966) for the church's account of this history. The figure is from the Committee on Publication's 1989 paper "An Empirical Analysis of Medical Evidence in Christian Science Testimonies of Healing 1969–1988," First Church of Christ, Scientist, 175 Huntington Avenue; Boston, Mass. 02115.

33. Talbot, "Position of the Christian Science Church," 1642.

34. See, e.g., Daniel Kahneman, Paul Slovic, and Amos Tversky, eds., *Judgment Under Uncertainty: Heuristics and Biases* (Cambridge: Cambridge University Press, 1982).

35. Nudelman, "The Maintenance of Christian Science in a Scientific Society," 49.

36. Base-rate and related information could presumably be accumulated if Christian Scientists as well as non-Scientists were routinely examined and diagnosed by physicians and if medical records of all procedures as well as records of healing by prayer were kept. Of course, this is not generally the case. Neither could the kind of persuasive evidence supplied by controlled clinical trials be obtained on the efficacy of Christian Science healing since it would not be possible to *randomize* subjects into groups, one of which would (sincerely) perform Christian Science prayer and the other of which would not pray but have

confidence in conventional medicine alone. The closest one could come to designing such a trial would be to randomize believing Scientists into groups that use prayer and those that, denied the services of a Christian Science practitioner, are offered only conventional treatment or to randomize nonbelievers into those who use conventional medical treatment and those who go through the motions of prayer.

A study cited in the *Hastings Center Report* (vol. 19, no. 3, May/June 1989, pp. 2–3) reports a randomized, double-blind study of the effects of intercessory prayer on hospitalized patients ("Positive Therapeutic Effects of Intercessory Prayer in a Coronary Care Unit Population," *Southern Medical Journal* 81(7): 826–29 [1988]). Of course, this study did not randomize patients who prayed for themselves, but patients who were prayed for by others; nevertheless, it did conclude that the group prayed for exhibited fewer complications than the control group.

37. Nicholas Rescher, *Risk: A Philosophical Introduction to the Theory of Risk Evaluation and Management* (Washington, D.C.: University of Press of America, 1983), 132.

38. Lois O'Brien, "Prayer's Not a Gamble," letter in *U.S. News & World Report,* April 28, 1986, 81.

39. Contrast the symposium articles in the *New England Journal of Medicine* 310(19): 1257–60 (May 10, 1984), with subsequent letters to the editor.

40. Rita Swan, letter to the editor, *New England Journal of Medicine* 310(19):1260 (May 10, 1984).

41. George Mills and Richard Grove, *Lucifer and the Crucifer: The Enigma of the Penitentes* (Colorado Springs Fine Arts Center, The Westerners, 1956), 21, citing Mary Austin.

42. Rev. Rodney Dorsey, Pocatalico Community Full Gospel Church, Sissonville, West Virginia, telephone communication with author, Sept. 20, 1989.

43. Pelton and Carden, *Snake Handlers,* unnumbered last page of Appendix.

44. Charles Fried, *Medical Experimentation, Personal Integrity and Social Policy* (New York: American Elsevier Publishing Co., 1974), 33.

45. By the turn of the century, Christian Science was viewed by the medical establishment as an alternative (and bogus) school of medicine, not as a religion. See Johnsen, "Christian Scientists and the Medical Profession," 72.

46. Johnsen, "Christian Scientists and the Medical Profession," 73. As Johnsen also notes, a unanimous opinion of the Rhode Island Supreme Court affirmed in 1898 that prayer in Christian Science could not be mistaken for the practice of medicine in any "ordinary sense and meaning" of the term.

47. Alan Brinkley, "The Oral Majority," *New Republic* (Sept. 29, 1986), 31.

10

Terminal Procedure

Much is not clear about the way the dogs died. Events on the periphery of the deaths, like points on undulating, outward-moving circles, recede into liquid uncertainty. The origins of the event are obscure, and its effects dwindle onward into indeterminacy. Causality cannot be established, and responsibility becomes a meaningless conceit, of no concern and no question.

Yet at the center remains the event itself, and it is fully clear: the dogs died.

Phase 1

If we look, we can see the place where the dogs died: a small laboratory, assigned to an associate named Boaz, in a sprawling research institute. The place has not changed; it is the same simple, almost square room, hidden in an obscure wing of an old building far to one side of the institute's grounds. We see the usual furniture of science: two bulky wooden desks, an untidy bookcase, and a flimsy file cabinet cramped together on one wall; on the other side of the room, flanked by its recording and control apparatus, the soundproof experimental box. On the floor beside the box, centered on a stained and yellowed newspaper, is a small tin water dish.

The lab has not changed since the dogs died there, except that the stack of data tapes grows no higher, and a half cup of black coffee left in a mug marked Maia has dried into a thick brown crust. And there is a small stain, left by a few drops of blood-tinged fluid on the tile floor, which the janitor, if he has come at all, must have missed.

The lab has not changed. There is no one there now, but if we look back we can distinguish two figures: the researcher Boaz, and his assistant, a girl named Maia. They move, they talk, they look together at the clock, though that is all we see; the causes are obscure. We cannot tell, for instance, what brought Boaz to neuropsychological research: whether he was groomed, as the eldest, most promising son of a well-established family, in the finest schools for an eminent career in science; whether he was impelled to the study of mental phenomena by a scrupulously sublimated attraction to a particular professor; whether he chose psychology simply to spite his nervous mother; or whether his penchant for experimentation was born in the alley, nailing half-conscious rats to the boards of a tenement fence. Nor does it matter: he is here. We can watch him in his laboratory, though his past be indeterminate and his future uncertain: we see him not as the product of any painstaking development, nor as a process toward some ineffable goal, but simply as himself.

We see what Boaz does before the dogs die: we see him in his laboratory, shuffling through stacks of graphs, drawn meticulously on green-ruled paper, running his fingers down the index columns in the back of a thick black-bound book; we see him sprawling in a swivel chair, talking with his assistant, the girl Maia, or perhaps by telephone with his wife; he sprawls back, his hand hanging idly over the arm of the swivel chair. One of the dogs is sleeping beneath the chair; Boaz's hand finds the dog, and his fingers play beneath the rope lead around the dog's neck. The dog moves just enough so that Boaz's fingers can scratch all of its neck, no more.

There is only one window in the laboratory, and it is obscured at the top by an uneven venetian blind, at the bottom by an old and noisy air conditioner. They will turn the air conditioner on in the afternoon, Boaz and the girl Maia, even though it is not summer: it will grow hot in the small square room with the door closed, hot and heavy with the odors of the dogs. They will have to keep the door to the lab closed so that the office workers across the hall do not see, and so that the dogs do not break loose and escape down the long colorless corridors. And they will think too, that the throaty hum of the air conditioner will cover the noise of the dogs, so that the office workers across the hall do not hear.

But the office workers asked anyway, when Boaz and Maia came back afterward to the lab, what they had done to the dogs.

"We had to give them a little shot," said Boaz.

"Oh," said the office workers. Uncertainly, some of them smoothed thick hands across the flat planks of their girdles. "We thought something was wrong."

"Nothing is wrong. It was just a little shot," repeated Boaz.

"They don't seem to like it very much," said the worker whose office door is just to the right across the hall from the lab. The worker whose office is directly across the hall is ill; her door has remained closed for a month now, maybe more. "They made a lot of noise."

"It's not getting the shot they mind so much," counters Boaz, his hand involuntarily pulling at his chin. "It's what's in the shot. When the fluid is forced into the tissue, it creates pressure. . . ."

The office workers understand. Some of them remember from the inoculations they had to have when they went to Europe, or from the preoperative injections given them when they had their root canals or their hysterectomies. They are not sure just how they know, but each is certain of the prick-pain of the needle itself, then the slow hard swelling within the flesh . . . yes, they understand, the needle does not hurt so much as the fluid. That is why the dogs made so much noise.

The office workers nod, and turn back into their separate rooms.

Phase 2

There we have it, some of the scene the afternoon the dogs died. We saw the researcher, Boaz, as he parried the anxious questions of the women who work across the hall, but we missed the girl Maia, his assistant. Perhaps she had just stepped out, down the long corridor to the bathroom, to comb her straight black hair back out of her face—when she came to work that morning her hair was hanging loose, but by the time the dogs were dead she had bound it back, severely, with a thin rubber band—or perhaps when we looked she was hidden by the door of the soundproof experimental box. The box, after all, is very large, a double-walled cube of steel, insulated so well that even a dog, whose sense of hearing is much more acute than any man's, can hear nothing, nothing at all outside the box, nor can anyone outside hear even the loudest noise of a dog within. Maia might have easily been standing behind the box. Beside the box is the recording and control apparatus, a complex construction of knobs and dials and levers, displaying a small oscilloscope screen and twin reels of recording tape. She might have been watching from behind the apparatus, peering out between its irregular protrusions. Or perhaps she had stepped behind the box to put the rubber band in her hair, for she is always just a little shy of Boaz's gaze and is not eager to invite any intimacies. In any case, she was there the afternoon the dogs died.

Of course she was there: it was part of her job. She must have known; she must have been told when she was hired to be Boaz's assistant what would happen to the dogs. Surely the institute's personnel officer, a conscientious man exactingly aware of the protective regulations, had felt obliged to tell her that the job involved handling experimental animals on which terminal neurological studies were to be performed. Or maybe Boaz had told her.

"Sit down, Maia," Boaz may have said, a gruff edge exposed in his low voice. "I am going to tell you exactly what these experiments are about, so you won't have any questions and so you won't say I didn't tell you."

She sat, crossing her thin legs, in the swivel chair, and smiled just slightly at him.

"The man in Personnel said you were doing basic research in comparative conditioning. Using dogs. My job would be to take care of the dogs and run the conditioning experiments. That's all he said."

"Let me explain," Boaz begins, rather stiffly. "There has been a lot of neuro-logical research done on how the brain codes things. And there's been a lot of research on how animals react and learn in particular situations, but that kind of behavioral research says nothing about what happens in the brain. Not many at-tempts have been made to correlate a specific behavioral event with a neural event."

"And that's what you're trying to do."

"Yes," said Boaz. "It's worth doing."

She tosses her head lightly. "Well, I'm glad of *that*," she says, a little fliply.

He leans forward in the swivel chair. "You must understand that this research is significant," he warns, "and that it's important that we do it just this way."

She does not answer, and he begins again to explain. "What we're trying to find out is what patterns of electrical activity occur in the brain during certain types of conditioning or learning. So we have electrodes implanted in the dog's brain, and then we record the population of neural cells that fire while the dog is being conditioned."

Boaz must have watched her as he talked; he must have noticed how small a girl she is, small and slender, made smaller by the large swivel chair. Perhaps she was wearing her thin black hair free that beginning day, or perhaps it was knotted up with a long paisley scarf, but surely Boaz must have noticed her eyes: wide eyes rimmed in black mascara, eyes so wide she looked as if she might cry at any moment.

"Each dog spends an hour in the experimental box every third day, learning how to react to a given stimulus situation. It will take the dogs three or four months, maybe longer, to complete their conditioning, and then—" He hesitates, watching her wide eyes.

She looks at him, saying nothing.

"Stereotaxic implantation is very difficult," he says distantly, "because you never can be sure just where the electrodes are."

She sits silent, listening.

"An electrode is nothing but a piece of conductive wire, inserted directly into the brain through a tiny hole bored in the skull. The shaft end is cemented to a terminal for the monitoring equipment, called a pedestal, and the pedestal itself is affixed to the skull directly over the cortex region. The pedestal anchors the elec-trodes, and—"

"Do they hurt?" Maia interrupts.

"What?" he stops, a little annoyed.

"The electrodes. Do they hurt the dog?"

"There are no pain receptors in the brain," Boaz answers flatly. "Does it bother you?"

"No, I just wanted to know." She pulls a long strand of hair out of her face. "I just wanted to know, that's all. Go on with your story."

"This is not a story, Maia."

"I know," she answers quickly. "I'm sorry."

"The problem," he begins again, "is to determine just where the electrodes are. It's not easy to implant them precisely, and there's only one way to determine exactly where they are."

"What's that?"

"By direct inspection of the neural region." He talks more quickly, enunciating the syllables almost too clearly, as if to conceal in scientific jargon something he does not quite want her to understand.

She sits still, saying nothing.

"The procedure is terminal," he says at last.

"I knew that," she says flatly, and Boaz realizes that she is not going to cry, that her eyes are wide all the time.

"I am going to tell you how we are going to do the termination," he says, "just so you'll know."

Maia sits motionless. "All right."

"After the dog has completed its conditioning program, we give it a double or triple dose of anesthetic. Then we open the chest cavity while circulation is still functioning, and by inserting a tube directly into the heart, we can pump fluids up into the capillaries in the brain. We use a saline solution first to flush the blood out, and then a Formalin fixative. The Formalin prevents decomposition."

"Keeps it from spoiling," Maia translates, partly to herself and partly so that Boaz will know she understands.

"Then we remove the head, and put it in a preservative. Anytime after that we can remove and section the brain."

Maia sits quietly, as if forming questions. "Do you do all this?" she asks finally.

"No, no indeed," says Boaz, almost amused by her suggestion, "not when there are people around the institute who are really experienced at that sort of thing—"

"Who?"

"Some physiologists in the animal-surgery laboratory, over on the other side of the institute. It's all arranged."

"All we do is bring the dogs?"

"That's all."

She still sits quietly, though her fingers comb unevenly through her long thin hair, or twist the ends of the paisley scarf.

"Why are you telling me all this?" she asks, after a long time, her voice even and clear. "Not just so I'll know."

"Yes," he said, "so you'll know. So you won't ever have to say you didn't know what we were doing."

"I'm not a coward," she says slowly, deliberately.

"Good," says Boaz, his mouth achieving a smile.

She smiles easily back.

It is possible that sometime after the experiments were terminated and the dogs were dead Maia came back to the lab, perhaps still employed, to help Boaz write up the results of the experiments, or just to retrieve the little china pot she had used to brew coffee. Perhaps she came for no reason at all, just wandering in, opening the door by chance, to see the small square room again. Her eyes must have traveled over the walls, over the neat graphs Boaz had drawn of the dogs' performance in the box, graphs he had tacked to the walls, graphs with the dogs' names. Mustard, Monroe, Eggyolk, Isabel, graphs with the dogs' names. Frenchfry, Faulkner, Yoghurt, Trotsky, Theresa, 23 dogs, 23 names, Hubert, Pablo, Pianissimo;

her eyes must have wandered over the untidy bookcase, the flimsy file cabinet holding old research proposals and reprints of other neuropsychological studies on dogs, mostly brown mongrel dogs, dogs with names, for it is customary in the biological sciences to name laboratory dogs, though cats and rats and mice are given only numbers, over the cabinet full of electronic scraps, bits of electrode wire and odd-numbered dials and snipped lengths of exposed film, over the old brown desks where she and Boaz had sat, talking or not talking while the dogs ran their trials in the experimental box. And when she came back, Maia may have stepped across the stained floor to the soundproof box, put a thin hand out to touch the metal sides of the huge box; she may have opened first the outer door, pressed the heavy handle down, and then the inner door, as heavy as the first, and perhaps she stepped inside the box, as she would have with a dog, any dog, with Mustard or Muffin or Petunia, to see one last time the stout canvas harness in which she would have strapped the dog, Pablo, maybe, or Theresa, the dangling wires ready to connect to the pedestal cemented to the center of the skull, and other wires to be taped to the dog's wrist to administer graduated levels of electric shock; perhaps she would finger the slender bar to which the dog's foreleg would be tied so that when the dog lifted its leg in the response expected of it, the bar would move and record the leg lift on the dual spools of tape turning slowly at the top of the recording apparatus outside. Perhaps Maia, her eyes still rimmed in black and her hair falling free, would sit motionless in the soundproof silence of the box, or perhaps she simply turns away, steps down out of the empty box, and lets the door bang heavily shut behind her.

Or perhaps she did not come back.

Still later, much later, Maia shows someone a photograph, though the circumstances are so remote from the center that almost none of the details are clear. It may be in responding to the courtship of a new lover that Maia takes the small, square photograph, its corners bent, from her purse, as if by that one picture to explain herself; or perhaps she reminisces with her family, leafing through a dusty album of her single years. Perhaps she shows the photo to a colleague, laughing over cocktails at a convention of neuropsychologists, where Boaz will be honored for his work; or perhaps she sits alone, on the hard edge of a hospital bed, and shows the picture to herself. But the photograph itself, since it was taken much closer to the center, is quite clear; it is a snapshot, taken presumably by Boaz, of Maia on the lawn behind the lab, running in from the kennels with two of the dogs. The dogs strain ahead on their leads, their noses to the ground, but Maia is only allowing herself to be tugged, her head tossed back, her hair loose in the wind, her face laughing.

As she studies the photograph, Maia binds her black hair back with a rubber band. But she is too far from the center now, and we cannot see if there is any expression on her face.

Phase 3

Still, some things are already clear. It is certain, for instance, that both Boaz and the girl knew what they were doing. Boaz knows because he designed the experiments, or at the very least took them over from some other researcher; in any case he knows: exact determination of the location of the electrodes is essential to correct analysis of the experimental data. That is what he knows.

And Maia knows too, knows that the dogs she runs through the experiments will eventually be put to sleep, have fluids perfused through their brains, have their heads severed, soaked in preservative, and their brains removed. But Maia also knows that however protracted the surgeries, the dogs will feel none of it; their conscious end will be swift, sleepy, painless. She finds nothing wrong with the plan.

And the dogs? Do they know? No, they are just dogs; they do not know anything more complex than immediate attention or actual pain. They are just dogs, common mongrel dogs, their coats dull and their markings irregular. Their breath is sour from the standard kennel diet, and the electrode pedestals protrude like plastic cancers from their heads. But their tails beat against the sides of the wooden desks when Maia brings them in from the kennel and one jumps up to lick her hand.

Ah, yes, the one that licks her hand is Mustard. He is just a little smaller than most of the dogs, but smarter, sharper, and his coat is an almost yellowish brown— which is why, of course, Maia named him Mustard. She has just brought him into the lab; they have run breathless together across the wide green lawn, and after his hour in the box, they will run back again, loping free across the green grass to the kennel. But now Maia has looped the rope lead through the handle of the file drawer. Mustard paces nervously, keeping as far from the experimental box as possible; the rope pulls the file drawer out, then back, then out again. Annoyed, Boaz drums on the surface of his desk.

Maia presses a button on the recording apparatus; she speaks into it, her voice small but clear: "Now running Mustard. Avoidance conditioning. Number of trials: 50. Prestimulus interval 2.0, poststimulus interval 5.0 seconds." As she speaks, she twists the numbered dials on the face of the control apparatus, setting it to sound the stimulus tone and record the dog's behavior. "Shock duration .5, shock intensity 2.25 milliamps . . ." Then it is ready, and she turns toward Mustard.

She loosens the rope lead from the file cabinet, and pulls the dog toward the box. He struggles back, but the rope lead tightens, like a choke, and he has no choice. Maia lifts him up onto the platform inside the box; he struggles, but she is stronger, and she straps the canvas harness around his body. He struggles still, but now he cannot escape. She ties his right foreleg to the movable leg-lift bar; he pulls on it a few times, as if he remembers what response is expected of him, and the bar makes a little clicking noise outside the box.

Then Maia reaches for a thin coil of wire hanging from the ceiling of the box; there is a flat patch at the end of it, a sensor to measure electromyogram potentials in the muscles, and with adhesive tape she fixes the patch to a shaved area on the side of Mustard's leg. Finally, she tapes two small silver disks, attached to the end of a red wire, to the wrist joint of Mustard's foreleg, just above the footpad and below the dewclaw. It is the terminal that will give him the shock. She tightens the stomach strap.

"Good doggie," she murmurs, and she rubs the underside of his neck, just for a moment, before she puts the head restraint on him. Finally, when the restraining collar is in place and his head is secured so that he cannot move it, she plugs the wire leads into the pedestal in his head.

She stands back, checking: Mustard is strapped firmly in position, unable to move anything except his right foreleg and his tail.

"Good doggie," she says to him again. He is the cleverest of all the dogs. "Do a good job, Mustard, and you'll be the first one through." She hesitates, suddenly aware of her own words, and looks at Boaz. He looks back, as if to call her bluff.

She takes it. "Do a good job, Mustard," she promises, "and you'll be the first one to get your head cut off."

Boaz smiles into his papers, and Maia closes the inner door of the box. Mustard barks, but the sound is very flat, muffled by the door; after Maia has closed the outer door, she can hear nothing more. She looks in through the triple-thick window; Mustard, she can see, is still barking, but the straps are holding well. She turns to the control panel; it is all set, and she flips a single switch. The two tape reels at the top of the recording apparatus begin to turn, in unison, and the conditioned stimulus, a single clear tone, sounds. Then there is a clicking noise, the noise made by the bar as Mustard lifts his leg, and finally the rapid clatter of the printer, recording the data of the trial.

Then it is quiet. If we look in through the window, we will see Mustard standing motionless, his tail still and his eyes fixed dully on the wall of the box in front of him. The tone sounds again; this time he fails to lift his leg, and after precisely five seconds the shock is presented. He jerks his leg rapidly, since that is the only movement he can make, and then holds his leg up, unaware that the terminal is taped to his wrist and cannot be avoided. He struggles in the harness, but the canvas is tough, unyielding, and he cannot free himself. He drools heavily.

It is difficult to tell just how much more time elapsed before the end came, though surely Maia could figure it out from the dogs' records, from the protocol sheets or the data tapes or even the learning graphs taped to the walls. And it is hard to say just when they realized that the end had come: that some of the dogs had learned as much as the design of the experiment required, and that the experimental data on them was complete.

It may have been Boaz, sitting engrossed over long columns of figures recorded by the apparatus, who sees first that three of the dogs are finished. Or it may have been Maia, watching each of her dogs through the thick window of the box, who sees the end: Mustard, frail Theresa, and Pablo. Or perhaps they did not realize it at all; perhaps Boaz simply telephoned the animal surgery laboratory.

He swivels outward from the telephone. "Tomorrow," he says to Maia, "be here early. We'll do them first thing in the morning."

She is puzzled. "I thought you said the physiologists were going to do it."

"They will," Boaz assures her, "all except for the anesthetic. We do that, here."

"How can we do it here? Wouldn't it be easier to do it there, then we wouldn't have to carry them . . . ?"

"No. Besides, that's the way we made the arrangements. We anesthetize the dogs here, and once they're out, put them in my car, drive over to the main building, and load them on a gurney at the shipping door. That way the physiology people won't have live dogs running around their sterile laboratory, and they won't have to waste a lot of time waiting for the anesthetic to take effect. It doesn't always work, you know."

"Why not?"

"You calculate the dosage according to the weight and condition of the dog. But you have to be sure not to give it too much, otherwise you'll kill it outright, so sometimes you end up giving it not quite enough."

"What happens then?"

Boaz smiles, tolerant of her question. "You just start all over again, that's all. That's another reason we're doing it here, in case we have to do any of the dogs twice."

Maia thinks for a moment. "I suppose it's nicer for the dogs to let them go to sleep in a place that's familiar, not with a lot of strange people standing around," she muses.

"I suppose so," says Boaz, without interest.

"Do I have to go with you to the surgery?"

He looks at her, and his gaze is suddenly kind. "No, Maia, you don't, not if you don't want to. I'll just need you here in the morning to help with the anesthetic."

She does not respond.

"Just hold some paws, that's all. It's just one little shot."

"All right," she says finally.

You see that they were quite calm about it beforehand, Boaz and the girl. After all, there was nothing unusual about the situation; their procedures were perfectly routine in experimental psychology, and they were executing these procedures as well as they could.

But afterward, after they had anesthetized the dogs and loaded them into the back seat of the car, Boaz saw that his hands were shaking.

Maia too may have seen his hands tremble, but she said nothing; she sat beside Boaz, immobile and silent. He knew the roads of the institute grounds well, and he had tried the great curve down the hill at every speed from 30 to 80, but his hands shook too much, he did not really see the road, he missed the turn. The car spun back off the road and slid, tilted, into a ditch; as it stopped Boaz heard a sliding noise, and then the heavy thump of a body falling to the floor. He turned quickly; it was Theresa, her leg bent back double beneath her body. He lurched over the seat to help her, but then he realized it made no difference. And he realized that Maia had not moved during the accident, not at all; she sat unmoving, her eyes glassy and hollow.

At the same moment Boaz saw a car pull off the road behind them, to help. He leapt out, strangely alarmed, as the car pulled up toward them. No, he thought, go away, and he ran toward the approaching car, "I'm all right," he yelled, his voice cracking, to the would-be samaritan, "I'm all right," his arms flailing, "go away, I'm all right," flailing, beating off the samaritan, and then, just for a moment, he saw himself: a madman, protecting an almost catatonic girl and three half-dead dogs.

Then he caught himself. "Thank you," he said to the driver, a bewildered student. "I think I can get it out of the ditch myself."

The record does not show how they get to the surgery lab: whether the student towed them out of the ditch, or whether Boaz scraped together branches from the woods and forced them into the mud under the wheels for traction; it is not important whether they took the usual route or another, back behind the pond; it is not clear how long Maia's state lasted, or when Boaz's hands stopped shaking, but the chief physiologist, a severe woman, said later that they were both present for the perfusion and termination procedure. She did say, when asked, that they were both rather quiet during the procedure, that she had expected Boaz, in particular, to be more interested in the findings—though of course they would all be recorded in detail and he would be able to study them later. She had attributed their silence to the natural squeamishness of those not accustomed to observing surgery, she said, and she quite understood. Besides, she guessed that Maia had grown fond of the dogs.

Phase 4

It seems, then that something must have upset them. Boaz was calm beforehand, calm and completely scientific, but afterward he ran his car off the road—a road he knew well—in broad daylight, without speeding.

And Maia? Wasn't she calm? She had been calm with the dogs that morning: she had done nothing unusual. She went out to the kennels, out behind the building, just as usual, quietly stepping through the early grass; the dogs heard her coming, and all 23 began to bark. She opened the wooden gate to the fence surrounding the kennels; the dogs leapt up, each in its own wire pen, to greet her. She began her duties at once, going from one pen to the next with the long-handled shovel, scooping out the little piles of excrement; then she hosed out the floors of the cages. Last she filled the dishes with water and with food, though she did not fill the dishes in the cages of Mustard, or Theresa, or Pablo. She walked the three back, each tugging in a different direction on its leash, across the lawn to the laboratory.

But Boaz was not ready. He had not been able to find the right kind of needle for the syringe. He had left a note for Maia, saying he'd gone over to the surgery lab to get a new needle. He might not be back until after lunch: she should wait.

So Maia was alone in the laboratory, with Mustard and Theresa and Pablo. She opened the drawer of her desk, and took out her sandwich. Ham sandwich, made from ham she had baked for someone, her boyfriend perhaps, or her father, or just herself. She folded out the square of waxed paper, opened the sandwich. Three slices of ham. Three heavy slices of thick, old ham, mottled with sinews that seemed to shimmer green. She wasn't hungry. Maybe the ham was spoiled; maybe the dark yellow mayonnaise was spoiled too. It would make her sick; no, she would not eat the ham, she would give it to the dogs; it would make them sick too, it would make no difference. She wasn't hungry, not at all.

She was suddenly aware of a dog's head in her lap. It was Pablo, nuzzling in between her knees, attracted by the sandwich. He was not an affectionate dog, but now he nuzzled up, his long flat head in her lap, his limp ears falling loosely over her knees. His smell surrounded her, the thick, sour smell of unclean animal. His eyes stared at hers, as if to plead for the sandwich, and her own eyes fixed on the pedestal in his forehead. Her hand moved up through the dirty fur to stroke the back of his head, but her eyes remained on the pedestal: a plastic cap as big around as a dime, protruding almost an inch from his skull. The skin had been slit length-wise along his head, but it had not healed well; it had remained spread apart, like half-open lips, for about four inches. She could see the sloping base of the pedestal, where it was cemented to the exposed skull; she could see edges of light-red flesh beneath the retracted skin. Pablo had had several infections, and even now a thin yellow pus oozed out from beneath the open skin, collecting in dirty black clots at the edges of the wound. She had tried to keep the opening as clear as she could, and from habit she reminded herself to put on more of the antibiotic ointment, but she realized there was no point in it: within an hour, or at the most two, she would see Pablo's head sitting not in her lap but in a stainless steel basin.

Almost reluctant to touch them, she lifts the slices of ham from her sandwich. She gives one to Pablo, the second to Theresa; Mustard jumps up and snatches his from the desk. She steadies herself against its edge, unwilling now to scold.

She considers the bread of her sandwich, not the ham, just the bread; she wonders if she ought to eat the bread, if she ought to eat something, so that she won't feel weak later on, later on at the surgery lab, when they are cutting into the chests of the dogs, when they are inserting the thin tube into the heart, still beating, into the heart still beating, so that it can pump the fluids into the brain, beating, beating slowly . . . she must eat the bread, she decides, so that she won't feel weak, so that . . .

Then she hears Boaz returning. Her stomach knots sharply, and she is glad she has eaten nothing. She gives the bread, too, to the dogs.

Boaz brings the new needle. He unwraps it, fits it carefully onto the syringe, and from his pocket takes a small rubber-sealed bottle: Nembutal. He has already calculated the dosage; it will be three times the normal amount. He picks the bottle up in one hand, inverts it, and pierces the needle upward through the rubber seal; he draws the plunger out, watching the syringe fill slowly with the clear fluid. When it is full, he withdraws the needle from the bottle, and puts them both on his desk.

"Ready, Maia?"

She looks at him; his face is firm, impassive, strange, and she wonders if she has ever seen him before. She wonders suddenly where he came from, if he was a rich child or a tramp, whether he could conjugate a Latin verb or skin a rat, whether he ever thought of death, and if he ever had a dog.

"Ready, Maia?"

She starts. "Yes, I'm ready," she answers, and together they begin. It is not easy; Maia must hold the dog, while Boaz injects the anesthetic. They do Theresa first, as if to practice on the weakest of the dogs, then Pablo and finally Mustard, and by the time they have finished with Mustard, the drug is already beginning to affect Theresa.

Afterward, there is nothing to do but watch; Maia pours two mugs of coffee from the little china pot, and she and Boaz sit in the chairs at their desks, swiveled outward. The dogs move free around the room, though always at a distance from the experimental box, as if they do not understand why they are not tied to the file drawer or harnessed up inside the box. Theresa is already distinctly slower, as if burdened by some weight; she lies for a moment on a pile of rags in the corner, and Mustard sniffs uncertainly beneath her tail. She struggles up again, but her hind legs drag; she pulls herself forward a little, then turns and drags her legs back toward the pile of rags. She does not reach it. Maia sees her fall; unsure, she stands, aware that Boaz is watching her, and pulls Theresa gently over to the rags, so that her head and forepaws rest upon them. Maia looks into the dog's eyes, as if perhaps expecting gratitude, but they are growing glassy. Theresa pulls for breath in short small shallow gasps, but as the drug overcomes her, her breaths grow long and wholly automatic. She does not move again.

"One down," observes Boaz, his voice flat.

"And two to go," answers Maia, her tone equally artificial. They do not look at each other.

Mustard and Pablo, heavier, healthier dogs, take longer to succumb; they stumble and dance, they slide down and fight back up, their legs slipping out from under them as they stagger sideways; they slurp water from the tin dish until they can no longer control their tongues, they whimper and thrash their tails and roll their heads, and in the end they too go down in motionless forms, their eyes glazed, their tongues hanging thick and still, their respiration so slow and even that it can barely be detected.

"Let's go," says Boaz finally, and Maia says nothing. She moves mechanically to open the door of the lab, and Boaz carries first Theresa, then Pablo, and then Mustard past the open doors of the office workers, outside to his car.

Phase 5

Wait. We saw, fairly clearly, what happened just beforehand: how Boaz got the right needle for the syringe and Maia fed her sandwich to the dogs, and we observed them together afterward, sitting silent in the lab, watching the dogs struggle down. But we have missed something between; we must have flinched, as one does in the face of the sun, letting our eyes close and turn away. If we are to see clearly, we must look back one last time.

We have seen them moving toward the center, Boaz and the girl, Maia. They have glanced at the clock, though they have not read it; it is early afternoon now, and on the other side of the campus people are waiting for them. Maia has loosened Theresa's leash from the drawer of the file cabinet; she has stood for a moment, uncertainly, in the middle of the room; now she sits, slowly, on the floor beside the dog. The filled syringe lies waiting on the desk; Boaz takes it and squats on the floor beside them. He puts the syringe on the floor, aware there is no need for sterile precautions, and looks just once at Maia. Together, they turn Theresa over so that she is lying on her back, Maia at her head, Boaz at her tail. Maia places her own thin leg over the dog's chest, to pin her down, and grasps her forelegs tightly, just above the elbow joint. Boaz shifts, uneasily, from squatting to kneeling, and picks the syringe up from the floor.

Watch: we see Boaz at the center now, as he kneels over Theresa, positioning the syringe over her belly. We see his back first, clearly; a small red mole on the back of his neck, then the fine creases of adult skin; we see the cross-woven threads of his cotton work shirt. We circle around his collar, and we count three anomalous whiskers, not more than an eighth of an inch long, that his razor has missed this morning. We see each separate stub of hair, closely shaven, we note the tiny pocks and minute lines of his skin, drawn in tight lines toward his mouth. We see small round beads of sweat across his upper lip, and others on his temples. If we are still, we sense the anxious pace of his heartbeat and feel the tight constriction of his breath. And then we see what he sees: the uneven edges of his fingernails, the coarse and calloused surfaces of his fingers, gripping the slim barrel of the syringe. He sees the slant-sharpened needle, poised. The drug must be injected directly into the peritoneum, he knows, and he chooses a place to the side of Theresa's abdomen and low, just above her back leg, where there are no internal organs that might be punctured. The hair on Theresa's belly is thin, and the needle rests directly on her pale skin. Her body moves a little as she struggles, but we see Maia holding her, her thin bare legs clamped across Theresa's chest, her small hands tight around the forelegs.

And we see Maia, too, we see the separate strands of her black hair, falling now into her face, into the face of the dog beneath her. It is thin hair, without curl or gloss. We see her round black-rimmed eyes, but they do not answer: they watch the floor, the cold tile floor, see the inexact angles of the edges of the tiles and the small fissures cracking between them; they study the scuffs and scratches, the streaks of dull gray color, the tiny pits and dents, the uneven seepages of mastic, the yellowed film of ancient wax. She looks once at Boaz and finds him watching her, his eyes wide, staring; her eyes recoil.

Her eyes recoil from his, and then she feels the dog jerk, she can almost feel the needle through the dog, the needle plunging into the soft belly, and she clamps her hands more tightly as the dog's throat arches back, yelping. She is afraid she will lose her grip, that the dog will struggle free and bite her, and she looks once more at Boaz, sees him fight to keep the dog's hind legs clamped between his knees, sees the syringe flap in the thrashing stomach, sees that it is still full, sees Boaz break, sweating heavily now, sees him break, lose hold of the syringe. It flaps wildly, and he grabs it, pulls it out.

The syringe is still full; the fluid is not in Theresa.

Boaz draws back, wipes his arm across his forehead. "I thought it would be easier," he says, unsure, afraid. His eyes plead.

But her eyes do not answer his. "Don't you know how to do this?" she asks, deliberately, almost coldly.

"Inject the anesthetic directly into the peritoneum," he recites mechanically, like a rote-learning schoolboy. "Be sure to avoid the internal organs. . . ."

"Haven't you done this before?" she asks, her voice kinder now.

"No."

"Then could we get somebody else to do it for us, somebody who knows how?" Maia's thin voice is hopeful.

Boaz turns on her. "I thought you weren't a coward."

She does not answer. She sees him pick the syringe up off the floor, the tip of its needle tinged with blood, and as she tightens her grip on the dog, she sees him hold it high, then thrust it hard into the abdomen. The dog howls again, hard and long. Maia's arms are suddenly weak, and she sees Boaz, his face sweating, his eyes narrow. She sees his hand move around on the syringe so that his thumb is on the plunger and he can press the fluid out of the syringe; she sees it, sees Boaz's thumb press the plunger, slowly, sees the Nembutal move slowly out of the syringe, through the needle, into Theresa, and she looks down into Theresa's face, sees the brown eyes wide and motionless with terror, feels the huge howl of pain welling up from her throat, from her bowels, a constant, motionless howl, frozen, frozen in pain, and Maia sees forever down in Theresa's open mouth, sees the brown-stained teeth and the flattened tongue, sees all the soft pale-red glistening surfaces of her throat, motionless in an eternity of pain.

No, much is not clear about the way the dogs died. Events on the periphery of the deaths, like points on outward-flowing circles, recede into ambiguity. The origins of the fact are obscure, its effects indeterminate. Causality has not been traced, at least not securely: dare we impute responsibility? Responsibility? To Boaz, or the thin girl Maia? No, responsibility is an empty conceit: of no concern, no consequence.

At the center there is only the fact: the dogs died.

Note

First published in *American Review* 22, 1975; reprinted in Martha Foley, ed., *The Best American Short Stories 1976* (Boston: Houghton Mifflin, 1976). © 1975 by M. Pabst Battin. Reprinted by permission.

11

The Ethics of Self-Sacrifice

What's Wrong with Suicide Bombing?

To cite just some of many examples, the Tamil Tigers have pursued a strategy of suicide attacks to pursue separatist aims in Sri Lanka; the Japanese kamikaze units used air and submarine suicide attacks during World War II; on September 11, 2001, al-Qaeda operatives used suicidal airplane crashes to destroy the World Trade Center and other targets in the United States; Palestinian militants have targeted Israeli civilians in tactical terrorist missions labeled *jihad*, and Iraqi defenders loyal to Saddam Hussein have tried to target U.S. military invaders. Most prolonged in the Palestine/Israel conflict, such missions have typically involved using young people strapped with explosives, dispatched as ordinary pedestrians to outdoor cafés, buses, seaside resorts, university commons, or anywhere civilians could be killed, on what the West called *suicide bombings* but which the militants themselves understood as *martyrdom*. In these remarks, I'd like to explore the deeper conceptual and ethical significance of tactical suicide missions within the context of more general issues about suicide, self-sacrifice, heroism, martyrdom, and other forms of self-caused death. What, exactly, accounts for the heightened moral repugnance with which these missions are viewed, compared to other resistance, military, and guerilla tactics? Is there adequate moral ground for this heightened repugnance—dubbed with the particularly pejorative label of "suicide"—or is it merely a matter of ideological prejudice?

Questions of *tactical* suicide and self-sacrifice arise in many practices around the globe, including situations like deliberate self-starvation in northern Ireland, fatal hunger strikes in Turkey, and self-immolation for reasons of social protest in Vietnam and Japan. Questions of tactical or goal-oriented suicide and self-sacrifice are also relevant to widely debated domestic questions of death and dying in terminal illness, severe disability, and extreme old age as well, where suicide may be undertaken in order to avoid pain, alleviate one's suffering, reduce health care costs, or spare one's family the anguish of watching a difficult death. Indeed, such issues are relevant in a great many contexts, among them literature—for example, in figures from Sophocles' Ajax to Goethe's Werther; philosophy—for example, in accounts from Plato to Hume; in theology, as in writings from Thomas Aquinas to Dietrich Bonhoeffer, and many, many more. The conceptual and ethical issues I wish to explore here about tactical suicide in political contexts, exhibited particularly vividly in the Israel/Palestine conflict, are not only questions about military strategy but at a deeper level issues about the role of the individual in bringing about his or her own death and equality in defending oneself from death.

Background Cultural Traditions

Virtually all major world traditions involve conceptual tension over the issue of self-caused death. In what is known as the Judeo-Christian tradition, suicide comes to be rejected (at least by the time of Augustine) as sinful, but is often conceptually difficult to distinguish from voluntary martyrdom—death accepted and in many cases sought or embraced to attest to one's faith and perhaps to seek salvation. In contrast, the tradition that begins with Hinduism and comes to include Buddhism includes many currents that emphasize release from self and from cycles of birth and rebirth: one seeks *not* to be reborn. Conceptual and moral tension is also evident in accounts of other forms of tactical suicide, for example Japan's use of kamikaze aircraft and submarine attacks toward the end of World War II, or the self-immolation of Buddhist monks and nuns to protest the policies of the Diem government during the Vietnam war. Similarly, current suicide bombing attacks by Palestinian militants and some few Iraqi loyalists must also be understood against a set of cultural and religious backgrounds, including Islam's uncompromising prohibition of suicide as well as its simultaneous embrace of voluntary martyrdom in the defense of the faith. But background cultural traditions are hardly the whole story, and conversance with them does not reveal the full depth of the moral issues—though in the end I think background cultural traditions will play a major role in the explanation of what is wrong.

Scientific Theories of Suicide, Biological, Psychological, and Sociological

Scientific theories of suicide beginning with Durkheim, Freud, and other figures at the beginning of the twentieth century variously understand the phenomenon of suicide as the product of specific forms of social organization, or as the product of ubiquitous human traits—for example, the expression of a deep-seated "death wish" or the product of psychopathology, as in depression or other mental illness, and in many other ways. Current research in suicidology further identifies epidemiological patterns of suicide, psychological profiles and traits that are held to characterize heightened suicide risk, and biochemical markers that are associated with suicide. Under contemporary scientific theories that attempt to understand suicidal behavior like self-starvation, self-immolation, and suicide bombing, an adequate account must uncover the psychopathology involved, including that brought about by the oppressed situation of political groups. The Palestinians' turn to suicide bombing, many contemporary analyses suggest, results from the desperate situation of the populace, particularly among young people growing up angry and hopeless, some of them naively idealistic and some of them manipulated for political ends by the group's military strategists.

There is a great deal of truth in these claims. The Palestinian populace is desperate. Its young people are angry and hopeless. The idealism of some is manipulated by military strategists, and families respond to inducements like large cash payments. Just the same, I think there is a great deal more to say about the ethical issues in such practices, and it cannot be assumed that they are simply a matter of psychopathology.

The (Im)morality of Suicide Bombing

A number of different reasons may be advanced to show that suicide bombing is immoral, and indeed of heightened or, one might say, aggravated immorality.

1. First—and most obviously—tactical suicide bombing kills people. As it has been employed in the Israel/Palestine conflict, it targets civilians: noncombatants who are killed indiscriminately but in ways designed to maximize public fear and outrage. These include bystanders, bus passengers, people at leisure, people at parties and celebrations, off-duty soldiers, children, and so on, but generally not officials, on-duty military personnel, or other military targets. Clearly, much of the repugnance of the practice is associated with its homicidal character: it is a strategy used to kill people. However, the ways of killing people used by other parties in political conflicts—howitzers, F-16s, bombs lobbed over borders or dropped from the air—also kill people, and while these actions too are considered homicide, they do not seem to arouse the same sort of special moral repugnance that suicide bombing does.

   However, suicide bombing also kills the suicide bomber himself or herself. This latter fact is sometimes used to account for the heightened moral repugnance of suicide bombing compared to other forms of political or military aggression: if the loss of life of a suicide-bombing attack is compared to that in a conventional attack of equal force, suicide bombing kills one more: the bomber him or herself. But this crude enumeration of lives lost is unable to account for what is widely perceived as the heightened, indeed aggravated immorality of suicide bombing.
2. Suicide bombing is often said to be of heightened moral repugnance be-

cause it is duplicitous. The suicide bomber can look his or her victims in the eyes, then violate that act of humanity by blowing them up. Furthermore, the gaze is one-sided: the suicide bomber arrives at the scene disguised, seemingly an everyday pedestrian, with the explosive material hidden under clothes; the purpose too is disguised, and the about-to-be-victim has no chance to see through the duplicity involved. The bomber smiles the "smile of joy," *bassamat al-Farah,* said to symbolize the joy of martyrdom,[1] but it is not recognized as such by the Westernized victims. When the first few female suicide bombers acted, the sense of duplicity was underscored: no one on the target side had expected women to play such roles.

3. Suicide bombing is also sometimes said to be of heightened moral repugnance because it involves *suicide,* and suicide is in itself wrong. The fact of suicide thus compounds the wrongness involved in targeting and killing civilians and other wrong-making features of this practice. But, of course, this is to assume, not prove, that suicide is wrong, or that it is wrong in this context. The history of both Western and non-Western thought involves extensive reflection on the question of whether suicide is wrong in itself, with some thinkers—notably those associated with monotheistic religious traditions (like Augustine, Thomas, Muhammad) or with deontological, principle-based ethical systems (like Kant)—holding that it is always wrong, while non-Western religious systems (especially Hinduism, Buddhism, and various traditional oral cultures) and somewhat more consequentialist and situation-relevant ethical thinkers have typically maintained that while suicide is morally wrong in some contexts, it is morally permitted or even obligatory in others (e.g., the Stoics, Hume, Nietzsche). Thus, the claim that suicide bombing is wrong because it involves *suicide* does not succeed without challenge.

4. Then, too, it may be argued that suicide bombing is morally problematic because the perpetrator cannot be held accountable; he or she is dead. Of course, many combatants in conventional combat also end up dead, and thus not able to be held accountable; but there is a certain sense in which one's posthumous reputation and memory can be held accountable. It is true that the perpetrator does not have to live with the negative consequences of the deed (in fact, perpetrators are said to believe that they will go to paradise), but the lack of individual accountability hardly seems to account in full for the heightened immorality of the deed. Nor is it clear that suicide bombing would somehow be less problematic if the perpetrator did get away alive; some argue that this would be still worse.

5. Finally, the 'tactical' feature of the suicide may seem to be problematic. While ordinary suicides of depression or remorse or unrequited love may have some dyadic features, aimed as they may be at changing the relationship between the victim and some other person, in tactical suicide bombing the suicide itself *is* the tactic. It does not so clearly exhibit the personal suffering of the person who commits suicide, and it is not just a

suicide, but something else. What is an ordinary expression of individual, personal crisis is warped, detractors might say, into a purposive tactic with an immense human cost.

But while this line of thinking points to one of the central characteristics of suicide bombing, its tactical character, it does not without further argument account for the heightened immorality of the practice.

The (A)morality of Suicide Bombing

A further line of thinking about the moral issues in suicide bombing does not try to establish its immorality directly, but challenges the notion that such suicides are voluntary, rational acts for which direct ethical assessment is appropriate. This line of thinking construes suicide not so much as *wrong,* but as *sick:* in keeping with contemporary clinical understandings of suicide and suicidal behavior, it sees suicide as pathological. It is thus not subject to moral assessment in ordinary terms; it is essentially amoral, to be condemned because it kills individuals (and the bomber) but not an appropriate subject for blame.

This line of thought is patently anemic. While there is truth in it too and while many of the suicide bombers are surely under intense psychological pressures, are subject to depression, have other mental illnesses, are forced into it in ways that violate autonomy, and so on, it is clear from accounts the bombers have left, videotapes they have made, notes they have written, and observations by others that their choice to engage in this activity was largely voluntary in a robust sense. True, some of those who have acted were still virtually children. But the same cannot be said of, for example, the pilots who trained for the suicide bombing of the Trade Centers, the driver of the van loaded with explosives that drove into the U.S. Embassy in Beirut in 1983, or the Palestinians who schooled themselves long in advance for suicide attacks and competed to be chosen. Nor do external incentives like large payments to surviving family necessarily play a choice-compromising role. What evidence there is suggests that the choices of the suicide bombers have often—though certainly not in every case—been precisely that—choices—and hence appropriate targets for moral assessment. Unlike some (but not all) ordinary suicides, they do not appear to be the product primarily of mental illness; to suggest that suicide bombing is *amoral* rather than *immoral* would be to fail to see one of the central characteristics of this act. Suicide bombing involves electing to die for a cause. As Fathi Shikaki, the spiritual leader of Islamic Jihad who was assassinated in Malta in 1995 had told reporters, he didn't personally choose suicide bombers: "Some of the youths insist that they want to lead a suicide operation—perhaps because they are influenced by the teachings of Islamic Jihad. My orders are to persuade them not to go, to test them. If they still insist they are chosen."[2]

The Morality of Suicide Bombing

Suicide bombing is seen as immoral, and indeed of heightened moral repugnance, by the side that is attacked or has been scheduled to be attacked—Israelis and

Americans, as well as many others in the industrially developed, traditionally Judeo-Christian nations. However, in the areas and nations from which the practice emanates, suicide bombers are seen as morally exemplary agents. They are martyrs, not suicides; their actions are heroic, their self-sacrifice noble and supreme, supported by interpretations of the Quran and Islamic history that date back to at least the seventh-century Battle of Karbala.[3] While it is true that the Quran itself implies that suicide is prohibited and the autobiography of Muhammad clearly rejects it, martyrdom and self-sacrifice in defense of Islam are just as clearly celebrated. To the extent that what the West calls suicide bombers are viewed as martyrs by the Islamic Middle East, they are admired, emulated, venerated.

Just as there is more to say about the rejection of suicide by Christianity and to a large extent by Judaism, while at the same time both traditions accept and celebrate martyrdom and self-sacrifice, there is more to say about these issues in the context of Islam as well. Clearly, the line between suicide and martyrdom is not drawn in quite the same place in these traditions. Contemporary vocabularies used to discuss these issues—vocabularies, especially scientific ones, for the analysis of suicide, and vocabularies, especially religious ones, for the celebration of martyrdom—tend to obscure these distinctions. But I want to look at a somewhat different issue in trying to tease out what, at least from the point of view of the West, accounts for the heightened moral repugnance of suicide bombing, and what may well account (though I am a good deal less sure about this) for the heightened moral esteem it earns within some factions within Islam.

The Central Moral Core of Suicide Bombing

I think the central feature of suicide bombing, in al-Qaeda attacks on the World Trade Center, in Iraqi loyalist attacks on U.S. soldiers, and especially in the attacks of Palestinian militants disguised as pedestrians crossing into Israel, has to do with the apparent violations of tacit presumptions of equality in mortal combat, including war and other forms of combat and aggression. It is, at root, an issue of fairness, one with disturbing implications.

Consider a variety of adages that serve to regulate individual behavior in aggression and combat: "Don't hit a man when he's down." "Don't stab someone in the back." Adages of this sort serve to promote relatively equal circumstances in fighting: you may hit another only when he is "up," that is, standing and not already seriously injured, and thus still in a position to hit you. Similarly, the second adage directs, you may stab a person only when he is facing you, hence able to see what's coming and thus able to prepare for and return the blow; it would be unfair to take advantage of a person by killing him unannounced and from behind, without fair warning. I think adages such as these operate, albeit usually tacitly, in much of our thinking about fighting, combat, aggression, and war. What the use of suicide bombing does is to violate this tacit assumption of equality in combat: suicide bombing confers unfair advantage. The party that employs suicide bombing has a weapon—the stealth and ability to penetrate invisibly into target situations—the other side doesn't. It can generate terror of a distinctive sort, possible precisely because of the tactic's capacity for intimate, unnoticed infiltration. It hits when someone is down, or at least defenseless; it stabs from behind, unexpected, unseen.

This argument may seem utterly facile in the context of the Israel/Palestine conflict. Unfair advantage? Even if the Palestinians have a weapon the Israelis don't—namely, suicide bombing—the Israelis have many, many weapons the Palestinians don't: tanks, F-16s, and, although they haven't used them yet, nuclear weapons. In contrast, the Palestinians, inhabitants of a controlled and occupied zone, have virtually no advanced military hardware at all. To suggest that what is central to the issue of suicide bombing is the notion of unfair advantage may seem insensitive, absurd, or worse.

However, what constitutes an "unfair advantage" is not merely a question of what weapons are currently available, but what one side or the other *could* use. The Palestinians do have the weapon in question, the tactic of suicide bombing—a tactic that, compared to other forms of political resistance, seems to be efficient, effective, and to maximize public notice—and the Israelis do not. However, this is not to say that the Israelis could not use such a tactic and thus, so to speak, even the score. Of course, it could be argued that the Israelis would be controlled in a way that prevents the acquisition of this advantage-conferring weapon, suicide bombing, if for instance international codes of war were to prohibit such tactics, just as the Palestinians are controlled in a way that prevents the acquisition of another set of advantage-conferring weapons, namely tanks, fighter jets, and the like; but while the codes of war prohibit commanders from sending soldiers on clearly suicidal missions, they do not prohibit soldiers from volunteering for high-risk missions.

But there is I think a much more interesting argument about the violation of the presumption of equality in such situations. This issue can be perhaps best explored by asking what sort of response to tactical suicide is justifiable, either by individuals or governments. Could, or should, the Israelis, the Americans, and the industrialized West that is the target of *jihad* actions adopt the same sorts of tactics in return? After all, these tactics have been visible and effective in achieving much of the Palestinian aims, with, as is often pointed out, comparatively little loss of life compared to conventional military forms of conflict resolution; they have been described as "the Palestinian H-bomb."[4] The question is not just whether such strategies could happen in other parts of the world as well, either occasionally or as a routine method of pursuing particular political agendas, but whether they should. To be sure, Israel has used a tactic of stealth-based assassinations of Hamas leaders and others believed responsible for the Palestinian uprising and suicide bombings, but these have been actions largely targeted at military figures, not bystander civilians. Americans killed hundreds of thousands of fleeing Iraqis during the first Gulf War; these are repugnant actions outside the realm of what is understood as permissible in war. Israelis, Americans, Europeans, and others have all sent their soldiers, sailors, pilots, and other combatants on missions from which there was only minuscule chance that they would return. But neither Israel nor the U.S. nor the Europeans have used suicide bombings or other forms of deliberately tactical suicide, as if there were something distinctively wrong with the deliberate use of *suicide,* somehow more problematic, more wrong than the other ugly actions of war.

But it is precisely here that the answer about what accounts for perceptions that suicide bombing is of heightened moral repugnance begins to emerge. It is not that the Israelis and the industrialized West do not use such tactics; it is that they *cannot* use them. This, I venture to suggest, is because the long cultural traditions of what has been called Judeo-Christianity not only revile suicide, but draw the line between suicide and martyrdom in a way that would preclude suicide bombing of the sort employed by the Palestinians and others. It is not that the West does not have this weapon; rather it cannot have it and cannot use it, because its cultural underpinnings provide no respect for it at all. It is, in a deep sense, unthinkable for the West. That is not to say that there might not be some volunteers who would be prepared to sacrifice themselves in this way for a cause they thought worthy, but that there would be little or no cultural support for suicide-based action at all. It could not be conducted as a routine strategy, it could not be counted on for a supply of willing volunteers, and it would not receive the elaborate sorts of social support, including adulation and financial reward, that Palestinian martyrs enjoy.

I think this is at least what makes the Palestinian use of tactical suicide so repugnant to the West. Palestinians can do this with eagerness and seeming ease; but the West cannot respond by flying its airplanes into buildings or sending young volunteers strapped with explosives into Palestinian markets, buses, or cafés. This is a moral inhibition, not a technical one, but a very real one nonetheless.

Suicide bombing, thus, exposes what the West experiences as a weakness in the face of an unfair advantage—"they" can fight in a way "we" cannot. The real issue is whether the use of tactical suicide is indeed morally repugnant, and should be used by neither side in any conflict, or whether its moral legitimacy in combat and war is a function of background cultural ideology: all right for "them," not all right for "us." This is why, I think, the West labels this practice "suicide" (one of the West's most negative, completely pejorative terms), why it refuses to see these actions as defensible cases of martyrdom, and why in general it does not try to think through the morality of the practice, but rejects it out of hand. Clearly, a practice that involves killing is repugnant in that fact alone, but whether it is a practice of heightened, aggravated immorality is the issue that remains to be further explored.

Notes

From *Archives of Suicide Research* 8(1):29–36 (2004). © International Academy for Suicide Research. Reprinted by permission.

1. Kushner, H. W. (1996) "Suicide bombers: Business as usual." *Studies in Conflict & Terrorism, 19,* 329–37, p. 331.
2. Kushner, "Suicide Bombers," p. 33, quoting L. Beyer and D. Fischer (1995), "Can Peace Survive?" *Time* 145:32.
3. Peters, R. (1996). *Jihad in classical and modern Islam.* Princeton: Markus Wiener.
4. Luft, G. "The Palestinian H-bomb: Terror's winning strategy." *Foreign Affairs* (2002, July/August): 2–7.

DILEMMAS ABOUT DYING
IN A GLOBAL FUTURE

12

Genetic Information and Knowing When You Will Die

The Size of Our Lives

Most of us, whether we like it or not, already have some rough idea of the likely size and shape of our lives—how long we will live, in what state of health, and what we will eventually die of. We live in an age in which life expectancy patterns for populations and subgroups of populations are known and predictable. We know the frequencies of the principal causes of death and the ages at which they are most likely to prove fatal. We know accident rates, risk ratios, and predictive factors for high-risk behaviors. Most important, we know that the age and cause of death of our own parents is the best predictor of our own mortality. Of course, we cannot for the most part tell if we as individuals will actually contract a specific disease, or become the victim of an accident, or succumb to some other cause of death. Furthermore, we often deceive ourselves about the ways our own health mainte-nance habits (or lack thereof) influence our expectable lifespan. Nevertheless, in general, in an extremely rough, often inchoate, not fully recognized way, we have a sense of what to expect about our own deaths and the periods of morbidity that may precede them: what is likely to happen to us, more or less, and about when, at what age, and for what reasons it will occur. If our ancestors all lived into their nineties and died of "old age," that is, of conditions that occur primarily at very advanced ages, we have a pretty good chance of doing so too; if they died of heart attacks in their fifties or cancer in their sixties, our anxieties mount when we reach these ages.

Many factors—improved actuarial computation techniques, better recordkeeping of mortality and cause-of-death statistics, better inter- and intrapopulation comparison data, better prediction of the emergence of new pathogens like viruses and flu strains, and so on, are likely to contribute to a change in this picture. Most of them are likely to make the picture sharper and clearer. But the biggest factor in changing this picture will be the increased possibilities of genetic analysis, coupled with clinical and epidemiological data that make possible both population-wide and individual prognostication. As it becomes increasingly informative to trace an individual's genetic legacy and thus to identify inherited disorders and diseases, physiological characteristics, and disease susceptibilities, it will become increasingly possible to make more and more accurate predictions about how long a person is likely to live, in what condition and with what degree of function, and when and how that individual is likely to die. Of course, as the possibility of prediction increases, so will the possibility of treatment, but people will still eventually die—in more predictable, forseeable ways.

This is the matter I want to explore. While I think human awareness of eventual illness and death will involve gradual change, barely perceptible to most individuals, I also think we must recognize that this is a process of change already well underway. This change will constitute a substantial transition from the present, and a huge departure from the past. What lies at the center of this change, I want to show, is the increasingly informative possibility of genetic prognostication (something of which we are already partly aware) about the size—the length, health characteristics, and cause of demise—of an individual's life.

I'm not the only one who wants to explore this possibility; Hollywood does too. Just the issue I want to explore has been very alarmingly raised—though I think trivialized in the most simple-minded reductionist way—in the science-fiction film *GATTACA,* released in 1997.[1] I take the box-office success of this film as a symptom that the general public may be sensitive to this issue too, at least at a superficial level, and I even imagine that this sensitivity may itself be a sign of the changes I want to describe.

Death in the Future: A Conjecture

Let us, then, jump to the future—the fairly near future, a world we already see on the horizon, not so awfully far away—maybe 20, maybe 50, maybe 100 years away at most. It will be a world, we may foresee, in which not only has the human genome been fully mapped but comprehensive correlation with clinical and epidemiological data has been already been carried out on a very broad scale. Genetic diagnosis and treatment have become routine, largely noncontroversial parts of the medical armamentarium. It will be a world in which familial patterns of disease are readily identifiable, and outcomes of both untreated and treated disease are known. It will be a world in which patterns of susceptibility to workplace toxins, environmental influences, ambient parasites, bacteria, and viruses, and other external factors, wherever these are controlled or influenced genetically, are also understood. In this not-so-distant future world, for example, it is possible to predict which miners are most likely to get black lung disease, which taxi drivers are most vulnerable to air pollution in urban environments, which women will probably suffer toxemia in pregnancy, who will get the flu, and which smokers will die early deaths. When new strains of viruses or new mutations in human genetic material appear, enhanced capabilities for detection and tracking will make it possible to understand these phenomena and their probable consequences for specific individuals quickly. Of course, all these things will involve an enormous amount of data collection and correlation with the findings of genetic research, including molecular genetics, genomics, and proteomics. It will be amplified by much greater scientific sophistication and the avoidance of simplistic assumptions about the genetic determination of human physiology and behavioral traits. Of course, it will reject the naïve radical genetic reductionism evident in Walter Gilbert's 1992 claim, "I think there will be a change in our philosophical understanding of ourselves . . . Three billion bases [of a human DNA sequence] can be put on a single compact disc (CD), and one will be able to pull a CD out of one's pocket and say, 'Here's a human being; it's me'!"[2] Rather, the application of advances in genetics will be the business of medicine, carried out with the aid of such specialized research fields as population genetics, epidemiology, and other areas of applied research. Its goal, scientifically challenging as it would be, is the complete "gene scan," routinely and easily made available for any individual human being.

Data too will be available for accidental risks, disaggregated finely over very small subgroups. While it will never be possible to anticipate what accidents will befall exactly which individuals, risk ratios for various groups, we may assume, will be known. We already know, for example, what subgroup is most likely to suffer fatal ski injuries (males ages 17–24), how often epileptics have fatal automobile accidents (very seldom, compared to adolescent males), how often condom breakage during sexual intercourse leads to the transmission of HIV. If genetic information becomes available about behavioral traits associated with, for instance, various forms of risk-taking behavior, including sports and adventure risks, sexual risks, and risks in impulsive and aggressive behaviors, this picture may also grow sharper and clearer.

Thus the future picture I want to explore is one in which many factors, but especially developments in genetics and related subfields, make it possible to prognosticate far more accurately about the cause and timing of an individual's death. What I want to ask is whether this will be a bad thing—yet another feature of some brave new world (like *GATTACA*) in which privacies are invaded and human meaning undermined—or whether it will be a good thing, still another product of advances in science that improve and enhance the human condition. I don't think this is an easy question to answer, and what I can say here will be but the barest sketch. But now let us return to the present, partway between the past and the future I wish to explore.

The Complexities of Genetic Prognostication

Some genetic prognostication about the size of life, though comparatively crude, is already possible. The child diagnosed with Tay-Sachs disease, for example, can be predicted to live only a couple of years—to age three or four, at the most. At the opposite extreme, the person whose parents died of Alzheimer's disease with onset in the eighties can with some degree of likelihood expect a similar demise at about a similar age, at least if his or her genetic makeup includes the relevant gene or genes from one—but only one—of these parents; if he or she has the gene or genes from both parents the likelihood is of onset and death at a much earlier age. Here, the likelihood that is genetically predictable includes both contracting Alzheimer's at that late age and not contracting any other fatal disease at an earlier age: if the parents did not, the offspring is less likely to do so either. People testing positive for Huntington's can, on the whole, expect the onset of symptoms in their mid-thirties to mid-forties, with death about ten to fifteen years later. Similarly, it appears that women with mutations in the BRCA1 gene associated with breast cancer have a 50/50 chance of developing the disease by age 50, and an 85% chance by age 70, though some women never contract the disease at all, and it may be—though we do not yet know—that the risk varies by population. With familial polyposis, colon cancer is most commonly diagnosed in the thirties and forties. Inherited cancers tend to be of earlier onset than those associated with sporadic mutations and those in which there is no known germline abnormality at all.

With a handful or two of exceptions like these, genetic prognostication about the size of life remains at the moment enormously crude. Furthermore, these exceptions are in themselves still quite crude. Many genetic conditions have reduced penetrance, and individuals without symptoms may have the same gene mutation as individuals who do have symptoms; we do not know how to predict this yet. Symptoms may be severe in one person but mild in another. It is often difficult to distinguish between early-onset versions of a disorder and late-onset forms, and whether, indeed, they are different forms at all. The predictive value of genetic information often depends on information about other affected family members, information that is not always available. The activity of some genes may counteract that of others, as do oncogenes and tumor-suppressor genes, and there may be other as-yet-undiscovered patterns. We have only a rudimentary understanding of "two-hit" conditions, abnormalities that must be present in two different alleles or two different genes affecting the same pathway for symptoms to occur, or of multifactorial conditions in which a genetic disposition results in disease only in the presence of specific environmental modifiers. We do not fully understand the function of genes that, in heterozygotes, protect against some conditions, like malaria but, in homozygotes, cause others, like sickle-cell anemia. Treatment may already substantially affect the outcomes of some genetic diseases, so that there are fewer cases available for observing their natural history. And, of course, our present capacities for genetic prognostication are limited by the fact that while the mapping of the human genome was officially completed in 2003, much more refinement is needed; not only have we not yet identified the genes involved in all single-gene mutation disorders, but disorders involving several interacting genes, genetic and epigenetic modifiers, and multifactorial disorders exacerbated by or associated with environmental factors, behavioral and personality traits, and many other factors have not yet been discovered.

But, let us assume, they will be. That is what a *complete* mapping of the human genome, coupled with comprehensive medical and epidemiologic study, would provide: this is the complete "gene scan." We cannot of course at the present moment know how far advances in genetic science, together with developments in medicine and epidemiology, will take us, or at what point we will know, so to speak, everything there is to know about the human genome and its implications for human health—or, indeed, whether we will ever reach that point. But we will certainly know a *great* deal more in the future than we do now, and it is crucial to anticipate what these changes in scientific and clinical knowledge will contribute to changes in human experience.

How It Used to Be

At all periods of human history up until the middle of the previous century, the length and character of the end-stages of an individual human life were far less predictable—indeed, virtually unpredictable—except perhaps for someone born in already compromised health and with obvious deficits: then, clearly, life would be short, though some individuals born apparently healthy would also live short lives while others much longer ones. In these earlier periods of human history, life expectancy fluctuated between about ages twenty and forty, depending primarily on the occurrence of famines and epidemics of infectious disease, particularly evident in high rates of infant mortality. These were interrelated: famine resulted in malnutrition and hence increased vulnerability of the individual to infectious and parasitic disease; epidemics of infectious and parasitic disease affected food supplies, including crops and animals; and epidemics affecting crops and animal food supplies, together with variations in the weather, increased the chance of famine for humans. The specific occupations or roles of individuals might enhance their risks: soldiers suffered an increased risk of death due to infected battle wounds (a bigger killer in most wars than outright trauma), and women in childbirth were far more vulnerable to generalized sepsis. To some degree, the aristocracy in nearly every society was protected from some of the risks the peasantry faced, at least by virtue of better nutrition, better sanitation, and freedom from the risks of physical labor, but the aristocracy were not entirely protected. They too succumbed to infectious and parasitic disease. In all these previous eras of human history, death could occur at any time, largely without much warning, and largely without the physician being able to do much to prevent it. While it might have been possible to predict life expectancies for population groups and subgroups in various circumstances (though no societies had adequate datakeeping methods for doing so), there was little one could predict about the fate of a given individual. If a person got an infection, he or she might or might not survive; if the plague was raging, some individuals but not others who were exposed would live through it. There was little or no way to predict which ones. Similarly, some soldiers but not others would die of seemingly equally infected battle wounds; some women but not others would become septic in childbirth. Beyond appraising such matters as nutritional status, age, and the presence or absence of other concurrent diseases, it would be hard to predict of any individual with any potentially but not uniformly fatal disease or condition just what the outcome would be, survival or death.

Some of this mortality, we may assume, was associated with heritable diseases. Much more of it, we may also assume, was associated with varying degrees of susceptibility to endemic bacteria, toxins, viruses, and parasites, and these varying degrees of susceptibility, we may suspect, will also have been due at least to some degree to heritable patterns. But while many of these societies recognized notions of family traits—similarities of facial appearance and physical characteristics within a lineage—and also had extensive empirical experience in the practice of animal husbandry, they had no well-developed notion of genetic science. Heritable conditions and diseases in humans could be recognized as "running in the family" only after they became symptomatic; and the notion of a genetic pattern fixed at conception was completely unknown. Adopted children and people whose parents had been killed in accidents or war early in life had little way of knowing their own family health traits at all.

Even with a conception of family traits, people in societies prior to the development of genetic science would be prone to various sorts of error in predicting the likely course of their own lives. Each individual has two genetic parents, four genetic grandparents, and eight genetic great-grandparents, typically with different disease and mortality histories. Without the mechanisms of genetic diagnosis, that individual has little reliable way of telling which "family traits," from which side of the family, he or she receives. Of course, there is often an enormous amount of speculation within a family about which ancestors an offspring "takes after" that might provide the basis for speculation about the size of that offspring's life, but this of course would trade on the unfounded assumption that a child with resemblances to a given parent in facial appearance or other externally observable characteristics will therefore inherit the same health traits as that ancestor, including as yet asymptomatic diseases and disease suceptibilities. This is a form of rudimentary genetic prognostication, but it is not very reliable at all.

But that picture is changing, for two principal reasons. First, beginning around the middle of the nineteenth century, with the development of the germ theory of disease and associated improvements in public sanitation, antisepsis, immunization, and, in the twentieth century, the development of antibiotics and other resources for controlling infectious and parasitic disease both in humans and in their food sources, the principal causes of death have changed. Now, in the developed world of the twenty-first century, most people die of degenerative diseases—heart disease, cancer, various types of organ failure, neurological diseases, and so on, which are the product not so much of external causes like bacteria, viruses, and parasites as of internal breakdown. To be sure, some of this breakdown is associated with or caused by external factors, as liver disease is associated with alcohol consumption, or lung disease with smoking and environmental conditions. Some we're not sure about, for example, the possible associations of Alzheimer's disease with a virus. But by and large, the contemporary causes of death are different in kind from those of our earlier world. To put it most simply, in earlier periods of human history, most people were killed by germs and worms; now most people in the developed world fall apart from malfunctioning of their own systems.

In contrast to the infectious and parasitic diseases of which people typically died in all earlier ages of human history, the diseases of which we die now tend to have onsets at comparatively predictable ages and exhibit comparatively predictable courses. With germs and worms, you could never really predict when they would kill you, though certain situations—agricultural labor, military service, childbirth—provided much greater invitation. In contrast, the principal contemporary causes of death in the developed world are degenerative diseases—heart and circulatory disease, cancer, organ system disease, and neurological diseases that, even when associated with viral or bacterial factors, are far more predictable: once a "terminal" illness is underway, we have some idea about the way it will go and about the duration of the downhill course. Furthermore, this is true for most contemporary dying in the developed world: heart disease and cancer, both clusters of degenerative conditions with comparatively predictable characteristic courses, account for about two-thirds of deaths. Only a minority of deaths in the modern world are completely unforeseen and unpredictable.

That picture is also changing because of our greater alertness to the importance of genetic information. As Bob Cook-Deegan suggests (personal communication), we are probably the first generation to care about what happens to our parents not just from affection and filial loyalty but in part because we realize in an informed way that it is predictive of our own personal futures. The greater predictability of degenerative disease over infectious disease is further enhanced as genetic diagnosis makes it increasingly possible to detect heritable versions of these conditions and susceptibilities to disease. For the first time in human history, we now sometimes reliably know what to expect even in advance of the appearance of symptoms. Thus, not only do we die of more predictable diseases at more predictable ages than did human beings in the past, but genetic diagnosis also makes it possible in many cases to say which disease specific individuals are likely to die of, and thus, what the timing and conditions of their deaths are likely to be. This is not, of course, guaranteed; but it is *likely*. In short, we already know far more about the likely circumstances of the ends of our own lives than have human beings at any earlier age. This, I believe, has already subtly begun to change the way we see death.

The Complexities of Genetic Prognostication, Continued

But although we now know far more about the probabilities in the character and timing of our own deaths than have human beings in the past, we must not oversimplify this claim. There is an enormous amount we do not and cannot yet know.

Take, for instance, what we can now predict about the lifespan of someone who tests positive for the Huntington's disease (HD) gene mutation. In the first place, we must admit that this claim itself is not certain; there is a small chance—though less than 1%—of lab error. Second, we cannot say for certain in a more general metaphysical sense that this person will *ever* develop the symptoms of Huntington's; there is always the possibility that life will be interrupted in some other say, say by an unrelated fatal disease, accident, or other cause of death, even though this individual would have contracted HD if he or she had remained alive.

Even the predictions we do make are rough at best. Although we can predict, for the person testing positive for the genetic mutation associated with Hunting-ton's, an onset of symptoms somewhere between the ages of 35 and 45, a subse-quent life expectancy somewhere around 12–15 years, a course that declines into pronounced disability due to chronic progressive chorea and dementia, and death of secondary infection, aspiration, or heart failure, none of these predictions are exact. For one thing, they are all based on statistical distributions. For example, although the onset of symptoms typically occurs between ages 35 and 45 (with younger-onset cases typically having affected fathers), there is a bell-shaped tail extending away from the mode on either side, with a few cases far earlier—children as young as 2, and some later, at 50, 60, and even a few at 80. Life expectancy after onset is also a statistical claim: although average life expectancy is about 12–15 years, some people die of Huntington's (not other causes) within a few years of the first appearance of symptoms, and some live for quite a number of years, especially in late-onset families; some are relatively mildly affected and only be-come symptomatic at later ages, increasing the likelihood that other factors will be the cause of death. Typical life expectancy for HD children is shorter, about 8–12 years, but this too is a bell-shaped modal prediction with tails on both sides. The nature of the symptoms is also variable. Although for most people with HD the chorea or tremor is the most pronounced physical symptom, in some individuals the disease involves progressive rigidity, not choreic movement. And death can occur in a variety of ways, not just the most frequent forms listed here.

To be sure, some of this variation itself may be predictable. For example, although some Huntington's families are comparatively late-onset families and oth-ers early-onset ones, and although some families exhibit less, others greater, amounts of variation within the family, much of this variability is accounted for by the number of expanded repeats in the IT 15 gene on chromosome 4. While variability remains wide, where there is a CAG repeat size of more than 60, for example, the disease tends to have become symptomatic before age 40, while in-dividuals with lower numbers of repeats tend to have onsets at later ages as well as more variability in age of onset.

In short, just having the Huntington's gene doesn't entail that a person will develop specific symptoms at a certain age and die a fixed number of years later—that would be a common misperception rooted in overly simplistic genetic deter-minism. Nevertheless, HD is one of the best current examples of a heritable con-dition in which the identification of a gene mutation makes it possible to say—not precisely, but roughly, very roughly—how long a person will live and what he or she will die of—that is, what the approximate size of his or her life will be.

This picture is far from exact. While Huntington's is currently one of the most predictable known late-onset genetic diseases, the predictions now possible are so far from exact that most HD testing centers caution against using data to make specific predictions about the life expectancy of a given individual at all. Never-theless, even if this prognostic picture is far from exact, it is far more specific than the kind of prognostic picture an individual could have made prior to 1983, the year the markers were identified and linkage data became available. Before 1983, the best guess you could make, if you had a parent with HD, was that you had a 50/50 chance of having HD yourself and a greater chance of earlier onset if that parent was your father rather than your mother; but if you did not have an HD parent, you had virtually no chance of developing HD.[3] That was *all* you could know. And this prognostic picture of just a little more than a decade ago was in turn already far more specific than what had been available in the more remote past, before it was known that Huntington's involves an autosomal dominant gene. We can speculate about how an autosomal-dominant disease like Huntington's might have appeared to a prescientific, pre-Mendelian tribe (though the disease was not described until 1872): a scourge that afflicts some of the children of a person afflicted by it—perhaps the manifestation of divine revenge for wrong behavior or a curse upon a particular lineage—but skips other children of the same parent. With just this information, the children of an affected parent might themselves wonder whether they would get it, but would have no explanation for why it might be themselves and not their siblings. To a group that knew nothing of genetics, autosomal recessive conditions would surely have appeared even more erratic, more mysterious in their manifestations, explanable only as a curse or scourge the gods could inflict on anyone at any time, but without much warning at all. Even now, people symptomatic for recessive conditions often protest, "but it never showed up in my family before."

Genetic prognostication, even in its inexact present, must take into account other factors as well: for example, the changing risks as avoidance of conception, selective abortion, and somatic and/or germline therapy are used. For example, another of the currently best predictive examples is Tay-Sachs disease, a heritable condition in which symptoms lead to death within a fairly narrow range of ages: a Tay-Sachs child typically dies by age 3 or 4. However, due to widespread, well-accepted screening, Tay-Sachs is very rapidly disappearing as a disease among the population formerly at highest risk, Ashkenazi Jews, though the prevalence of the genetic mutation is not reduced by parental choices to abort or not to reproduce at all, since their affected children would in any case not themselves have reproduced. While it is not likely that this disease will disappear altogether from human experience, its prevalence is already dropping dramatically, and with it one of the conditions in which the predictability of the size of life was highest.

Improvements in treatment will influence predictability as well. For example, variability of outcome appears to be increasing among patients with cystic fibrosis (CF). Not long ago virtually all classical CF victims died by the time they were teenagers; now, many people with CF live longer lifespans. To some degree, this may reflect greater ability to diagnose mutations associated with milder forms of the disease, but it is certainly also a function of substantial gains in effective treatment. Similarly, untreated hemochromatosis characteristically produces organ deterioration beginning in the thirties and forties and death in the early fifties in males (though iron overload is not typically a problem in females until after menopause), but with early, presymptomatic treatment, life expectancy rises to normal. Predictability may seem to be reduced by this greater spread of possible outcomes for diseases like cystic fibrosis and hemochromatosis, though what we are actually seeing is in part the spread in outcome among untreated, routinely treated, and expertly treated disease: cases in each group would be increasingly predictable.

In the long run, advances in genetic diagnosis, together with advances in treatment of genetic diseases and disorders, may work to make the size of life more nearly uniform for all individuals. Heritable conditions involving very young onset age and uniform lethality, like Tay-Sachs, anencephaly, and some of the trisomies will, I think, be virtually eliminated as diseases altogether, as screening programs and risk analysis dissuade parents from conceiving infants who will with certainty be affected in these ways. Improved therapy will delay the onset, increase the survival rate, and in other ways increase life expectancy for those with later-onset or later-mortality conditions. Of course, we cannot know whether advances in genetic diagnosis and therapy will also work to increase the life expectancy of the oldest old, so that human lifespans will still vary substantially in size, or whether the length of life—increased for those who would have died earlier of heritable conditions—will approach and eventually equal those who now die at the oldest ages. We also cannot know how our health-care institutions will change and what their degree of commitment will be to treatment of these conditions, and in general whether people will have uniform access to these advances. But whether or not individuals' lifespans continue to grow more nearly equal (as they already have in the industrialized nations), the predictability of them, whether short or long, is certain to increase.

The Future: More Predictable Death

Will it be a good thing to inhabit a future world in which, routinely, we know our complete genetic makeup and hence—as is my specific conjecture here—have a far more concrete idea of the likely size and shape of our lives? We will never know in advance a specific date of death, of course, but we may well know when it is likely to occur within a far narrower range. Will this be a harm, either to specific individuals, to their family members and social groupings, or to society as a whole? And will it be a loss both of human innocence and of something central in human experience, something at the root of deepest human meaning? Or will the future mean relief from uncertainty, a waning of background anxiety over death, or the end of chronic, though suppressed, terror over impending doom? If we are now partway between a past in which human beings had little way of guessing when they would die and a future in which human beings will routinely almost all know more or less what to expect, is this progress in human experience, or a loss?

A science-fiction social-issues film like *GATTACA* tries to answer just this question, but does it in a perfectly predictable way. Like many other such films, including, for example, *A Clockwork Orange* and *Soylent Green, GATTACA* works on a tacit "slippery-slope" model, taking a possible future technological change (whether sophisticated operant conditioning or genetic diagnosis and prenatal genetic engineering) and positing extreme negative social consequences that would ensue—usually suppression of individual liberty, the development of intrusive social constraints, and tyranny by the technological elite. Such films' plots work by focusing on one or two innocents who resist such a society, and in the process, typically, fall in love. What is glossed over in such films are the questions about why such a society might develop, and what other consequences might be foreseen for the particular technological changes imagined. Hollywood needs challenge, threat, crisis, and the small forces of good against a huge, entrenched evil to make a powerful plot; but philosophers may want to look at the issues in a more open and informed way.

Would the world we can foresee be a better one, or not? This is a complex question, with a number of interrelated issues to be explored. Some initial objections might be entered to assembling information about a person's overall genetic makeup or to divulging it to people in a routine way. For example, it might be argued that divulging such information to people would be undesirable because it would alter their risk-taking and health-maintenance behavior: believing they will live to 90, they will not protect themselves in their twenties. But such behavior would involve a logical error: that someone expects to die of Alzheimer's disease in her nineties does not mean that she cannot die of a skydiving accident in her twenties. On the other hand, at least some health-maintenance behavior would, presumably, be altered favorably to try to arrest the course of a known though not yet symptomatic disease—people testing positive for hemochromatosis, for example, would refrain from eating iron-rich foods.

It might also be argued that routine assembling and divulging of such information would undercut people's insurability. Certainly, information about genetic risk could constitute a real liability if it were disclosed to a health insurer—and if the insurer were legally permitted to act on it.[4] But in a world in which assessment of individuals' entire genetic makeup is routine—perhaps routinely disclosed, for example, to schools, employers, the military, the justice system—insurance as we now know it cannot exist, since both the prospective insureds and the insurers would have the same information, and cream-skimming—selective coverage of people with better health risks but denial of coverage to those with worse risks—would be impossible. People with long expected lifespans and low expected morbidity would not need much health insurance, except coverage for accidents, though insurers would be willing to sell it to them; people with short expected lifespans and/or long periods of expected morbidity would seek health insurance but find it impossible to purchase at any reasonable fee. Thus, the entire system of health insurance would be undercut. Presumably, health insurance would be replaced by some form of universal-access program of care, and life insurance, trading as it does on risk, would virtually cease to exist at all.

Greater predictability of medical and behavioral characteristics of individuals will raise many other questions as well. Workplace exclusion policies are already heavily debated, both publicly and in the courts: should employers be able to exclude from jobs workers who exhibit genetically demonstrable higher susceptibility to diseases associated with various workplace toxins and environmental factors? May mining companies refuse to hire miners at greater risk for black lung disease, or taxi licensure boards refuse medallions to drivers more vulnerable to air pollution? May the school system or the military or the criminal justice system track individuals on the basis of genetically based behavioral predictions? Or suppose musical talent turns out to be genetically based: minimal endowment in this area may provide a reason not to save a child a place at the conservatory, but would it be sufficient reason to exclude him or her from the high school band? And there is *GATTACA's* practical question: may people with greater risk of heart conditions be excluded from eligibility for a space-flight program?

These questions and objections aside, the real issue concerns what sorts of changes might occur in the human experiential condition. How will we feel about knowing so nearly the likely character of our final illnesses and the time of our dying? Of course, not all deaths are due to heritable diseases, disease susceptibilities, or causes influenced by inherited or sporadic genetic mutations: some people will still be hit by lightning or be run over by trucks. But except for unpredicted trauma, including some but not all homicide and suicide (some of which may be associated with genetically based behavioral traits, like aggressiveness), we may conjecture that genetic factors control or at least influence most deaths. This includes both deaths from infectious and parasitic disease and also deaths from degenerative disease, but since degenerative disease is itself more predictable in time of onset and in its terminal course once begun, predictability is far greater here. Thus, newly available genetic information, sophisticated in its background science and linked with advances in epidemiology and other data-correlating fields, will give rise to a dramatically new prognosticative picture. We cannot be sure of the details; but we can be sure that huge changes are coming, and indeed are already underway.

How will we feel about the far greater predictability this information will bring? Predicting how people will respond and behave in such a world is, of course, sheer conjecture; but it is not entirely uninformed. Here are some things to consider about how people now react to genetic diagnoses that may suggest how people will respond to new capacities for prognostication in the future. For one thing, as one genetic counselor currently puts it, people measure their plight in terms of everybody else.[5] If a person believes (albeit falsely) that most people live to the average life expectancy, now nearly 73, but discovers that because of a genetic disorder he is likely to die at 30, he experiences this as deprivation compared to everybody else—he "loses" more than forty years. Furthermore, it seems to him that it is only he who has discovered that his life will be short; other people do not have such specific knowledge about when or of what they are likely to die. He is doomed, it seems, and they are not. He also loses the capacity they have to believe they will live long lives, even if it is not likely to turn out to be true.

How people react to the news about a future disability or death also depends on how everybody else reacts, or how that a person believes others will react: if they expect others to react to the news about genetic disease with horror, disgust, rejection, accusations of taint, and so on, that person's own reaction is likely to be that much worse. Furthermore, many people (and their doctors) do not process risk information very well: what does 1:200 mean? 1:5000? 1:2, if you still cannot tell what this means for sure about your own specific case? Some people avoid genetic testing because, they fear, this would take away hope (they sometimes forget that the test result could be negative); others, even when they have a positive test result, continue to hope—not that they will not develop the disease, but that they will have a very-late-onset case, or a mild case, or that a cure is developed. It may also be that people seem primarily concerned with potential symptoms, disability, and the experiences of other affected family members when they are confronted with the possibility of genetic disorders, but these may also mask concerns about illness as the process that leads to death. We see all these responses to what is regarded as "premature" death; we also see them even for many individuals who live well past the average life expectancy, since even the latter deaths seem unpredictable and often, thus, somehow unfair when they do occur.

An Impossible Future: Knowing the Date of One's Death

Check one box:
__ I'd like to know the exact date, time, and cause of my death now.
__ I would not like to know the date, time, or cause of my death in advance, at least not now.

Barring astonishing developments in clairvoyance, human awareness of death— regardless of the sophistication of genetic and other prognostication—will never be so good as to be able to predict the precise date, time, and cause of an individual's death. But what people say in response to this forced-choice question provides some indication of how they might respond to substantially increased possibilities of genetic prognostication about the likely size of one's life. Here's what some people say:

1. Yes, then I could take care of my business and plan for the end.
2. No, it would ruin my life; I'd be worrying about it all the time.
3. I'd only like to know if the date isn't within five years.
4. I wouldn't like to know now; but I would like to know if, in general, everybody else knows the dates of their own deaths.
5. I'd rather know about my own parents' deaths than my own.
6. I don't want to know, and I want to convince myself that it doesn't matter.
7. I'd like to know only if my death would be sudden, so that I can say goodbye to people first. [Note that accidental deaths not associated with a genetically based behavioral trait are the one sort that would not be predictable on the basis of genetic information.]
8. I wouldn't want to *know*, but I would want to have the predictive capacity to change my circumstances.
9. Yes, I'd want to know, just because it's *my* death.
10. I wouldn't like to know, because I'd give it away by acting differently even if I didn't actually tell anyone, and they'd treat me differently as a result.
11. I don't care so much about when I die, but how, and about what this would do to my relatives.
12. I don't care about the date of my *death*. What I care about is the date of my incapacitation—would I be in a coma for 20 years before death?

The question to which these answers are responses, "Would you want to know the exact date, time, and cause of your death now?" is a crystal-ball question, an impossible question to which we will never be able to provide real answers. But the responses people give to it allow us to discern what we can expect would be two quite different patterns of response to the prospect of knowing much more nearly the *likely* time-range and cause of one's death: not just yes-or-no answers, but two basically different types of answers: instrumental and noninstrumental forms. This difference between instrumental and noninstrumental responses to the prospect of knowing the crystal-ball date and cause of one's death allows us to begin to answer the question of how our world will change—and whether these changes will be good or bad—as increasing capacities for genetic prognostication actually do make it far more possible than at any period in human history to know the approximate date and cause of one's own death—not just shortly beforehand but for most of one's life, even, perhaps, from childhood on.

The Genetic Future: Knowing the Size of Our Lives

Knowing the size of our lives, at least approximately so, will, we can predict, elicit both instrumental and noninstrumental responses. But they are very different.

Instrumental responses

Instrumental responses to the prospect of knowing something point to the uses that can be made of that information. If the information concerns the approximate timing and cause of one's death, known far in advance, we can imagine at least three areas in which this information might be used.

PREVENTION AND TREATMENT OPTIONS

In some cases (for example, hemochromatosis), presymptomatic knowledge of a genetic disease permits the choice of prevention and treatment options—here, the prevention of iron accumulation, or treatment by flushing out of iron accumulation—that can radically alter one's prospects for life. Of course, one does not have to know the approximate timing of one's death in order to select prevention or treatment options, but one does have to know one's disease status, and with this, in the future I am exploring, comes at least some knowledge of the approximate timing of one's death.

PLANNING

Pragmatic planning of many everyday matters may hinge on knowing the approximate timing and cause of one's death: for example, whether to purchase life insurance, if risk-rated insurance remains available at all (important if you have dependents and expect to die young; a waste of money if you expect to die in old age); whether to take out disability insurance or long-term care insurance (important in conditions like Alzheimer's and Huntington's); whether to take out a 30-year mortgage, whether to sign up for a long tour of duty in a country with an inadequate health-care system, whether to explore with one's physician the possibility of eventual assistance in suicide, and so on. Of course, it may be hard to predict whether knowing in advance will enhance or undermine an individual's psychological capacity for planning, and whether in particular those with predicted shorter lives are more likely to live in unplanned, "fast-lane" ways just because they expect to die young. It may also be hard to predict whether individuals will respond in rational or irrational ways to advance notice about their own deaths. But some individuals will see it, as an economist might put it, as an opportunity for allocating resources prudentially over one's expected lifespan, and hence maximizing benefit without risking loss.

COMMUNICATING

Prognostic knowledge of the likely cause and timing of death may facilitate communication among family members, both in order to begin saying goodbye and to prepare family members for the kinds of terminal illnesses to be expected. These patterns already occur among, for example, people at risk for Huntington's; their experience (though not necessarily the fear of such a difficult end) might be far more widely replicated among individuals generally. Communicating about these matters might of course generate its own moral dilemmas: if you fall in love, are you obligated to tell the person you love that you expect a lifespan of, say, only five or ten years? Should you undertake parenthood if you do not expect to live another twenty, until a child reaches adulthood? Should you enter a partnership or make a contract you do not expect to be able to maintain over time? Of course, these are dilemmas already faced by people with some genetically based conditions; in the future, they would be faced by nearly everybody as they neared the end of their projected lifespans, on a far broader scale.

Life Choices

Basic life choices also might ride on knowing the approximate size of one's life. These life choices can involve such basic matters as career choices, mate selection, emotional investment in long-term projects and goals, and so on. For example, the smart kid who expects a comparatively short life might choose to be a mathematician, on the grounds that most advances in mathematics are made by people at very young ages—the late teens, early twenties; the same smart kid who foresees a very long life might instead choose a field (perhaps philosophy) where maturity of thought counts for a great deal. Similarly, knowing the approximate size of one's life might invite one to think more carefully about selecting a mate with the same sorts of prospects, about reproductive choices and whether and when to have children, and so on. And one will, presumably, select life-commitments and life-projects in accord with some more realistic notion of whether one will be able to see them through, and not be interrupted by an "untimely" death. These basic life choices are perhaps best conceptualized as a more profound sort of planning and communicating, but a sort that is only possible now in the most rudimentary, unreliable sort of way.

Noninstrumental Responses

Noninstrumental responses to knowing information about the likely end of one's life are far harder to understand. These are situations in which knowing information is significant, though not because it is to be put to any practical use. Where the information is information about one's own genetic makeup and so information about the likely cause and timing of one's death, this may contribute, in some intangible way, to one's sense of self, of who one is, what sort of person one is, what one's life is like. Self-knowledge is often painful, and this form of self-knowledge may be so as well. But it may also contribute to what we think of as the quintessential way of being human in the world. It is far harder to talk about the value of being able to comprehend and reflect about one's own circumstances as a human being, and there is even disagreement about whether it is a value or a disvalue (though the maxim "better Socrates dissatisfied than a pig satisfied" still rings in our ears), but it is the really important issue here. Advances in genetic science will presumably also make it possible for us to perform the same sort of prognostication about the length of life for individual animals and plants of various species, but animals and plants cannot comprehend this information and do not, we assume, have a sense of self, something usually held to be possible only for humans. For humans, the possibilities of genetic prognostication, I think, will bring something new to the sense of self an individual has, something we now have only in the most inchoate ways: the sense of myself as a person with a certain size of life, whether short or long.

How will knowing oneself as a person with a probably short lifespan, or a probably long lifespan, change us? Will knowing this from childhood on be more or less like knowing—something that will also become possible—whether one will be tall or short, something that, for the most part, an individual eventually must just accept? After all, the capacity to know in advance is likely to precede the capacity to do anything about changing it. Do we adapt better to the circumstances of our lives if we know what they are going to be?

The barest evidence from studies of responses of people taking diagnostic tests for Huntington's disease invites us to conjecture that knowing one's genetic makeup and hence knowing in advance the probable timing and cause of one's death will lead to a decrease in anxiety and stress. Of subjects measured before and after undergoing diagnostic analysis, those who received good news (negative for the Huntington's mutation) and those who received bad news (positive for the mutation) both experienced decreases in anxiety and stress; subjects whose results were inconclusive remained at higher anxiety and stress levels.[6] There are reasons not to draw too heavily on this study; for one thing, it was flawed by the design of the control group, which included some subjects who were not tested at all, and, for another, it examined people who got news comparatively suddenly, after a test, about a matter they had been in the dark about for their whole lives. It has not been replicated for BRCA1 testing. And in any case, it is a big leap from this one small study of one disease condition to a generalization about what it would be like for human beings to be routinely aware of their own genetic makeup and of the approximate size of their lives. Yet it is a tempting leap anyway: we may speculate, at least, that human beings would experience less anxiety about death, less open-ended, free-floating *angst*. At the same time we can predict that that knowledge will be painful for some, namely, those who must expect short lives. And anxiety may increase for all individuals as the age range in which they can expect the onset of the disease or condition that is likely to kill them approaches. And, of course, there can be no guarantees; the prognostications that genetic science increasingly makes possible do not ensure that some accident, violence, or unrelated disease will not interrupt life earlier, or that there will not be mistakes in prognostication. But it may well undercut our tendency to avoid issues of death altogether, to refuse to prepare for it in any but the most superficial ways, and to treat death as an existential unknown, when in fact it is becoming something that can be increasingly foreseen.

It is impossible to deny that we are already involved in a process of profound change, from the human past—say, the sixteenth century—in which a person could have very little realistic idea of when or how he or she would die, through the present, in which more of us have some rudimentary, inchoate idea of our own fates, into a future in which it will be possible to prognosticate increasingly accurately about the cause and timing of each individual's death. Of course, we cannot now say with certainty how accurate or complete our capacities for genetically based prognostication will eventually be. But we can already begin to ask the ethically important questions: will this be a bad thing—yet another feature of same brave new world, the *GATTACA* dystopia, in which privacies are invaded and human meaning undermined, or will it be a good thing, yet another product of advances in science that improve and enhance the human condition? I myself see it as closer to the latter, but then I am someone who would (I think) choose to know now, if I could, the date and cause of my own death. Yet many—maybe most—readers of this essay will have answered the forced-choice test question the other way. This suggests they will see the answer to the ethical issue raised here the other way around too. But whether one would want to know or not, whether one sees this change as good or bad, we cannot deny that it is a change that is coming in the human future, and that, compared to the human past, we are already partway along in a huge transformation, but one for which it is difficult for us to see that it is already well underway.

Notes

From Alison K. Thompson and Ruth F. Chadwick, eds, *Genetic Information: Acquisition, Access, and Control,* New York and Dordrecht: Kluwer Academic/Plenum Publishers, 1999, pp. 219–233. © 1999 Kluwer Academic/Plenum Publishers. Reprinted by permission.

For comments on earlier versions of this paper, I'd like to thank several of my temporary colleagues in March 1996 at the Green Center for the Study of Science and Society, University of Texas at Dallas, especially Robert Cook-Deegan and Gail Geller, as well as students and participants in a seminar at the Green Center; I'd also like to thank a number of my current and former colleagues at the University of Utah, including Bonnie Baty, Jeff Botkin, David Green, Leslie Francis, Jan VanRiper, Chris Grammes, Tom Stillinger, and Lenny Moss.

1. It may interest some readers to know that, except for direct references to the film, this paper was written before GATTACA appeared.

2. W. Gilbert, "A Vision of the Grail," in Kevles, DJ and Hood, L, eds., *The Code of Codes*. Cambridge, MA: Harvard University Press, 1992, p. 96, as quoted by Sahotra Sarkar in "From Genes as Determinants to DNA as Resources: Historical Notes on Development, Genetics, and Evolution," ch. 14, p. 24.

3. A 2001 study reported that some HD families in British Columbia have no family history of HD. This was explained by "intermediate repeats" that do not themselves cause HD, but can expand in children. This is a higher "new mutation rate" than previously reported. Almqvist EW, Elterman D. S., MacLeod P. M., Hayden M. R. (2001). "High incidence rate and absent family histories in one quarter of patients newly diagnosed with Huntington disease in British Columbia." *Clinical Genetics* 60, 198–205.

4. Robert J. Sawyer's science-fiction novel *Frameshift* (New York: Tom Doherty, 1997) provides a lively example of speculation about unscrupulous health insurers.

5. I thank Bonnie Baty for this point, and for many other contributions to this paper.

6. Wiggins S., Whyte P., Huggins M., et al. (1992), "The psychological consequences of predictive testing for Huntington's disease." *The New England Journal of Medicine* 327: 1401–5.

13

Extra Long Life

Ethical Aspects of Increased Life Span

The prospect of extra-long life spawns a bloom of ethical issues, among them how to achieve intergenerational equity; how to balance health care entitlements with rising costs for the elderly; how to divide years of life between work and retirement; how to assign the responsibilities of young family members for care of the old; and how to answer philosophical questions about the meaning of life, the "naturalness" of the human life span, and the wisdom of "tampering" with nature. Many writers on life-extension touch on these issues and in doing so share a common assumption: if extra-long life becomes possible, people will actually live it. This assumption is central not only to ethical issues but also to economic and social policy forecasts. Yet this assumption is valid only under unlikely scenarios of how the human life span might come to be extra long; it is clearly faulty under other scenarios, and it is weak under the most plausible scenarios, the very ones we should be using in such forecasts.

Three Scenarios of Extra-Long Life

At least three scenarios of extra-long life can be imagined for future generations proximate to our own. In the most optimistic of these scenarios, *the longer-health scenario,* people will normally live substantially longer and will be in relatively good health until just before their death. The duration of healthy adult years increases, but the period of debility before death will not increase and may shorten. In the most pessimistic scenario, *the longer-dying scenario,* most or all of the extension of the human life span will consist in physical disintegration and severe debility. What is now the unfortunate plight of some would become normal for most: a protracted preterminal and terminal period. Intermediate between these two scenarios is *the longer-decline scenario,* in which an increase in longevity will involve an extended descent from good health to death, during which physical and mental deterioration is spread out over a sustained period of time.

Contemplating these different possible futures, a pressing ethical issue confronts our own generation: whether to pursue medical techniques that would foreseeably lengthen the human life span. Are such efforts wise? That is, would benefits exceed costs, and would the outcome be distributively just? The answer hinges on the foregoing central assumption, and it is thus imperative that we explore this assumption in the light of well-founded projections about the future.

Means of Extending the Human Life Span

The human life span might be expanded in many ways. Improved disease prevention; life-style regulation; dietary matching of individual needs with available foodstuffs; understanding of human physiology and the way it is affected by exercise, stress, and caloric intake; and better management of depression and mental illness might all contribute to longer life. So might improved supportive care, including better management of cardiac dysfunction, respiratory support techniques, management of electrolyte imbalances, and repair of nervous system function. Specific advances in disease prevention and treatment can be anticipated, and some are already on their way, including improved regulation of sugar metabolism and the prevention of diabetes, better control of blood pressure, vaccines for cancer, more precise targeting of therapeutic drug regimens, and improved imaging in diagnostics and treatment.

The point so easily ignored is this: Not all ways of extending the life span point toward the same outcome scenario. Some—improved disease prevention, better diet, and better understanding of exercise, stress, and mental illness—herald the scenario of longer health. On the other hand, if longer life is realized through medical techniques that are invasive or that use drugs with serious side effects, longer dying may be the outcome. The implications of some potential technologies are unclear: Stem-cell-farmed replacement organs, for example, could lead either to longer health (if the function of multiple interactive organ systems is improved by the replacement of one or more parts) or to longer dying (if repeated surgeries required to replace various failing organs contribute to an overall decline in health).

Advances in genetics offer additional routes to extended life spans but may also point to different outcomes. Genetic diagnosis—beginning with carrier screening before conception, continuing with prenatal diagnosis and early childhood examination, and extending to early-adult diagnosis—will make it possible to identify and avoid genetic traits that lead to early death. For some conditions this promise has been realized. The incidence of Tay-Sachs disease, a condition that causes death in early childhood, has already been reduced among Ashkenazi Jews to below the rate for the general population. Genes have also been identified for cystic fibrosis, breast cancer, and early-onset Alzheimer's disease. Deselection of such disease genes, although it would reduce mortality among the young and thus lengthen life expectancy of populations as a whole, does not affect end-of-life scenarios for those who reach adulthood. Other genetic interventions, however, might be used to favor genes predisposing for longevity; or for reduced susceptibility to environmental toxins; or for avoiding life-threatening social behaviors; or for preventing aging-related telomere shortening.

The human life span is also sensitive to external factors (climate, air, soil, background radiation, and infectious disease). Many changes in these factors could decrease human longevity, but others could operate to extend it: for example, warming trends that made available a range of new foodstuffs or atmospheric changes that counteracted human-caused pollutants. Unlike at least initial developments in medicine or genetic technology, changes in these factors, if they occur, are likely to operate on a very large scale, and yet it is difficult to say whether they would herald longer health or longer dying.

What Will Future Generations Know?

People of proximate coming generations are likely to be reasonably conversant with their world, to have adequate information about their own health and health prospects, and to understand why their life expectancy has increased. They will also know what past human existence was like. Our successors will be at least as knowledgeable as we are about, for example, the processes of human psychology, the reasoning powers of the human mind, and characteristic human errors in reasoning, like the tendency to argue from anecdotal cases rather than base-rate information, to overemphasize recent evidence, and to use seemingly irrational discount rates. They will know how optimism embellishes perception of the future and how fear can infect their choices. In short, they will be in general moderately self-aware, reasonably rational creatures capable of making choices—sometimes good ones, sometimes not so good—about their lives.

Let us also imagine our successors as culturally literate, familiar with writings in history, literature, sociology, and theology that bear on issues about length of life. For example, they will have read Cicero's *On Old Age*. They will know the views of both Seneca, who supports suicide as the responsible act of the wise man, and Thomas Aquinas, who denounces suicide as the worst of sins. They will have read Jonathan Swift's account in *Gulliver's Travels* of the Struldbruggs, who were lucky enough to be immortal—or so Gulliver thought, until it turned out that immortality meant perpetual, unceasing decay. People in future generations—at least some of them—will also be philosophically sophisticated: For instance, they will know Bernard Williams's account of the Makropulos case and his reflections on "the tedium of immortality"; they will know Daniel Callahan's writings on the overuse of health care at the end of life; and they will understand Norman Daniels's Rawlsian reconstructions of justice in health care. They will have seen plays, films, and other works of past generations such as *Whose Life Is It, Anyway?* and *Soylent Green*. And they will have read plenty of trashy novels about treachery and stealth and evil physicians who make a mockery of death and dying. Of course, they will also have read accounts of triumph over illness, disability, aging, and the like. They will know the hopeful literature and the grimly realistic as well.

In short, they will know what we know and more. Thus, because we know at least part of what they know, we have some basis for predicting how they might behave when facing the prospect of extra-long life.

Questioning the Central Assumption

To restate the central assumption: If extra-long life becomes possible, people will actually live it. But it is possible that future generations will not, after all, live the "extra-long" part of their potentially extra-long lives. To see why, it is instructive to compare the different scenarios of possible extra-long life.

Suppose that longer life usually yields longer health. Under this scenario, neither the wisdom (in cost-benefit terms) nor the justice (in distributive terms) of extra-long life will be at issue. Added life will be a clear benefit. People not only will live longer but will also be able to work longer. They will thus not impose increased burdens on the young, either directly or through publicly supported pensions or health care programs. Although there will be many old people, most of them will be old only in number of years, not in health status. To be sure, the population structure will change, as family structure becomes more vertical, but this change will not mean added burdens for the younger generations.

If longer health is the scenario of the future, people can be predicted to choose to live extra-long lives, and no party or institution will try to keep them from doing so since there will be virtually no negative social impact. This scenario provides an answer to the moral question, Should we pursue the techniques that will lengthen life? If those techniques promise longer health, the answer seems to be a resounding yes.

Suppose, however, that longer life usually takes the form of longer dying, that most people will face a protracted period of preterminal and terminal decline— say, an extra twenty or thirty years in a hospital wing or a nursing home or the back bedroom of an overburdened, resentful family member's house, reduced in physical and intellectual capacity, limited in activities of daily living, perhaps unable for extended periods to engage in social interaction or to recognize family members or to experience life's pleasures. The early and middle years of life might be much the same as they are for us now, but life would conclude with a far more extended period of senescence and medical dependency. The cost-benefit balance will be negative; issues of justice will be exacerbated as the many, many very old strain societal resources and consume ever greater shares of the health care pie. If this longer-dying scenario is the picture of the future, the answer to the moral question about whether techniques for extending life expectancy should be developed seems to be a clear-cut no.

But suppose techniques for extending the human life span are developed anyway or that increases in longevity result from exogenous processes. What can we predict about whether these potentially extra-long lives will actually be lived? While it might seem that such a question can be answered only with sheer speculation, we already know how the present generation behaves in more limited versions of such situations, and we can assume that proximate future generations will have some of the same self-perceptions and cultural backgrounds and, hence, be likely to act in much the same way.

This leads us to expect that future generations will use some of the same mechanisms for avoiding overly prolonged life that the present generation does—and for the same reasons: to avoid suffering, indignity, loss of control, and pain. For example, among the mechanisms now used to avoid overly prolonged life in situations of terminal illness are living wills and durable powers of attorney for health care—two types of advance directive, legally recognized in virtually all states, that allow people to reject in advance certain life-prolonging treatments or to designate a surrogate with legal powers to act on their behalf. With both directives competent patients can decide, before they become incompetent, that their lives are not to be prolonged even though it is technically possible to do so. These instructions may direct the physician to issue a "do not resuscitate" (DNR) order; they may stipulate that specific treatments such as dialysis or the use of a respirator are to be withheld or withdrawn; or they may be used to accept pain control but refuse antibiotics, or accept antibiotics but refuse surgery, and so on. While advance directives are at times used to request rather than reject treatment, they are used primarily to curtail rather than extend life.

Paid control measures, especially opiates, are also often used in a way believed to hasten death, though there is some controversy about the pharmacology. Escalating doses of morphine, for example, are used under the principle of double effect to control pain, despite the foreseen but unintended possibility that they will eventually suppress respiration and bring about death. In 1997 the U.S. Supreme Court explicitly acknowledged the legality of this use of pain medication.[1] Although data is not as readily available on decisions about dying in the United States that involve the alleviation of symptoms with possible life-shortening effect, about 20 percent of deaths in the Netherlands occur in this way.[2] In the United States and elsewhere, terminal sedation is also sometimes used for patients in intractable pain: The patient is sedated into unconsciousness and artificial nutrition and hydration are withheld, with the result that the patient dies.[3]

Patients sometimes seek direct means of ending life. During the first six years after the legalization of physician-assisted suicide in Oregon, 171 people used this means of hastening their deaths.[4] A physician may provide a competent, terminally ill patient who has requested it, under legal safeguards, with a prescription for a lethal drug. In the Netherlands, where physician-assisted suicide and voluntary active euthanasia have long been legally tolerated and are now legal, an estimated 2.4 percent of annual mortality is attributable to voluntary active euthanasia provided by the physician at the request of the patient; 0.2 percent is attributable to physician-assisted suicide.[5] In the United States, a national study shows that a substantial proportion of physicians report that they receive requests for physician-assisted suicide and euthanasia and that about 6 percent have complied with such requests at least once.[6] Another study estimates that one in five physicians have received at least one request for assistance in helping a terminally ill patient die and that, despite the fact that doing so has not been legalized in any state except Oregon, between 3 percent and 18 percent of these physicians acceded to these requests.[7]

To anticipate how many people in the future will fail to live as long as they can, one must also anticipate how they will be treated by others—that is, how often other parties will choose shorter lives for them. Contemporary medicine routinely includes DNR orders, the withholding or withdrawing of medical life-support, the use of opiates under the principle of double effect, and both legal and clandestine assisted suicide and euthanasia. In some cases, the patient is aware of and requests or accepts these practices, but in other cases the patient is incompetent, confused, not informed, or otherwise unaware of them, and decisions are made on the patient's behalf by others: family members, physicians, or designated surrogates. Thus some of these practices are voluntary on the part of the patient, some are nonvoluntary, and many occupy a gray zone in between. Although many very ill and old people seem to want to hang on to life indefinitely, resisting death, nevertheless the majority of deaths occurring in institutions in this country (and the majority of deaths do occur in institutions) are "negotiated" in a way that involves a shorter life than would otherwise have been possible for that person. The medical and legal euphemism is that these patients are "allowed to die."

How frequent such decisions are is difficult to determine. In the United States it has been estimated that some 70 percent of deaths in institutional settings involve some form of negotiated strategy.[8] The most recent comprehensive Dutch study, covering a six-year period ending in 2001, finds that of all deaths in the Netherlands, about 20.2 percent involved the withholding or withdrawing of life-sustaining treatment; in another 20.1 percent, pain and symptoms were alleviated with doses of opioids that may have shortened life. The ending of life without a current explicit request, a violation of Dutch law, occurred in about 0.7 percent of all deaths (though in virtually all cases with the prior request of the patient or when the patient was no longer capable of communication). Altogether, some 43.7 percent of all deaths—a figure approaching half—appear to have involved decisions that probably or certainly allowed or caused death to occur sooner in order to avoid a dying process regarded as worse.[9] Roughly similar pictures are believed to be true of other advanced industrial democracies in Europe, Australia, and elsewhere.[10] A study of six European countries released in 2003 reveals that the frequency of end-of-life decisions (including decisions about withholding or withdrawing care, alleviation of pain and suffering in a way that might foreseeably hasten death, euthanasia, physician-assisted suicide, and direct termination of life without an explicit current request) ranged from a low of 23 percent in Italy to a high of 51 percent in Switzerland.[11] The ending of life without the patient's explicit request happened more frequently than voluntary active euthanasia in five of the six countries studied (Belgium, Denmark, Italy, Sweden, and Switzerland; all except the Netherlands) and was the only form of doctor-assisted death recorded in Sweden.

Thus even now lives are often less long than they could be. To be sure, they are not very much less long. In the Netherlands, the best-studied site of these end-of-life practices, relatively little life is forgone; in about 50 percent of cases of euthanasia, physician-assisted suicide, and life shortening without explicit request, life is shortened by an estimated twenty-four hours or less; in another 30 percent, life is shortened by less than a week, and only about 9 percent involve shortening life by more than a month.[12] A generously estimated average by which life is curtailed by direct termination of life, practices that account for about 3 percent of total deaths, is 3.3 weeks.[13]

Clearly, abbreviations of this modest sort have little impact on overall longevity; an extra-long life that is shorter on average by 3.3 weeks is still extra long. However, the amount of possible life not actually lived by future generations might be much greater. Not only does the estimated sacrifice of 3.3 weeks by today's Netherlanders not include deaths that occur earlier as a result of "allowing to die," but today's Dutch, like inhabitants of advanced nations generally, face a comparatively short preterminal and terminal phase. Proximate future generations for whom extra-long life becomes possible could face the scenario of longer dying, a protracted period no better in quality of life than that which some contemporary people now seek to avoid. Although measures to curtail or terminate life may now be used sparingly in advanced nations, they are already in place and are used, with professional and public knowledge and acceptance, to spare people deaths that could be much worse than the deliberately chosen death.

Although some such measures doubtless are rooted in self-interest or greed, second-party decisions to allow a patient to die or to assist in causing death are not typically malevolent. Rather, they are seen as benevolent choices made by concerned family members, physicians, or others to spare the patient a much worse death. It is rapidly becoming a culturally accepted view that when all that remains is a painful process of dying, it may not be in the patient's interests to continue living; the patient may refuse to continue to live; or if not able to make that choice, others may do so on his or her behalf.

Thus if medical, genetic, and environmental science produces a longer-dying scenario, we should expect both that people will find the likely end periods of their lives not worth living and voluntarily elect not to continue them, and also that others will make such choices on their behalf. Under the longer-dying scenario, the amount of life forgone will likely be greater than it is now. We should also anticipate that medical, legal, and social attitudes and policies will conform to the view that longer dying is not acceptable. To anticipate that individual behavior and social institutions will evolve in this fashion is not to put forth a slippery-slope argument, which predicts wholesale nonvoluntary deaths; rather, it is to argue that the very considerations that underwrite currently accepted practices—that it is a good thing to spare people bad deaths—will find application in the future if generally bad deaths strung out over extended periods of time—that is, longer dying—is what they face.

The present provides a basis for predictions about the future. Few people now enjoy longer health—that is, a long life span with good health until right before death. Instead, the vast majority of people in the United States, and indeed in the developed world in general, die of degenerative diseases (especially heart disease, cancer, and stroke), which often exhibit long terminal declines.[14] However, few people now suffer the much longer terminal decline that would characterize the longer-dying scenario of the future. Good ends today are not always as good as they could be if longer health were genuinely the case—that is what contemporary medical science tries to achieve; and bad ends today are shorter and easier than what longer dying might impose. Yet we already often forgo these even shorter end stages. Would not the members of proximate future generations behave in much the same way? If longer health were the norm, it would be enthusiastically lived; if longer dying were the norm, it would likely not be lived at all.

These predictions also provide some basis for speculating about the impact of future scenarios of extra-long life on economic and social policy issues. If longer health is the scenario, people will live extra-long lives but constitute no extra burden. If longer dying is the scenario, their very extensive care, social security, and health care costs could constitute a real burden, but they are unlikely to be willing to live such lives or, for that matter, be allowed to live such lives. Thus the impact of longer health and longer dying on social institutions and programs might be similar. Exactly how much future generations may choose to curtail life if they face longer dying is unclear, but we cannot rule out the possibility that they would shorten life enough to call current economic forecasts into question, especially those that see the social costs of extra-long life as an immense, unsupportable burden about to spiral out of control. The assumption at the heart of such forecasts—that if extra-long life becomes possible people will actually live it—is persuasive only under one scenario, that of longer health. It is unpersuasive under the alternative that predicts these huge burdens, longer dying.

Longer Decline, the Plausible Scenario

I have so far explored two stark alternative future scenarios in order to highlight the ubiquitous problematic assumption that runs throughout discussions of extra-long life: the scenario of longer health, attractive in all ways and a burden to none; and the scenario of longer dying, attractive in no way and a burden to all. The more probable outcome, however, of mixed advances in medical science, genetics, environmental science, and other new fields we cannot yet anticipate—variously exacerbating and offsetting each others' advantages and disadvantages—is the longer-decline scenario. This intermediate scenario is the most plausible but, paradoxically, yields the least secure predictions. If longer decline materializes, we cannot reliably predict whether future generations will elect to live out whatever extra-long life becomes possible for them. Nor will it be an easy choice for the them or for their caretakers, medical managers, or policymakers. Unlike longer health and longer dying, longer decline bodes an uncertain demographic future.

Notes

From Henry J. Aaron and William B. Schwartz, eds., *Coping With Methuselah: The Impact of Molecular Biology on Medicine and Society*. Washington D.C.: Brookings Institution Press, 2004, pp. 235–246. This piece was originally a comment on Alex Capron's "Ethical Aspects of Major Increases in Life Span and Life Expectancy." © 2004 The Brookings Institution. Reprinted with permission.

1. *Vacco v. Quill,* 521 U.S. 793 (1997); *Washington v. Glucksberg,* 521 U.S. 702 (1997); decided jointly.
2. Van der Wal and others (2003), table 1.
3. Bernat, Gert, and Mogielnicki (1993).
4. Oregon Department of Human Services (2004).
5. Onwuteaka-Philipsen and others (2003).
6. Meier and others (1998).
7. Meier and others (2003), p. 1537.
8. Stell (1998), citing the amicus curiae brief filed by the American Hospital Association in *Cruzan v. Director, Missouri Department of Health,* 497 U.S. 261 (1990).
9. van der Wal and others (2003); Onwuteaka-Philipsen and others (2003).
10. Deliens and others (2000); Kuhse and others (1997); van der Heide and others (2003).
11. van der Heide and others (2003), p. 3.
12. Onwuteaka-Philipsen and others (2003).
13. Emanuel and Battin (1998).
14. Field and Cassel (1997), chap. 2.

References

Arrow, Kenneth J. 1951. *Social Choice and Individual Values.* Yale University Press.

Avorn, Jerry. 1984. "Benefit and Cost Analysis in Geriatric Care: Turning Age Discrimination into Health Policy." *New England Journal of Medicine* 310 (20): 1294–301.

Beauchamp, Tom L., and James F. Childress. 2001. *Principles of Biomedical Ethics,* 5th ed. Oxford University Press.

Bernat, James L., Bernard Gert, and R. Peter Mogielnicki. 1993. "Patient Refusal of Hydration and Nutrition: An Alternative to Physician-Assisted Suicide or Voluntary Active Euthanasia." *Archives of Internal Medicine* 153: 2723–8.

Callahan, Daniel. 1987. *Setting Limits: Medical Goals in an Aging Society.* Simon and Schuster.

———. 1990. *What Kind of Life? The Limits of Medical Progress.* Simon and Schuster.

Daniels, Norman. 1985. *Just Health Care.* Cambridge University Press.

———. 1988. *Am I My Parents' Keeper? An Essay on Justice between the Young and the Old.* Oxford University Press.

Deliens, Luc, and others. 2000. "End-of-Life Decisions in Medical Practice in Flanders, Belgium: A Nationwide Survey." *Lancet* 356 (9244): 1806–11.

Elliott, Carl. 2003. *Better than Well: When Modern Medicine Meets the American Dream.* W. W. Norton.

Emanuel, Ezekiel J., and Margaret P. Battin. 1998. "What Are the Potential Cost Savings from Legalizing Physician-Assisted Suicide?" *New England Journal of Medicine* 339 (3): 167–172.

Evert, Jessica, Elizabeth Lawler, Hazel Bogan, and Thomas Perls. 2003. "Morbidity Profiles of Centenarians: Survivors, Delayers, and Escapers." *Journals of Gerontology Series A: Biological Sciences and Medical Sciences* 58: M232–7.

Field, Marilyn J., and Christine K. Cassel, eds. 1997. *Approaching Death: Improving Care at the End of Life.* Washington: National Academy Press.

Fries, James F. 1983. "The Compression of Morbidity." *Milbank Memorial Fund Quarterly* 61 (Summer): 347–419.

Fuchs, Victor. 1984. "Though Much Is Taken: Reflections on Aging, Health, and Medical Care." *Milbank Memorial Fund Quarterly* 62 (Spring): 143–66.

Fukuyama, Francis. 2002. *Our Posthuman Future: Consequences of the Biotechnology Revolution.* Farrar, Straus, and Giroux.

Ginzberg, Eli. 1984. "The Elderly Are at Risk." *Inquiry* 21 (4): 301–2.

Hedberg, Katrina, David Hopkins, and Melvin Kohn. 2003. "Five Years of Legal Physician-Assisted Suicide in Oregon." *New England Journal of Medicine* 348 (10): 961–4.

Holden, Constance. 2002. "The Quest to Reverse Time's Toll." *Science* 295 (February 8): 1032–3.

Holmes, Oliver Wendell. 1858. "The Deacon's Masterpiece; Or, The Wonderful One-Hoss Shay: A Logical Story." In *Autocrat of the Breakfast-Table.*

Jonas, Hans. 1984. *The Imperative of Responsibility.* University of Chicago Press.

Kass, Leon R. 1985. *Toward a More Natural Science: Biology and Human Affairs.* Free Press.

———. 2003. "Ageless Bodies, Happy Souls." *New Atlantis* 1 (Spring): 9–28.

Kuhse, Helga, and others. 1997. "End-of-Life Decisions in Australian Medical Practice." *Medical Journal of Australia* 166: 91–6.

Lubitz, James, and Ronald Prihoda. 1984. "The Use and Costs of Medicare Services in the Last Two Years of Life." *Health Care Financing Review* 5 (3): 117–31.

McKibben, Bill. 2003. *Enough: Staying Human in an Engineered Age.* Times Books.

Meier, Diane, and others. 1998. "A National Survey of Physician-Assisted Suicide and Euthanasia in the United States." *New England Journal of Medicine* 338 (17): 1193–201.

———. 2003. "Characteristics of Patients Requesting and Receiving Physician-Assisted Death." *Archives of Internal Medicine* 163: 1537–42.

National Commission for the Protection of Human Subjects of Biomedical and Behavioral Research. 1978. *The Belmont Report: Ethical Principles and Guidelines for the Protection of Human Subjects of Research.* Government Printing Office.

Okarma, Thomas B. 2000. "Prospects for Cellular Therapies in the Treatment of Chronic Disease." *Journal of Commercial Biotechnology* 6 (Spring): 300–7.

Onwuteaka-Philipsen, Bregje D., and others. 2003. "Euthanasia and Other End-of-Life Decisions in the Netherlands in 1990, 1995, and 2001." *Lancet* 362 (9381): 395–9.

Oregon Department of Human Services, *Sixth Annual Report on Oregon's Death with Dignity Act*, March 10, 2004. www.dhs.state.or.us/publichealth/chs/pas/ar-index/cfm.

Perls, Thomas, and Dellara Terry. 2003. "Genetics of Exceptional Longevity." *Experimental Gerontology* 38: 725–30.

President's Commission for the Study of Ethical Problems in Medicine and Biomedical and Behavioral Research. 1983. *Securing Access to Health Care.* Government Printing Office.

Rawls, John A. 1971. *A Theory of Justice.* Harvard University Press.

Schwartz, William B. 1998. *Life without Disease: The Pursuit of Medical Utopia.* University of California Press.

Scitovsky, Anne, and Alexander M. Capron. 1986. "Medical Care at the End of Life: The Interaction of Economics and Ethics." *Annual Review of Public Health* 7: 59–75.

Stell, Lance. 1998. "Physician Assisted Suicide: To Decriminalize or to Legalize, That Is the Question." In *Physician Assisted Suicide: Expanding the Debate,* edited by Margaret P. Battin, Rosamond Rhodes, and Anita Silvers. Routledge.

ter Meulen, Ruud H. J. 1995. "Solidarity with the Elderly and the Allocation of Resources." In *A World Growing Old: The Coming Health Care Challenges,* edited by Daniel Callahan, Ruud H. J. ter Meulen, and Eva Topinková, 73–74. Georgetown University Press.

van der Heide, Agnes, and others. 2003. "End-of-Life Decision-Making in Six European Countries: Descriptive Study." On behalf of the EURELD Consortium. *Lancet* 362 (9381): 345–50.

van der Wal, Gerrit, and others. 2003. *Medische besluitvorming aan het einde van het leven.* Utrecht, Netherlands: Uitgeverij De Tijdstroom. Summary in English in Onwuteaka-Philipsen and others (2003).

Wade, Nicholas. 2001. *Life Script: How the Human Genome Discoveries Will Transform Medicine and Enhance Your Health.* Simon and Schuster.

World Health Organization. 2002. *Ethical Choices in Long-Term Care: What Does Justice Require?* Geneva.

14

Global Life Expectancies and International Justice

A Reemergence of the Duty to Die?

Is there a duty to die? This inflammatory question, often originally attributed to then-Governor of Colorado Richard Lamm, was being explored some years ago within the context of American health care, but lately has dropped out of sight—whether because it seemed to have no purchase in the light of new, globalized issues about justice in health care, or because the conclusion was so unpalatable it is hard to so. In either case, I want to revive it. Why? Simple. If the strongest argument for the existence of a duty to die, rooted in Norman Daniels' early Rawlsian reconstruction, is supplemented by Allen Buchanan's distinctive approach to issues of international justice, it is possible that a new, stronger duty to die might emerge from this conjunction. If so, we ought to recognize it, however difficult that might be; and if not, we still ought to recognize what might lead to its coming to be the case. This "duty to die" is, I predict, sneaking up on us as we explore multilateralist, cosmopolitan accounts of global relations.

In some familiar senses, we already recognize a variety of "duties to die"—including obligations to allow oneself to die, to risk dying, to let oneself be killed, or kill oneself—in a wide range of traditional circumstances. Some of these are role-dependent—for example in military and police services, medical services that may involve exposure to deadly communicable diseases during times of plague or contemporary viruses, or the spy with secret information. Some are less so: rescue missions and capital punishment, for example. Duties to die or to allow oneself to die are sometimes put forward as obligations in religious traditions, for example in Buddhist obligations of self-sacrifice or in the Catholic "higher way" of allowing oneself to die or be killed rather than have an abortion or kill another human being even in self-defense. But the particular duty to die at issue here is one based in distributive issues, where it is considerations of justice and equality that motivate the claim that one better-off party may have a duty to die to enhance the prospects of a worse-off one.

The issue of whether there is a distributively based duty to die has been argued both as a personal issue and as a societal one. Dan Callahan, who in *Setting Limits* and his later books[1] set the stage for the discussion by calling for restraint on the part of the elderly in the use of life-prolonging medicine, developed a view that would appear to underwrite a passive, though not active, duty to die. Some years later, drawing in part on work by Norman Daniels, I posed the question of the duty to die in an impersonal, social context about the choices one might rationally make under conditions of moderate scarcity in access to health care.[2] More recently, John Hardwig has posed the same question again in the highly personal context of a troubling rumination about duties to his own family—duties he says he willingly accepts not to burden them with obligations of excessive expense or care as he succumbs to extreme old age or terminal illness.[3] It is Hardwig who has made the argument most vivid. But neither Callahan nor Daniels nor Hardwig nor I have explored the question in a still larger context, that context in which it may seem to be both least persuasive to some but most troubling to others. This is the context of global justice.

Is there a duty to die? Consider the stark differences in life expectancy around the world. In the rich, industrially developed nations, where human development indices are high, average life expectancy at birth ranges roughly between 72-80 for both sexes, with Japan, Canada, Iceland, Australia, and the Netherlands at the top end of the range.[4] In the poorest, not-yet-developed agrarian nations of the so-called third world, where human development indices are low, life expectancy ranges downward from 60 to 40, and in some countries, like Malawi, Zambia, Mozambique, Zimbabwe, and Sierra Leone, at 40 or below. A child born in Sierra Leona today has a life expectancy of just 34.5 years. Although life expectancy has been increasing in most nations, in some, like Russia in the post-Soviet years, it has been plummeting, down from 69.2 in the five-year period 1985–90 to an estimated 64.4 for 1995–2000, with men dropping to 58.0.

There are also stark global differences in access to health care. The high-income countries (those with per capita annual incomes above $8,500) get almost all the health care made available in the world. In 1994, for example, the rich countries accounted for 89% of global health expenditures, even though they comprise only 16% of the global population.[5] The United States has 5% of the global population, but accounts for 50% of health spending. Furthermore, of the estimated 1.4 trillion disability-adjusted years of life that were lost to disease in that year, the inhabitants of the rich nations suffered just 7% of them.[6] People in rich countries live far longer, far healthier lives, and die much much later than people in poor parts of the globe.[7]

Can these differences serve to raise a question about a duty to *die?* Perhaps, like most other readers of these remarks, you will reject the question out of hand, even if moved by the plight of distant peoples around the globe. A *duty* to die? While life expectancies may be unequal, you will no doubt say, this hardly establishes that they are inequitable, or that those with longer lifespan expectancies have any duty to those with short life expectancies to even things out. To recognize that life expectancies, like rates of infant mortality and incidence rates for various diseases, are comparatively crude measures of morbidity and mortality, and that there are other far more sophisticated measures of health status and well-being, may still not persuade you that there is any inequity in health between the rich and poor nations that we ought to remedy. Even if there are great disparities, we do not, you may say, *owe* them anything at all.[8] No doubt you will agree that it is unfortunate that inhabitants of the poor countries receive less health care, experience much worse health, and lose far more years of life; but even if you grant that it is unfortunate, you will be less likely to see it as unfair, and in any case you almost certainly do not think that global differences in patterns of life expectancy can impose a duty to *die* on the residents of more fortunate nations.

However, if we look at the various arguments that Callahan, Daniels, Hardwig and I have made directly or indirectly about whether there might be a duty to die in what we all assumed was a Western, first-world, American context, we may see that when supplemented by a plausible additional premise, these arguments have implications reaching far beyond our borders—implications yielding troubling results in a global context—and perhaps bad news for you and me.

Arguments about the Duty to Die

The distributively-based arguments for a duty to die put forward in recent years fall into two general camps—"interactionist" arguments, of which Hardwig's is the best current example, and (for want of a better term) "early-Rawlsian" arguments like my own (drawing on Norm Daniels) and, to some extent, Dan Callahan's.

Hardwig's Argument

Hardwig argues that an individual who is terminally ill or in need of extensive care may have a duty not only to decline this care, but to die, in order to avoid imposing overly heavy burdens of care and support on family members or loved ones—even if they would willingly bear these burdens. This duty Hardwig sees as stronger for people who are older and who have already lived full lives, especially if they are facing dementing disease like Alzheimer's or Huntington's, whose loved ones have had difficult lives or have already made sacrifices for them; in such conditions, they can no longer hope to make significant contributions to the lives of their loved ones. An individual in this situation—and Hardwig clearly accepts the prospect that he may someday find himself in this position—ought to be willing to die in order to avoid "stealing the futures" of his loved ones, who would otherwise shoulder duties of care to him, rather than buying a little more time for himself.[9]

This is a complex argument, one that has generated vigorous controversy.[10] But given that it addresses obligations only to immediate family members and loved ones who are directly and severely affected by one's remaining alive, Hardwig's argument would seem to have no implications concerning distant peoples, remote residents of the world whom one does not know, with whom one does not interact, and who inhabit utterly different cultural, social, and religious spheres from one's immediate family. There are no personal ties here, no relationships of mutual affection, no obligations assumed in marriage or in traditional filial relationships, not even any relationships of co-nationality, and while we think it might be a good thing, a decent thing to contribute some of one's assets to help these unfortunate people, there is certainly no duty to sacrifice one's life.

Battin's Argument, Drawing on Daniels

My own argument about the duty to die has not been driven by sentiments of affection or concern for family members, nor is it confined to the orbit of the intimate family situation.[11] Rather, one might say, this argument has been driven by cold self-interest, at least of a theoretical sort. I had claimed that rational self-interest maximizers in the Original Position (whom one might recognize from the early Rawls)[12] choosing principles that would govern a society characterized by moderate scarcity of health care resources, would (as Norman Daniels had argued[13] recognize that health care resources spent earlier in life—that is, on people in younger age groups—would both be more efficient and would raise the chances of survival in early life (a precondition for later life), thus (except in the first generation of such a policy) enhancing one's chances of longer, better survival at a later stage of life. Thus parties in the Original Position would rationally reallocate health care away from the oldest ranges toward the youngest ranges, and because they would agree to this policy (recognizing that it would enhance their own interests as well, by increasing their chances of a longer lifespan), age-rationing policies would therefore count as just. At a minimum, this would mean—as Callahan and Hardwig both see—refraining from demanding or accepting expensive, high-tech health care—not only respirators, tubes, and machines, but elaborate diagnostic procedures, prolonged hospitalization, and so on—in a last-ditch effort to prolong their lives. But if there were a duty to refrain from using resources in terminal illness or extreme old age that might be more justly be allocated to the care of younger people, I then argued, given the potentially cruel consequences of living without adequate care, many rational self-interest maximizers in the Rawlsian Original Position would welcome social policies recognizing elective assisted suicide or active voluntary euthanasia—not obligatory or forced, not age-tagged, and certainly not secret, but available for those who might choose them. Thus there would not be a duty to cause oneself to die, but if there were an obligation to refrain from receiving care, causing oneself to die rather than merely being disenfranchised from care might seem the preferable choice. Thus policies permitting or even encouraging voluntary choices of an earlier, more humane but also more resource-conserving death, if supported in the Original Position, would then be just.

This argument too may seem to have little or no relevance to the global context. After all, it is not clear how voluntary choices of an earlier death, including those involving physician-assisted suicide or physician-performed euthanasia, even if supported by social practices and expectations, would have real impact on global differences in life expectancy. Drawing on data from the Netherlands, we can expect that such choices, at least as made in a current world in which they are legally tolerated and fairly widely socially accepted, would mean forgoing only the last few weeks of life, that only comparatively few people would make them, and that the savings in health-care costs would be modest—by one calculation, less than 0.07 percent of annual total health-care expenditures in the United States.[14] Savings would have comparatively little impact on overall health care costs even in a developed nation that permitted assisted dying, and virtually no discernible impact on global differences in life expectancy of people in poor countries.

Callahan's Argument

Dan Callahan also employs arguments that, in their origins, are sympathetic to Daniels's view of age-rationing. Callahan's initial view was that the elderly should rethink the meaning of old age and refrain from claiming expensive healthcare resources in an attempt to prolong life indefinitely; he has expanded this view to insist that all of us reinspect our assumptions about health, disease, aging, and death, and abandon our relentless pursuit of medical "progress" in general, not only in old age.[15] We must stop assuming that we can conquer all disease, or indefinitely prolong life, and turn things over to the generation after us.

Does Callahan think there is a duty to die? He is staunchly opposed to any direct ending of life, and would certainly deny that there is any "duty to die" in the sense accepted straightforwardly by Hardwig or partially and obliquely by myself. However, he recognizes that the rethinking of cultural assumptions about medical progress and the meaning of life will often mean that death arrives earlier, and he clearly recognizes obligations in connection with the approach of death: this is a "passive" duty, the duty of restraint, an obligation to refrain from claiming expensive health-care resources that might postpone death and prolong one's life— but a duty nevertheless.

Of these three discussions of duties at the end of life, Callahan's alone is sensitive to global issues in health. He holds that greater equality in health circumstances ought to be brought about around the world. But he sees this simply as a matter of holding back in the first world from our unthinking dedication to so-called medical progress, holding back in a way that will allow us to achieve a "steady state" medicine, allowing the developing world to gradually catch up with the developed world so that global health-care equality will be more nearly achieved. But, like Hardwig, Daniels, and Battin, Callahan does not explore the more direct obligations that his view might seem to support.

The Global Analogy

These views about duties to die or to refrain from care may seem to have little to do with the global situation or with differences in life expectancies around the world, differences that persist (though not as starkly) even if high infant mortality rates and the AIDS pandemic are factored out. That some sub-Saharan Africans have life expectancies under 40 or Russian men have life expectancies that have dropped to 58 while those of Japanese women have climbed to 83.3 (more than double the 38.5 of people in Malawi) cannot, it may seem, generate obligations on the part of inhabitants of richer nations—especially not substantial, personal obligations like a duty to *die*. After all, the Hardwig, Battin, and Callahan views about duties to die, whether accepted, accepted obliquely, or rejected, are all predicated on the assumption that savings gained in the costs of care if someone dies sooner have effects in other contexts—for Hardwig, because they spare costs affecting the nonfinancial and financial futures of his family members, for Battin and Callahan because they can be utilized in care for younger generational age groups.

But as Daniels has pointed out, such arguments trade on the assumption that savings are made in a closed system, one in which savings in one part yield usable resources in another.[16] The Rawlsian argument as adapted by Daniels to the health-care setting, on which the Battin and Callahan arguments in particular trade, presupposes not only a background of just institutions, but redistributive mechanisms that would ensure that savings in one place, namely health care in old age, would be reallocated somewhere else, namely as health care for the young. Closed health-care financing systems like this are imperfectly in place in some nations, like Canada and like Britain before its National Health Service began to be partly dismantled, but not in some other developed nations, particularly the United States.

But the "first," "second," and "third" worlds—the developed, the post-Soviet, and the developing nations—do not jointly form a closed system, in which health care savings in one part of the world are realized as resources in another. To decline dialysis in England does not buy immunization against malaria in Brazil; to have one's physician assist in suicide before the end-stages of cancer in the United States does not curb tuberculosis in Russia or reduce perinatal mortality in India. To be sure, declining dialysis or committing suicide would have some impact in reducing consumption rates in the developed world, inasmuch as someone whose death occurs earlier no longer consumes food, energy, or natural resources, but the extent of this impact would be negligible in altering medical outlooks and life expectancies in the developing world. Nor are we participants in a well-developed global cooperative scheme, one that, as the later Rawls sees it, might generate obligations of mutual support for each other among the various inhabitants of the globe.[17] Thus duty-to-die arguments, even if plausible within a single nation-state with an interactive health-care system, seem to have no purchase in the global context, where on the contrary the connection between a patient in the developed world and distant peoples in the developing world is so remote that the effects of an earlier death in one place will be barely detectable if at all in the other—so infinitesimally small that it could hardly seem worth the sacrifice of a life. There is nothing special about health care here—the same could be said of housing, food, or other basic needs.

Of course, I might draw up a will conveying my estate to the residents of, say, a specific African village, but unless I do so, my death—whether earlier or later—will have no impact on the fates of these distant peoples. My own earlier death would not protect Russian men; nor for that matter would it do anything to slow the climb of Japanese women up the scale of long life expectancy. This is not to say that earlier, cheaper deaths cannot benefit others. John Hardwig's earlier death, if he can will himself to bring it about, as he argues, might well protect his family members from burdens of expense and care they would shoulder out of duty to him. So might my own earlier death benefit my own similarly immediate family and, depending on the particular sort of insurance system by which I am covered, other claimants for health-care within the same system as well. Callahan's refusal to claim life-prolonging resources and to succumb to the dream of indefinite medical progress, if he can persuade others as well as himself to do as he recommends, would benefit American society as a whole. All three of our earlier and thus less expensive, more resource-conserving deaths might save health-care resources for redistribution within the American health-care system, as least within the immediate insurance pools of which we are each part, to provide for health care for some younger persons and thus give them a greater chance of longer life. It does not make much difference for this argument whether the duty to die involves letting oneself die or causing oneself to die, unless one or the other would produce great psychological distress or other harm; the distributive argument is the same.

Yet nothing Hardwig or Callahan or I or Daniels, for that matter, might do in shortening our lives or letting them be shorter would seem to affect the welfare of people in distant countries, or in any way serve to decrease the disparity between their life spans and ours. Arguing that John or Dan or Norm or I or, for that matter, you, the reader of this paper, ought to die a little earlier to extend the lifespans of people in the poorer nations of Africa or Asia or Latin America may seem just as futile as insisting that we eat all the food on our plates to keep people from starving in Somalia or Sudan or whatever is our current Armenia.

There are of course many things John, Dan, Norm, you, and I could do besides shortening our lives to improve the life prospects of peoples with lower life expectancies than our own. Restraint in consumption in surely one: burn less fuel, eat less meat (always inefficiently produced), recycle things made from nonrenewable resources, and so on. Then there are positive contributions we might make to remedying the social and economic circumstances that contribute to early death: reduce malnutrition, fight poverty and endemic disease, quell civil warfare, control the sex trade, combat alcoholism, and reduce environmental toxins. Even more directly, we could send food, medical supplies, and other aid. All these things would certainly help, and one can certainly claim that it would be a good thing, indeed perhaps a duty, for us to do them.[18] Like Peter Singer, we could send 20% of our incomes to alleviate poverty in the third world,[19] a move that would have enormous effect on reducing the disease burden among the global poor. Substantial increases in first-world charity and aid would produce a fairer world in the sense that the life prospects of all global inhabitants would be more nearly equal.

But it is not clear that these things would be accomplished by any of us taking ourselves to have a *duty to die*, particularly since the apparent impact would be so small. Is there a "global" duty to die, a distributively based duty to end one's life or let it end for reasons of global health equity? Is seems that the answer is *no*.

But I think this answer lets us off the hook a bit too quickly. Neither Hardwig's vivid and disturbing reflections nor Battin's Daniels-flavored argument nor Callahan's thoughtful perceptions about the state of American health care appear to found a satisfactory argument about a duty to die, whether positive or negative, direct or indirect, that has any purchase in a global context. Just the same, exposing assumptions central to these arguments and then exposing these assumptions to globalist critique may suggest that they could, on the contrary, be stretched to global scope.

How These Arguments Could Cover the Globe

Extension of these arguments, which have originated primarily in contexts of national scope, to cover the globe is the issue here; but achieving international scope is not such a simple matter.

Stretching Hardwig's Interactionism to Cover the Globe

John Hardwig's argument that there is a duty to die is based in a version of Interactionism that makes the non-Kantian, non-Utilitarian, non-Rawlsian assumption that it is close, personal relationships that count and that generate duties to each other. As Allen Buchanan puts the Interactionist view in the context of global justice, relationships of justice only obtain among those who are engaged in cooperation with one another.[20] Interaction of the relevant sort, especially cooperation, typically (but not always) occurs within a family, but it can also occur globally, when individuals or groups or peoples or nations are bound together in interactive relationships involving legal, trade, regulatory, cultural, and other institutions. Thus if Interactionism has implications for issues concerning a "duty to die" in domestic contexts, could it not thus also have global implications as well?

Hardwig does not make this argument. His concern is not with social cooperation or generalized social justice; it is about close personal bonds. But consider, for example, an analogy between Hardwig's responsibilities for his own family and his responsibilities for members of another group with which he has been involved in some relevant form of interaction. Suppose, for example, that Hardwig (like the example he describes) were at age 87 to develop congestive heart failure, and his APACHE score predicts that he had less than a 50% chance to live for another six months.[21] He might beg for the most aggressive life-prolonging treatment possible, and indeed it might succeed in continuing his life for another two years. But this care costs, let us suppose, $100,000 a year and will impose immense burdens of care on his 55-year-old daughter. John is—in his own view—obliged to spare her this.[22] But now imagine the $200,000 for John's health care for the two years he, like his example, manages to survive, translated to, say, a village in Uganda, where it will purify the water supply, provide vaccines for all the village children, hire a health-care worker to treat wounds, provide emergency surgical and psychiatric care, rehydrate children with diarrhea, and provide family planning and reproductive health care. John's $200,000 would go a very long way here. He knows this, let us say, because he has visited the village multiple times, he knows its members well; some of them have received him in their homes, he has had long conversations with them about matters of personal as well as social importance; and when they last parted, they all asserted over and over again that they were all "like family."

Now let us suppose that the funds Hardwig might save could raise the life expectancy of these villagers by, say, 5 years on average; it is now 44.7, but with John's contribution it would reach almost 50 for the entire village. There are a hundred people in the village, let us say; the total life-years gained would be 500. John, on the other hand, sacrifices just 2. Should he do it? If he ought to die a little earlier to spare his 55-year-old daughter her savings, her home, her job, and her career (as he insists he should), shouldn't he do so to spare a hundred people from death five years earlier on average than it might otherwise occur? They are "like family." Exactly what difference does it make that one is his own genetically related daughter, the others are "like family" but live farther away? Is this just a challenge to the Interactionist's calculus of interchange, where distance—whether geographically, culturally, or emotionally—may attenuate the intertwinedness of the interaction? But while the villagers may be not as close in some respects, they may be closer in others, and in any case the gains for them are much, much greater as they are spread out over the entire village: on average, 5 years of additional life, we are assuming, for each person there.

Yet we resist the conclusion that 87-year-old John has an *obligation* to forgo the health care that would preserve his life for an additional 2 years and save the $200,000, even though we might believe it would be a good thing, a noble, heroic thing, if he did. "Domestic" Interactionism like this involving close familial relationships is the most intuitively compelling sort, but even this does not persuade. For one thing, it might be replied that Hardwig's argument has involved only sparing burdens, not providing benefits, or in the language of classroom bioethics, that duties of nonmaleficence are far stronger than those of beneficence. Hardwig does not directly address the question of providing benefits by dying earlier, but because he would require the dying person not to impose burdens that would prevent the same sorts of family disadvantages, the Interactionist's positive obligation may not be out of keeping with his view.

It could also be argued that, given the underlying picture of balancing burdens and benefits that informs Hardwig's conception of family discussions concerning whether one of its members ought indeed to die,[23] there is a more Utilitarian metric at work here than Hardwig acknowledges. If by dying a little earlier the terminally ill family member could, for example, release many thousands of dollars of life insurance just in time for a granddaughter who could not otherwise do so to go to college, or the surviving spouse to rescue a business that would otherwise fail, ought he do it?[24] On a pure Utilitarian view, oughtn't he do it for just anyone or any group of people, where the gains to that person or persons offset the costs to himself?

Yet, on an Interactionist view like Hardwig's own, we reject this conclusion. Of course, it may not be that we are resisting Interactionism itself, but just that we resist the conclusion because we are not persuaded that being "like family" is an interactive-enough relationship to be as strong as that of true family, or perhaps because the geographic and cultural differences are so great between the first-world United States and third-world Uganda that the Interactionist premise seems strained. Perhaps we are just bigots, incapable of recognizing any duty to distant, differently-colored people; or perhaps we just don't buy the Interactionist view in any context, domestic or global, at all. To be sure, were the "like family" relationship envisioned here not the case, Hardwig would have no general duty to die under the Interactionist premise even if he could raise life expectancy in this or any other village by 5 or 10 years or more. However, even if we do accept Interactionism as the basis of whatever requirements of global justice may exist, the answer to questions about a *global* "duty to die" is still *no:* even if this one Ugandan village is truly closely connected to an ailing 87-year-old American whose savings in health care costs might extend all of their lives, the rest of the global population does not stand in this intertwined, cooperative relationship with him, and he thus does not have such duties to it. Nondomestic Interactionism does not make a stronger case. No global "duty to die" arises here, and Hardwig's argument does not stretch to cover the globe.

Stretching Battin's Daniels-based Early Rawls to Cover the Globe

A second kind of challenge to the negative result so far—that we in the first world have no global "duty to die"—responds to arguments that can be found indirectly in Daniels's early Rawlsian applications to health care and directly in mine, and even to some extent in Callahan's. For the early Rawls, parties to the Original Position, under the veil of ignorance about their own characteristics acquired in the natural lottery, recognize that they might occupy any position in the society; this is why they do not favor social policies that disadvantage some (e.g., slaves) but benefit others (e.g., slaveholders); after all, they might turn out to be slaves rather than slavemasters. Rawls does not apply either his original or his later view to the issues of health or health care; that has been the contribution of Norman Daniels. But the original Rawlsian conjecture was conceived of as confined to a single society or nation-state, and not thought of in terms of the huge range of societies inhabiting the current world; this was primarily because the conjecture requires the possibility of a moral community in which the benefits and burdens of social co-operation are shared. Rawls also assumed a society under circumstances of justice, and some societies in the actual world may not meet even his minimal conditions. Failing these things, can this second challenge succeed?

For consider what would happen if we were to perform the Original Position thought-experiment the other way around—conjecture first, considerations of community second. Thus—although this is no part of Rawls's own view—it would be plausible to ask why the participants in an early Rawlsian Original Position addressed primarily to matters of health (as would be the case in Daniels's conjecture) could not reflect on whether they might be, say, Japanese, with a life expectancy of 81.3, or Ugandan with a life expectancy scarcely more than half that, 44.7. If they do so, Rawls would predict, they would surely elect principles of health care distribution and other health-related matters that more greatly favor Ugandans than

Japanese—this is what the rational self-interest maximizer under the veil of ignorance would choose.

Importantly, however, it would not be at all obvious exactly what these principles might be. Furthermore, they would necessarily be framed at a fairly high level of abstraction, reflecting only the fact that if one does not know whether he or she will be Ugandan or Japanese, they would select principles establishing policies that have the consequence that Japanese live a little less long *if* this permits Ugandans to live longer, thus giving the greatest benefit to the least well off and ensuring that one does not find oneself in a disadvantaged category. Perhaps they would also choose, at least if there were adequate protections against coercion and other sorts of abuse, policies that would both limit first-world individuals' access to expensive life-prolonging care (this is Callahan's concern) and perhaps also permit or even encourage voluntary physician-assisted suicide or euthanasia (this is the argument Battin explored).

But what concrete form, what practical, on-the-ground policies, would these principles take? Parties to the Original Position could certainly favor the abstraction: those with extra long-life expectancies ought not prolong their lives or have them prolonged so that those with very short life expectancies can lead longer lives, but the mechanism not only of life curtailment but reallocation is not specific. The principle "We ought to die sooner, so that they could live longer" may not seem unjust if you do not know who the "we" and the "they" are and which group you find yourself among, and as long as this principle contributes to a circumstances in which any inequalities work to the advantage of the least well off—as all persons having more nearly equal life spans would do—but this still does not give us the practical details.

But, you will surely say, this is preposterous. After all, not only would my sacrifice of my life be a clearly futile gesture, since it would have so little impact, but even Daniels's strategy of considering issues of justice over a life span doesn't work in the global case (as would no doubt be Rawls's response as well): abbreviating my own life would not provide the theoretical advantage, central in Daniels's argument, of having already increased my own chances of survival through all my earlier years, years that are prerequisite to my current existence, by allocating more health care to younger age cohorts. This cannot be the case in the kind of world we have, a world in which various nations' health-care systems are not closely interrelated, do not form a global basic health-related structure, and certainly do not participate in anything approaching a closed system in which the dimming of my prospects may directly enhance yours. It makes a difference whether there is a community of cooperation and what sorts of specific policies are under consideration; highly abstract principles in the absence of any working mechanism are not enough. But seeing this uncovers our central problematic assumption.

How Buchanan's "Natural Duty of Justice"
Can Cover the Globe

In his argument for the claim that justice is a morally obligatory goal of the international legal system, Allen Buchanan, rejecting Interactionism, appeals instead to what he takes to be a more defensible foundation, the "Natural Duty of Justice."[25] Buchanan thinks this duty holds that even in the absence of any global basic structure of cooperation or any form of interaction whatsoever among individuals across borders, we still have obligations of justice that are rooted in the very nature of persons themselves. This is an eminently plausible assumption. I owe you something just because you are a person and are to be respected as a person (this is an essentially Kantian notion). Presumably—though Buchanan does not explore the converse in similar detail—you owe something to me for the same reason: I am also a person and to be respected as a person, just as you are. To be sure, Buchanan's argument will fail to persuade those of libertarian and similar stripe, but in any case it permits us to see what our mistake has been in trying to globalize questions of whether there can be a duty to die.

The Missing Link for Covering the Globe

Our failure to find plausible an argument for a duty to die based on current differences in global life expectancies does not rest in an adequate philosophical objection. It does not undermine the assumptions of any of these arguments. Rather, it results from a failure of vision, of seeing accurately what is the case in the world—a partial or nearly total lack of adequate redistributive mechanisms that might convey the savings from one person's earlier death in the first world to fund health care and related measures that would increase life expectancies among the least well off, the global poor in the second and especially third world—and thus, under Daniels's early-Rawlsian conjecture, improve the prospects for all. This is a specific instance of what Buchanan, although he is not primarily concerned with redistributive mechanisms, would call "institutional incapacity."[26] Of course there are other obstacles: callous bureaucracies, corrupt governments, insensitive economic analyses, and so on, but it is the lack of redistributive mechanisms that is key. It is also the case that savings may result not just from one person's earlier death but from changes in many organizational features of a health-care system—for instance, more efficient ways of structuring a system, lower overhead costs, more comprehensive coverage. Yet reorganization of a system brings one-time savings; a person's not using expensive life-prolonging care, and thus dying earlier than need be, would represent a savings that is realized over and over again, each time a person dies of a terminal illness with a long, downhill slope—by some estimates, as much as 70% of all deaths in the developed world. Because this is a lack, an absence, it is harder to notice than if there were some more concrete obstacle to global health-care justice at hand.

Because of this lack, the early Rawlsian, Daniels-modified argument constructed here about a *global* duty to die cannot succeed now, in a world that does not have such structures, because it does not have mechanisms for reallocation of health-care savings to younger generations and thus cannot serve to enhance life expectancy for all. But it *could* have them—say, international healthcare structures that worked to redistribute health care resources from rich to poor nations and thus to more nearly equalize health care resources for all, in an effort to make the life-prospects of all humans more nearly equal. Of course libertarians and antiegalitarians will shrink at the suggestion of such redistributive structures, but egalitarians and both early and later Rawlsians will welcome them. After all, Rawls argues that, for societies now "burdened by unfavorable conditions" (he has in mind "the poorer and less technologically advanced societies" of the third world, often burdened by "oppressive government and corrupt elites, the subjection of women abetted by unreasonable religion, with overpopulation relative to what the economy of the society can decently sustain"[27]) the goal is that eventually each of these societies "should be raised to, or assisted toward, conditions that make a well-ordered society possible."[28] Indeed, in Rawls's view, the well-ordered and wealthier societies have duties and obligations to societies burdened by such conditions to aid in seeing that human rights are to be recognized and basic human needs are met; this is a "duty of assistance."[29] And, to extend Rawls's concern to the health-related issues that are my specific focus here, such duties of assistance—moral duties, but duties that might necessitate legal requirements if they are to have any effective force at all—would certainly include the provision of information, technology, and medical resources directly bearing on the health status and life prospects of the inhabitants of these poorer parts of the world.

Yet this isn't enough. Fortunately, Buchanan's globalizing view provides a way to address this lack—to make sure it is filled. On the extension of Buchanan's view as applied to health issues I'm pursuing here, what is asked of those in the best-off positions (those in the first world—Europeans, Americans, Australians, and as measured by life expectancy, especially Japanese) is not charity or duties of assistance in any straightforward sense; rather, what they would presumably have is a duty to work to establish the kinds of health-care-relevant institutions that would enable savings in health care costs in one generation and in one area of the globe to be reallocated to younger generations whose prospects are poorer—young Ugandans, for example, whose life expectancies would then be increased. Buchanan does not argue for the development of institutions that are specifically redistributive as much as for the development of institutions that do not create or exacerbate injustice, but in this extension of Buchanan's view, the Natural Duty of Justice entails that those in the first world ought to work not so much towards charity health care dispensed by the first world to the third, but towards developing those health-related structures of justice that would allow the Danielsesque savings to be realized: that health care savings in the first world could be reallocated to those in younger generations who need care in the third, thus (in Daniels's application of the Original-Position conjecture) increasing the life expectancies of those who would have died soonest and thus enhancing the prospects for all. Yet it is only actual, practical, politically workable structures and institutions, not merely abstract ones, that could make this reallocation possible.

For consider some of the inequities that currently affect life prospects of the first, second, and third worlds. In the developed countries, access to vaccines is nearly universal: children routinely receive immunizations against tetanus, measles, and polio; in the third world, these are not always available, and death rates from these preventable diseases are high. Or consider reproductive health care: for a large catalogue of reasons, maternal mortality is just 5 per 100,000 live births in Denmark, but 550 per 100,000 in Lesotho, 1,700 in Angola, and 2,000 per 100,000 in Sierra Leone.[30] Rabies exposure is treated with comparatively convenient, painless drugs in developed countries; in much of the third world, it has been treated with earlier, less effective drugs, involving much more frequent and painful injections with a much poorer outcome. Or yet again consider people with HIV or AIDS: patients in the developed countries are now routinely seeing their lives extended by protease inhibitors; those in the third world have until very recently had none, and even now only a small fraction of people who have HIV receive modern drug therapy. These inequalities all affect life expectancy in substantial ways. And many of the disease conditions involved in these inequalities affect—indeed, kill—children and younger people: average life expectancy for the society would be particularly greatly increased if they were to survive. On the reversed globalized Original Position conjecture, one must choose policies not knowing whether one inhabits Norway (life expectancy at birth 78.7) or the Dominican Republic (66.7) or Botswana (44.7), or Zambia (33.4), and so will favor policies that enhance the prospects (as measured here by life expectancy) of the least well off.

Of course, these health inequalities could not now be reduced if John's death occurred a little earlier and more cheaply, or if mine did too, since what neither of us could guarantee is that the savings we yielded would be translated into longer life for someone else who would otherwise have had dramatically less, like children and young people in the Dominican Republic, Botswana, or Zambia. As things currently are, any savings from our earlier deaths would not be large in the first world. But they would have immense impact if they were translated into resources in the third world, and they would have still greater impact in the kinds of enhanced structure of institutional cooperation Buchanan (as expanded by Daniels and Battin) has in mind. If global health care were indeed an interactive, interrelated global system, whether based in nation-states or other administrative bodies, and if the appropriate redistributive structures were in place, these tiny savings from first-world choices of earlier death would prove far more efficient in protecting and extending life in the third world: the costs of one expensive and not very effective unit of life-prolonging care in the first world, say a week in intensive care on life supports, buys many, many units of inexpensive and highly effective care in the second and especially third: oral rehydration, vaccination, basic reproductive health care. This is just the point about savings and efficiency that is so central to the redistributive claims here. Health care–relevant institutions of this sort would enable savings in health-care costs in one generation and in one area of the globe to enhance life expectancy in younger generations in areas where it is now shorter—future Ugandans, for example—an effort that would (except in the first generation of such a policy) serve the interests of all. This is Daniels, writ large.

The Missing Link: Global Basic Mutual
Health-Related Structures

Thus this argument depends on the existence of redistributive structures that function on a global scale, making it possible for savings in the first world to serve as resources in the third. We do not have these structures yet—at least, not in full.

But we do have rudimentary and partial systems—rudimentary and partial in that they cover only some conditions or some areas, or are financed in limited ways: such organizations as *Médecins Sans Frontières* and a wide range of other largely volunteer, charity-financed organizations like *Operation Smile International* and *Partners in Health* that bring first-world medical resources to the third world. Several major foundations, particularly the Rockefeller Foundation and the Bill and Melinda Gates Foundation, have supported international health initiatives generously. Health-related nongovernmental organizations (NGOs) are numerous. There are government-funded projects, like Swedish Hospital for Children in Hanoi: the government of Sweden built the hospital in 1975 after the Vietnam War and donated it and operating costs for a year to the people of Vietnam. And there are also quasi-governmental organizations, like the World Health Organization, that operate around the globe. These are all financed primarily by the first world; but they are not yet financed by health-care *savings* in the first world, and they do not form a closed system in which savings in one place can be realized as resources in another. The existence of such institutions would be crucial to the argument at hand.

The argument, which began with a Rawlsian framework but has moved beyond Rawls to the cosmopolitan view that justice involves relationships not only within and between nations but among the individuals who inhabit the globe as a whole, also depends on the assumption that there is a network of interrelated obligations of mutual support that can form the basis of a global cooperative scheme. Cooperation is important here; obligations of mutual support cannot be just one-way, and it cannot be the case that the rich nations have obligations to the poor nations or rich individuals to poor ones, but not the other way around. To suggest that people in the rich, first-world nations have health-related obligations to people in the second and third worlds that might be reflected in more nearly equalized life expectancies is thus to raise the issue of whether people in the second and third worlds have health-related obligations to those in the first world.

Mutual obligations? Most health-care support seems to flow one way, as charity from the rich nations to the poor. But I think we do, however inchoately, recognize poor-to-rich health *obligations* as well, though these are usually discussed in the context of environmentalism[31] and, increasingly, public health and specifically infectious disease. In particular those of us in the rich nations (though here we must speak with some shame) assume that the people of the poor nations ought not do things that potentially affect *our* health and perhaps survival, including both those that damage the environment and those that affect our health in more direct ways. Thus *we* insist that *they*—we mean the global poor—ought not cut down the rainforest; that they ought not use coal-fired manufacturing processes without adequate pollution controls; that they ought not dump pesticides into the sea; that they ought not eat bush meat that risks allowing new infectious diseases to jump from animals to humans; and that they ought not destroy environments which harbor rare species of plants and animals that might provide discoveries of enormous medical and pharmaceutical importance—importance to *our* health, that is, by reducing health-care costs and lengthening lives in the first as well as third world.

This may seem to be pure arrogance on the part of the rich, yet another imposition by the first world on the third. But there is another way to see these expectations: as the first glimmers of the emergence of global, reciprocal, cooperative health-related structures that make rational distribution of health care savings possible. In this picture, "they" expect help with infectious disease like AIDS, malaria, and polio, support for reproductive health care, and access to basic medical and public health measures like oral rehydration and parasite control; but we in turn expect changes in environment-affecting, health-related practices from them, not to mention cleaning up the corruption that interferes with the function of health and other infrastructure systems generally. It may sound like bargaining: "We'll make antiretroviral therapy for HIV available," we might say, "*if* you place tighter controls on emerging new diseases and work to eradicate or contain the ones— like multidrug-resistant tuberculosis or hepatitis B or SARS or West Nile virus— that might spread to us." Such expectations are not simply predictions of future behavior; rather, underneath them are moral claims: because health is of such paramount importance we expect you, and you expect us, to act in certain ways, and we and you have mutual claims that we each do so.

Of course, the people whom "we" take to have these obligations to us, the global poor, may not honor them very well in practice, but we understand that this is because observing them in practice would be so costly in terms of their own life prospects—after all, the global poor depend for survival on many of these health-affecting practices: clearing new tracts of land in the rainforest, burning cheap fuels, disposing of waste in casual ways, eating bush meat when there is no other protein source for survival. As things now stand, not doing these things would be even more costly for the global poor than sacrificing a modest amount of life, as in Hardwig's conjecture: for the global poor not doing these things may mean death in youth or middle age, not just forgoing the last year or two of a terminal illness in old age.

Yet if we take Buchanan's Natural Duty of Justice seriously in the context of these health-related facts, we see that the specific obligation it would generate when applied to health would be to create, or reform, health-related institutions that make such mutually health-favoring "bargains" possible. Of course, Buchanan is not talking about health or about redistributive mechanisms per se; his concern is with basic human rights—but we can translate his interpretation of the Natural Duty of Justice into this context. He writes,

> The Natural Duty of Justice as I understand it says that equal consideration for persons requires helping to ensure that they have access to institutions that protect their basic human rights. This will sometimes require creating new institutions and will often require reforming existing institutions.[32]

Of course, helping to ensure that there are global health-related institutions that could facilitate health-related global reallocation would on the whole require less reform of existing institutions and more creation of new institutions than in other areas like international commerce or global lending, since the lack of adequate health related institutions that could accomplish the Danielsesque redistribution is so severe—indeed, there are hardly any. (Indeed, this is the reason the reverse-order conjecture in the Original Position couldn't initially get off the ground.) The early glimmerings already mentioned—various charitable, nongovernmental, and semigovernmental organizations amid a loose network of mutual expectations—these early glimmerings cannot now be described as an effective, efficient redistributive health-related global structure, but they may nevertheless play a substantial role in bringing such structures into being, fostering institutions that can operationalize those interrelated rich-to-poor and poor-to-rich obligations of mutual health-related support, obligations that if mutually recognized would serve both not to damage one another's health or potential health but to provide positive measures for improving it. It may even be that global health-related structures of this sort are tacitly presupposed by the rights to health contained in several influential aspirational manifestos of international human rights, for example:

> *The Universal Declaration of Human Rights:*
> Everyone has the right to a standard of living adequate for the health and well-being of himself and of his family, including food, clothing, housing and medical care and necessary social services, and the right to security in the event of unemployment, sickness, disability, widowhood, old age . . .[33]

> *The International Covenant on Social, Economic, and Cultural Rights:*
> The States Parties to the present Convenant recognize the right of everyone to the enjoyment of the highest attainable standard of physical and mental health.
> The steps to be taken by the States Parties to the present Covenant to achieve the full realization of this right shall include those necessary for:
> (a) The provision for the reduction of the stillbirth-rate and of infant mortality and for the healthy development of this child;
> (b) The improvement of all aspects of environmental and industrial hygiene;
> (c) The prevention, treatment and control of epidemic, endemic, occupational and other diseases;
> (d) The creation of conditions which would assure to all medical service and medical attention in the event of sickness.[34]

But could such structures—operationalized mutual health-related expectations, one might call them—form a closed system, the key to the kind of rational savings-reallocation that make the Daniels conjecture first work? What counts as a "closed system" in the first place? We need not suppose that closed systems can only be formed by centralized funding schemes; there may be other ways of putting a robust network of mutual health-related expectations into practice. Leslie Francis suggests, for example, a "third-world drug tax" on all brand name drugs prescribed in the United States, the proceeds of which would finance drug availability in the third world and at the same time encourage use of generics in the first world.[35] At the moment, however, it is sufficient to observe that global health care does not even nearly form a closed system now.

The Reemergence of the Duty to Die?

With this "missing link" in place, a set of global health-related redistributive structures against a background of interrelated obligations of mutual health-related support in a cooperative scheme involving some form or other of closed system, however, the conditions would be satisfied within which a "duty to die" would become a reality. This duty would be the duty to conserve health-care resources by foregoing treatment or directly ending one's life in the interests of justice in health care, and it would be reflected in more nearly equal health prospects and life expectancies around the globe. This is not to supplant other duties like restraint in consumption; but these are explicitly health-related duties within a closed redistributive system. Perhaps it might even amount to something stronger than merely a duty to cease consuming medical resources; a positive duty to die, at least if the development of a global system of health care, responsive to a wide range of cultural values, involved radical changes in attitudes toward life prolongation and the meaning of extended illness or old age. This is what I was concerned with at the outset—whether even as the issue of the "duty to die" seemed to have dropped out of sight as issues about justice in global health have come to the fore, that a new, stronger duty to die might emerge. I think it could. Those who argue in their various ways as Hardwig, Battin in drawing on Daniels, and Callahan do may well be committed to the conclusion that having one's death occur earlier, whether directly caused or as the result of refraining from claiming expensive life-prolonging care, would even in a global world be the morally right thing—indeed, the globally just thing to do.

However, while the arguments Hardwig, Daniels, Callahan, and I have explored can all finally be extrapolated to the global case after all, this is true at the moment only in theory. It is *not* possible as a matter of actual practice under current global conditions. How could "we," the global rich, translate savings from our own earlier demises into health gains for "them," the global poor? Charity, yes, but genuine reallocation, no. And how could "their" restraint in traditional health-affecting practices be organized so that it improved "our" health without making "them" still worse off? Thus while we in the first world cannot now have a global duty to die— whether by declining life-prolonging care or ending life in more direct ways—in order to promote lifespan equity among the inhabitants of the world, we certainly do, as Buchanan might well exhort us, have an obligation to promote international structures of transfer and redistribution of health-care savings, against a background of mutual health-related obligations, which would mean that choices concerning dying in the first world would directly affect life-prospects in the second and third. Similarly, while they—the inhabitants of the poor nations of the globe—cannot now have a duty to us, the rich, to refrain from health-affecting practices that compromise first-world health, like forest-cutting and field-burning and bush-meat– eating, they too could come to do so in the future.

Here, then, is the message for the future: First and foremost, though I have not argued for it here: the overall disparity between global rich and global poor must be reduced dramatically. But failing this, what needs to be built are the structures for a world in which my health prospects affect yours and yours affect mine, so that we all come to have a mutual interest in making both of our prospects better. Curiously, too, this very project of putting mutual cooperation into practice may also foster some of the personal human interaction on which Interactionism is based, thus giving some plausibility to this argument in global health-related contexts too. Thus this argument is not so much about the duty to die in itself, but about noticing what hugely important social institutions just aren't there, and recognizing our obligation to create them. The emergence of the duty to die would be a kind of epiphenomenon, so to speak, a symptom that we're getting these institutions in place.

Is this overall argument a *reductio ad absurdum* of the Hardwig, Daniels, Battin, and Callahan views, or a genuine conclusion, albeit, as Peter Unger would put it, an "extremely demanding" one?[36] I'd like to predict that with time, and with growing recognition of the interconnectedness of the interests of the various peoples of the globe (including not only our obligations to other peoples but their obligations to us), we will come to see it not as a silly thought experiment, but as a real challenge to our moral selves to work to develop global health-related structures that form an effective, efficient closed system. It might seem to be bad news for those of us in the fortunate situations of the developed world now enjoying long lifespans, especially since the gains from such savings cannot be realized in the first generation, but, viewed from an early Rawlsian and perhaps even Interactionist perspective, it would promote the good of us all by producing a far more just health-related world in the long run. In the bargain we would see extended life expectancies in future generations for all. The good news is that as global inequalities in life expectancy are reduced, the obligation envisioned here becomes less and less burdensome, and may even seem to disappear as appropriate healthcare structures are in place and life expectancies even out.

Notes

Portions of this piece appeared in my "Global Life Expectancies and the Duty to Die," in James M. Humber and Robert F. Almeder, eds., *Is There a Duty To Die?* Special issue of *Biomedical Ethics Reviews* 1999, Totowa, NJ: Humana Press, 2000; used by permission of Humana Press.

I'd like to thank Ryan Spellecy, Leslie Francis, Erika George, and Chandran Kukathas for discussions of these issues or of this paper at various times in its composition.

1. Daniel Callahan, *The Tyranny of Survival* (Macmillan 1973); *Setting Limits* (1987); *What Kind of Life?* (1990); *The Troubled Dream of Life* (1993); and *False Hopes* (1998); except for the first, all published by Simon & Schuster.

2. Margaret P. Battin, "Age Rationing and the Just Distribution of Health Care: Is There a Duty to Die?" *Ethics* 97:2 (1987): 317–340. With slight modifications, this piece is also reprinted in my volume *The Least Worst Death: Essays in Bioethics on the End of Life* (New York and Oxford: Oxford University Press, 1994, pp. 58–79, under the title "Is There a Duty to Die? Age Rationing and the Just Distribution of Health Care."

3. John Hardwig, "Is There a Duty to Die?" *The Hastings Center Report* 27(2): 34–42 (March–April 1997).

4. Life expectancy data are for 2001, *Human Development Report 2003*.

5. John K. Iglehart, "The American Health Care System: Expenditures," *The New England Journal of Medicine* 340(1): 70–76 (Jan. 7, 1999), p. 72.

6. Ibid.

7. For an extended discussion, see Solomon R. Benatar, Abdallah S. Daar, and Peter A. Singer, "Global Health Ethics: The Rationale for Mutual Caring," *International Affairs* 79:1 (2003): 107–138.

8. Jan Narveson, "We Don't Owe Them a Thing!" Paper for the Pacific Division meetings of the American Philosophical Association, April 1999.

9. Hardwig, p. 301.

10. See, for example, the many papers in James M. Humber and Robert F. Almeder, eds., *Biomedical Ethics Reviews,* special issue "Is There a Duty to Die?" Totowa, NJ: Humana Press, 1999.

11. Margaret P. Battin, "Age-Rationing and the Just Distribution of Health Care: Is There a Duty to Die?" *Ethics,* Vol. 97, No. 2, January 1987; reprinted in Battin, *The Least Worst Death* (New York: Oxford University Press, 1994), pp. 58–79.

12. John Rawls, *A Theory of Justice* (Cambridge: Harvard University Press, 1971).

13. Norman Daniels, *Am I My Parents' Keeper? An Essay on Justice Between the Young and the Old* (New York: Oxford University Press, 1988).

14. Ezekiel J. Emanuel and Margaret P. Battin, "What are the Potential Cost Savings from Legalizing Physician-Assisted Suicide?" The New England Journal of Medicine 339(3): 167–172 1998).

15. Daniel Callahan, *False Hopes. Why America's Quest for Perfect Health is a Recipe for Failure* (New York: Simon & Schuster, 1998).

16. Daniels, "Why Saying No Is So Hard," in *Am I My Parents' Keeper?*

17. In the Rawlsian view, this is what would be required for the existence of such obligations. See John Rawls, "The Law of Peoples," pp. 41–82 in his *On Human Rights.* Oxford Amnesty Lectures. New York: Basic Books, 1993.

18. See the impassioned analysis by Peter Unger, *Living High and Letting Die: Our Illusion of Innocence* (New York: Oxford, 1996), and the work of Peter Singer.

19. Peter Singer, "The Singer Solution to World Poverty," *The New York Times Sunday Magazine,* September 5, 1999.

20. Allen Buchanan, *Justice, Legitimacy, and Self-Determination. Moral Foundations for International Law.* New York: Oxford University Press, 2004, p. 85.

21. Hardwig, "Is There a Duty to Die?" p. 37. APACHE (Acute Physiology and Chronic Health Evaluation) is a scoring system used to measure the severity of illness in patients who are critically ill or likely to die.

22. Ibid.

23. See Ryan B. Spellecy, "Dying For Others: Families, Altruism, and a Duty to Die," in James M. Humber and Robert F. Almeder, eds., *Biomedical Ethics Reviews,* special issue "Is There a Duty to Die?" Totowa, NJ: Humana Press, 1999.

24. Life insurance would not be invalidated by withholding or withdrawing medical treatment, even if the patient's intention were to die; suicide would invalidate it only within a stipulated period after purchase (in most states, 2 years) and reduce double-indemnity insurance to payment of the face amount. In Oregon, at the moment the only state permitting physician-assisted suicide, the law permitting a physician to provide a lethal prescription to a terminally ill patient at that person's express request stipulates that the act of using it shall not constitute a suicide.

25. Buchanan, *Justice, Legitimacy, and Self-Determination,* p. 85.

26. Ibid., pp. 202–203.

27. Rawls, "The Law of Peoples," pp. 52, 77.

28. Ibid., p. 75.

29. Ibid., p. 75.

30. 2001 data, *Human Development Report 2003.*

31. See for example Leslie Pickering Francis, "Global Systemic Problems and Interconnected Duties," *Environmental Ethics* 25 (Summer 2003): 115–28.

32. Buchanan, *Justice, Legitimacy, and Self-Determination,* p. 88.

33. Universal Declaration of Human Rights, Article 26, paragraph 1.

34. International Covenant on Social, Economic, and Cultural Rights, Article 12. I am grateful to Erika George for these two examples.

35. Leslie Francis, personal communication.

36. Unger, *Living High and Letting Die,* pp. 152–56.

15

New Life in the Assisted-
Death Debate

Scheduled Drugs versus NuTech

Change in the Issue of Physician-Assisted Suicide

In the years since Dr. Jack Kevorkian went to jail, public involvement with the issues of physician-assisted suicide and voluntary active euthanasia may seem to have subsided in the United States. Front-page stories less frequently raise the question; debates on talk shows have turned to other social issues like stem cell research and gay marriage; there seems to be less volatile, less frequent, less consuming public debate about hastened death and the right to die. Many other countries have been concerned with end-of-life issues—Canada, the Netherlands, Britain, Australia, Switzerland, Belgium, the Scandinavian countries, and others—and in some of them the debate seems to be in decline, but I think the change is most evident in the United States. The assisted-death debate may seem moribund, if not nearly completely dead.

Some of the apparent decline in the American public's interest in issues about physician-assisted suicide and active euthanasia may be attributed to the disappearance of Kevorkian from view—after all, "Dr. Death," as he was often called, was a master at knowing how to arouse the interest of the media. Now in prison on a sentence of 10-25 years, he is no longer even allowed to talk to the press in person. However, I think something else is at work as well. The dispute over hastened death is evolving, mutating, in a way that lends itself less easily to public debate, but at the same time is far more vulnerable to political manipulation. It is this current process of mutation in the debate, evident in the strategies of both proponents and opponents of legalization, that I want to explore here. While this process is occurring in many countries, I think it is most pronounced in the comparatively adversarial legal climate of the United States. I do not think the assisted death debate is dead at all.

I shall focus particular attention on the ways in which new strategies of political and legal activism on both sides are tending to escalate the debate, taking it first from populist appeals to state-law initiatives and counter initiatives, and then from state-level to federal-level maneuvres.[1] But this pattern is hardly complete. The opportunity for reasonably stable compromise seems to have failed, and the debate now stands at what may be an even more charged and polarized point than at any earlier moment, albeit more out of public view. It is the point, I think, at which the entire model of approach to end-of-life issues in the United States could change, even as the nation yields to pressures for greater liberalization, and it is not clear that this would be a change for the better. Yet while there is reason to think the situation could get still worse, there is also some slight reason, as I shall suggest, to imagine that it could take a turn for the better instead.

Political Escalation

Concern with end-of-life issues began to arise in the United States in the late 1960s and early 1970s, in part as a product of the civil-rights and rights-favoring movements that spoke not only for African-Americans but also for other disfavored groups: women, people from religious minorities, people with disabilities, and so on. Among those seeking to gain recognition of a larger range of rights were medical patients—people with illnesses, injuries, or other reasons for involvement with the health care system, and in particular people with terminal illnesses.

Some of the rights secured by patients with terminal illnesses were informally recognized rights established in professional practice, like the right to know one's diagnosis—something nearly universally withheld in the 1960s but now nearly universally provided, at least in the United States (though not, for example, Russia, Greece, or Japan). Many other sorts of rights pertaining to patients, especially patients with terminal illnesses, were legally codified—sometimes in legislative action, sometimes as a result of court decisions, but almost always with considerable social and legal dispute. Over a long period of years, patients, especially patients with terminal illnesses, sought and won not only the right to full information about their conditions and prognoses but also the right to refuse treatment, to discontinue treatment, to specify in advance what treatment they would and would not accept if they became incompetent, and to insist that they be treated only with their explicit, advance, or, in emergencies, implied consent.[2] Gradually the issues that came to light at the time of the passage of the California Natural Death Act of 1976, the first of the living-will statutes, developed into a full-blown dispute over the issue of direct control of the process of dying. This was the foundation, the floor, so to speak, from which has emerged a pattern of continuing escalation in the political disputes over physician-assisted suicide.

Populism and Its Alternatives

It was around this time, in the late 1970s and early 1980s, that back-and-forth political volleying over the issues of assisted dying, including physician-assisted suicide and voluntary active euthanasia, began in earnest. To be sure, the issue had been percolating for many years. But the first real efforts of proponents of physician aid-in-dying, including both those who believed that these practices should be recognized as ethically acceptable and those who believed they should be legalized, came as an effort to sway public opinion.

This was the first new step of what would be a long series of further escalations. There were many contributions to the effort to bring the issue of assisted dying to public attention, but perhaps the most visible of the early proponents of moral legitimization and legalization was the British journalist Derek Humphry, whose frank book *Jean's Way* described his own role in assisting the suicide of his first wife as she was dying of cancer. Humphry followed this with a second populist move, the establishment of the Hemlock Society (1980), a grassroots organization of people interested in personal choice for themselves in the matter of dying and with the legalization of such practices.[3] Still later, Humphry made a third, perhaps even more effectively populist, move: not only did he bring to the public instructions for using an ordinary plastic bag to bring about death, but in 1991 he published a book of hitherto professionally restricted information crucial in assisted suicide, the how-to manual *Final Exit*. This little book provided concrete, explicit factual information about lethal drugs for use by the terminally ill, a move so effective in reaching the public that the book hit the top of the *New York Times* how-to bestseller list and its title became a household phrase.

Humphry wasn't the only writer to address the public at large; a variety of novelists and memoir-writers had also been exploring personal experiences in the matter of the right to die, including Lael Tucker Wertenbacker, Jessamyn West, and Betty Rollin. Jack Kevorkian, M.D., also played to the public, exhibiting his considerable capacity to keep the issue of physician-assisted suicide before the public view: he made sure the press was called when the people he had assisted were found dead in Volkswagen buses, motel rooms, and the like. These early moves in the disputes over the right to die had the effect of escalating the debate by first bringing the issue out into the open, primarily by portraying a series of heartrending personal cases, then—still drawing on these cases—by establishing a constituency committed to change. Perhaps most important, it made crucial information public; now there could be no turning around.

Opponents took their case to the public too, though they used a quite different strategy. They also tried to appeal to the public through personal memoirs, interviews with the press, and by developing grassroots organizations, but they more frequently worked through or in concert with existing organizations, especially the Catholic Church, Hospice, disability rights groups, and the American Medical Association. Opponents of assisted dying urged these groups to take stands against legalization or to articulate their stands more forcefully and broadly. This strategy, while it also served to intensify the debate, had the advantage of suggesting that the bulwark institutions in society were opposed to expansions in the right to die, and that indeed society would be undermined if aid-in-dying legislation permitting physician-assisted suicide or voluntary euthanasia were allowed to pass.

State-Level Legislation

The next escalation in the dispute occurred in the mid-to-late l980's, as proponents sought change through state-level legislation to make physician-assisted suicide legal.[4] Proponents understood physician-assisted suicide largely in the "arm's-length" sense, favoring changes in the law that would permit a physician to provide his or her terminally ill patient who so requested with a prescription for a lethal drug. Proponents worked to bring referenda before the voters in a number of states, and succeeded in putting it on the ballot in Washington (1991), California (1992), Oregon (1994), Michigan (1998), and Maine (2000). This was an attempt to change not just public opinion but the law.

There were victories and losses for both sides in these events; every step of the way was contested, in a pattern of what Robert Kagan and other commentators have called "adversarial legalism."[5] Referenda failed in Washington, California, Michigan, and Maine, though in several of these states by very narrow margins. However, Oregon's initiative (known as Measure 16) passed—indeed, passed twice, first by a very narrow margin in 1994 and again in 1997 as the Oregon legislature returned the measure to the ballot box for a second vote, where it passed the second time by a much wider margin.

At each of these junctures in each state, but especially in Oregon, the tension between proponents and opponents increased, as did the amount of money flowing into campaign chests. The playing field had changed: though appeals to public opinion remained important, as they had from the outset of this debate, the real contest was now the battle for state law. There was no longer, if there ever had been, any sense that an influential, centralized governmental or moral authority could make policy acceptable to both sides, and the dispute became even more adversarial and politically charged.

Federal-Level Activity

Concurrently, a new escalation in the ongoing battle was also taking place, upping the ante still further, so to speak, to a new, federal level: in an effort to secure civil rights in courts that couldn't be attained legislatively (a strategy much like that which proponents of contraception and abortion had used), proponents succeeded in bringing a pair of cases, *Washington v. Glucksberg* (Ninth Circuit) and *Vacco v. Quill* (Second Circuit), before the Supreme Court. The Court's ruling in these cases, handed down jointly in 1997, held 9–0 that the state statutes in question in Washington and New York—statutes prohibiting assistance in suicide in general, without specific reference to physician-assisted suicide—were constitutional. Opponents claimed they had won the day: the high court had said there was no right to physician-assisted suicide. Proponents pointed out, however, that the Court had made it clear that states could adopt laws criminalizing assisted suicide if they wished, but that they could also refrain from adopting such laws or, in adopting them, could make an exception for physician assistance in the circumstances of terminal illness. Thus it would be equally legal, proponents reasoned, for a state to leave the issue of physician-assisted suicide open, as several states did, or to legalize it, as Measure 16 had done in Oregon. Indeed, there was reference in the Supreme Court's decision to the prospect of a "laboratory of the states," in which some states might legalize physician-assisted suicide while other states hung back, so to speak, to see how it would go.

Interlude: The Failure of Compromise

This picture, I think, shows us the moment in which real compromise between opponents and proponents of assisted dying might have been possible, and in which the series of escalatory moves—each upping the ante to a new level—might have ceased. This was the picture in which one state, Oregon, was willing to try legalized physician-assisted suicide under a series of careful controls and with state-mandated reporting, but the other 49 states either had no law (as was the case in just a handful) or (like the vast majority of states) prohibited assisted suicide. This was the picture the Supreme Court's decision almost seemed to recommend: opponents could hold the forces of change at bay, since physician-assisted suicide would not be legal in 49 out of 50 states, but proponents (and the entire country) would have the opportunity to see how such a practice might function where it had become legal. If it were legal, would there be only defensible, controlled use, free from pressures of all sorts? Or would it lead to the abuse of vulnerable patients, as both opponents and even some proponents feared? Time would be allowed to tell, and in those states where physician-assisted suicide was not legal (that is, almost all of them) such already legal measures as the heavy use of opiates under the principle of double effect and recourse to terminal sedation could still be used in the most difficult cases.

Of course, such a "compromise" did not satisfy real advocates of the right to assistance in dying, since it left dying people in 49 out of the 50 states without recourse to active help. Nor did it satisfy opponents either, since it accepted actual legalization, even if only in Oregon. It was just a compromise—not even a negotiated compromise, but one emerging from contrary political pressures. Yet it still might have seemed a desirable compromise, since it both remained open to further evidence about the effects of legalization and yet was given some limited validity by the Court's intimation that it would accept either further legalization by additional states or an end to legalization in the one state that had granted it.

But the political reality has, in the few years since the Supreme Court's decision, turned out to be quite otherwise. Despite some academics' and physicians' attempts to frame conciliatory positions, and despite real agreement among many parties on the importance of better techniques of pain control and greater access to pain management, there does not appear to be a stable political compromise emerging at all in the social and legal debates over assisted suicide, but rather, continuing political hostilities and further escalatory moves. Better pain manage-

306 DILEMMAS ABOUT DYING IN A GLOBAL FUTURE

ment is not the only answer; the dispute is still fueled by issues about personal vision and control (see chapter 17, this volume).

Escalation, Continued: The PRPA and NuTech

Seeing Oregon as the hole in the dike—the domino that would let many others fall—opponents sought from the moment Measure 16 first passed in 1994 to undercut it. The first attempts were pursued at the state level, a complex series of legal maneuvers challenging the referendum at every turn, delaying implementation so long that the Oregon legislature finally ordered the second vote. However, with the final implementation of Measure 16 as law, the Death with Dignity Act, in November 1997 (three full years after its original passage in 1994), opponents turned to a new tactic, seeking to scuttle Oregon's law by changing federal regulations. This move too further escalated the dispute.

Their first effort was to have the federal executive branch, specifically the Justice Department, override Oregon's law by preventing physicians from using scheduled drugs for "nonmedical" purposes. Attorney General Janet Reno rejected this move, and opponents then turned to a congressional measure. This second effort, pursued first under the label *Lethal Drug Abuse Prevention Act of 1998* and then as the *Pain Relief Promotion Act of 1999* (PRPA), sponsored by Representative Henry Hyde and then also Senator Don Nickles, was a measure that would amend the Federal Controlled Substances Act. The revised Act would "prohibit the dispensing or distribution of a controlled substance for the purpose of causing, or assisting in causing, the suicide or euthanasia of any individual." It would not make physician assistance in suicide illegal; instead, it would make illegal the use of scheduled drugs for the purpose of causing death. Thus, the very drugs that make it possible for physicians to induce a painless death without unwanted side effects like hallucinations or convulsions—the barbiturates and related drugs—would be unavailable to physicians; penalties for violations could range from loss of practice privileges at specific hospitals to a federal prison sentence of up to 20 years. Since the effect of Oregon's Death with Dignity Act was precisely to allow physicians to legally give patients a prescription for lethal drugs, the PRPA would effectively gut the Act, and—this is the specifically escalatory feature—any similar law that might pass in any other state in the future. Lesser measures, like triplicate prescription laws, computer-based prescription tracking, and state limitations on maximum doses of morphine, have something of the same deterrent effect. Although the PRPA died without action at the end the congressional session in 2000, partly because of opposition from palliative care specialists who pointed out that it would impair good pain relief in all 50 states, Attorney General John Ashcroft then renewed the effort by issuing a Directive that also interpreted the Controlled Substances Act to prohibit physicians from prescribing Schedule II substances like barbiturates to cause death, on the grounds that, among other things, such prescriptions served "no legitimate medical purpose." Ashcroft's move was rejected by the Ninth Circuit Court of Appeals in May 2004 and again in July 2004, but both sides had previously said they would appeal an unfavorable decision to the U.S. Supreme Court.

Even before this escalatory move by opponents had actually taken place, it had already elicited a further escalatory counter-move from proponents. Proponents (correctly) viewed the PRPA and subsequent federal efforts like the Ashcroft Directive to restrict scheduled drugs as directly aimed to undercut their gains so far, gains made in the arduous and expensive process of bringing one referendum and then another, and another, onto state ballots. What they needed was a strategy that could not be vetoed by a federal-level tactic like the PRPA or the Ashcroft Directive, which at one blow would raise the threat of erasing all their careful state-level work so far *and* precluding any such efforts in the future. Indeed, the PRPA and the Directive threatened even the quiet underground of physicians willing to help patients ease into death in a discreet way, since it would permit new surveillance of their activities. Some activists among the proponents (though not all) thus turned to a new sort of strategy. This new strategy involves the development of *nonmedical* means of bringing about death, means that are not subject to the restrictions imposed by the PRPA and the Directive. Ironically, this move represents a return to a broad-scale, populist approach, reminiscent in certain ways of the early days of the right-to-die movement.

What proponents are developing as a response to the PRPA, the Ashcroft Directive, and any similar federal measures that are intended to undercut state law legalizing physician-assisted suicide is a series of methods of producing death that can be employed without the assistance of a physician and without prescription-controlled drugs, though they will still assure a gentle, easy death. These techniques are generally referred to as "self-deliverance new technologies," or "NuTech." Under development by a group of researchers known as "the engineers" (especially centered in the Last Rights Publications group run by John Hofsess, with support from Hemlock, from Derek Humphry's organization Ergo! and from Philip Nitschke's Voluntary Euthanasia Research Foundation in Australia), NuTech involves a range of devices using a variety of mechanisms for causing death or, as NuTech supporters put it, "deathing" (like "birthing").[6] These include a customized plastic bag (the "Exit Bag") and a variety of delivery devices for various inert gasses, like helium, argon, and nitrogen, which have the effect of reducing the oxygen concentration in air and so causing asphyxia.[7] Among the devices is a hypoxic tent (known as the "Exit Tent"), available in a one- or two-person model, which uses the same techniques athletes use for reducing oxygen—that is, mimicking high-altitude training—but lowers the oxygen content to fatally low levels. Similarly, an apparatus known as a "Debreather" uses scuba technology to recirculate breathed air and so slowly reduce the oxygen level. Also under development are the use of toxic plants that are not federally scheduled, like hemlock (used in the execution of Socrates) and nicotine, methods of carotid artery occlusion, the toxic modification of existing pharmaceuticals, various veterinary euthanatics, and certain poisons.

This new move, the development of NuTech for use in suicide by terminally ill patients, still further escalates the dispute over physician aid in dying by taking the issue out of the hands of physicians altogether. None of these devices are illegal; indeed, anyone can buy a tank of helium, usually sold for inflating party balloons. The very purpose of NuTech is to develop "nonfelonious" ways of bringing about death, as Derek Humphry puts it, a "new technology for legal acts of self deliverance," or as Philip Nitschke puts it, "methods of self deliverance independent of mandatory expert assistance"—that is, "Practical strategies that allow a competent person to effectively and peacefully end their life."[8] While not illegal, these new technologies also leave little postmortem evidence on the body, so that if the devices themselves are disposed of effectively by friends or family members, the circumstances under which death occurred remain relatively secret.

Thus NuTech, responding to the PRPA's attempt to gut Oregon's law legalizing physician-assisted suicide, in effect undercuts the intent of the PRPA: it circumvents the need for scheduled drugs, and by taking physicians out of the picture altogether, renders irrelevant any attempt to restrict what their intentions may be in prescribing such drugs. The PRPA was intended to make it illegal for physicians to prescribe the drugs typically used in assisted suicide for the purpose of causing death, and thus to gut any state law that might legalize physician-assisted suicide, even though the Supreme Court had clearly intimated that such laws could pass constitutional muster. NuTech moves outside this picture altogether. It tries to do so by moving beyond the guns, ropes, bridges, razor blades, sleeping pills, and high buildings people have traditionally used for suicide by providing methods seen as less violent and more humane, but where control is still retained by the person in question. The PRPA and the Ashcroft Directive were intended to gut Oregon's Death with Dignity Act; NuTech in return aims to utterly disempower these federal measures. To be sure, it does invite alternative "deathing" counselors and providers into the market, like Caring Friends, Compassionate Chaplaincy, and Compassion in Dying, but these groups consist primarily of volunteers rather than professionals like physicians and do not have the problematic weight of institutions like health insurers and hospitals behind them.

To some observers, the various devices under development as NuTech seem ghoulish. The debreather involves a face mask placed over the nose and mouth of the patient. The Exit Tent is a closed space, somewhat like a backpacker's camping tent, rolled out on a bed or on the floor. The helium delivery system presents a difficult three-way tradeoff between technical reliability, privacy, and low cost: while a "party tank" of helium for filling balloons costs about $22 and can be purchased anonymously, it lacks a flow control mechanism; a professional high-pressure helium tank with a regulator not only requires registration for purchase but costs some $260.

Opponents have called these devices "human-zappers," like insect-zappers,[9] and many have pointed out the association with Nazi euthanasia practices that gas machines seem to evoke. Not all proponents of physician-assisted suicide support NuTech, and many of the more centrist organizations supporting legalization have shied away from it, insisting that what they seek is a change in the law to make physician-assisted suicide legal. Supporters of NuTech agree that it would be better to have *physician*-assisted suicide legalized and readily recognize that patients would rather have an oral drug, a simple, side-effect-free drug that could be taken easily without gadgetry and would ensure a gentle, painless death—but they point out that this is exactly what the PRPA, the Directive, or any federal-level administrative edict restricting scheduled drugs would render impossible. It is in this way, they say, that the disputes over aid-in-dying have been irrevocably altered. If patients cannot have legal physician-administered aid-in-dying, they must be able to do it for themselves.

NuTech is not yet widespread, if it ever will be, though by mid-2004 some 173 cases had been reported.[10] A few observers think that because NuTech's anoxic technologies are more immediately and reliably efficacious in producing death than oral medications, it will be preferred to barbiturates or other drugs, and they insist that it is not unpleasant: after all, as high-altitude climbers know, lack of oxygen produces euphoria. They also point out that because its use is hard to detect, families can be more directly involved. Derek Humphry has already issued a "Supplement to *Final Exit*" describing the use of helium inhalation and plastic bags. Nor is it clear whether NuTech will survive legal challenge. In Canada, 73-year-old Evelyn Martens was facing trial scheduled for September 2004 in a case that has constitutional implications for Canada's criminal prohibition of aiding suicide, and in Ireland the Rev. George Exoo has also been charged in connection with the use of NuTech methodologies. However, among those who support legalization, the more centrist groups continue to press for state-level and—as a long-term strategy—Supreme Court legalization of physician-assisted suicide.

It is far too early to tell whether the pattern of mutual escalation reflected in the PRPA and its successors and in NuTech will be the shape of the future (the next Supreme Court case that now seems inevitable will perhaps determine this), or whether the current picture of polarization and politicization represents a transitory blip of extremist but peripheral moves by both sides in an otherwise relatively smooth pattern of development toward eventual political and legal consensus. At the moment, the issue is whether any new sort of compromise could emerge.

Is a New Compromise Possible?

Although this goal has so far proved elusive, NuTech engineers have also begun working to develop a "suicide pill" that a patient could synthesize in the privacy of his or her own home out of readily available, nonrestricted ingredients that could not be banned. This is something quite far beyond the so-called "Drion Pill" (or "Last Will Pill") being discussed in the Netherlands, a hypothetical euthanatic drug named after the former member of the Dutch Supreme Court who launched a much-discussed conjecture about it.[11] Unlike the Drion Pill, the pill that the NuTech engineers envision—this is its particularly important feature—would be self-compoundable. A suicide pill (or drink) that could be synthesized at home out of easily available ingredients would give terminally ill patients irrevocable control over their circumstances by making them able to end their lives as they choose, the NuTech engineers point out, without being dependent on physicians for assistance in doing so. Nor would patients violate state or federal regulation in ending their own lives, since suicide itself is not illegal—though, of course, if interrupted in the act, they may be judged a danger to themselves and involuntarily committed for mental health treatment. In January 2005, Philip Nitschke, the Australian researcher who is the director of EXIT/Australia/New Zealand, plans to hold a series of workshops in outback Australia to instruct small groups in formulating a "Peaceful Pill" that can be manufactured at home with household ingredients.

Similarly, a Dutch group including the well-known figures of Pieter Admiraal and Boudewijn Chabot, responding to complaints that Dutch physicians withhold assistance in suicide and euthanasia too frequently from patients who desire it (only about 1 in 9 patients who make informal inquiries about aid in dying receive it, and only 1 in 3 patients who make explicit requests), have recently published a book *Informatie over Humane Zelfdoding*,[12] to appear in English in 2005 under the projected title *Information on a Humane Self-Chosen Death*. This volume details specific combinations of common drugs that will cause death, though they require following a very detailed set of procedures to ensure the desired outcome. The book is sent only to "doctors and to others involved in counseling and helping people with a well considered wish to die. . . . ,"[13] but it too makes self-help in dying possible even without a physician's cooperation.

If an oral euthanaticum of this self-compoundable NuTech sort continues to be developed (Nitschke has announced it several times previously, though less concretely, and as of this writing the "Peaceful Pill" had not yet been tested) and information about it is widely and publicly promulgated, this might seem to complete the series of escalating moves begun in the early days of the right-to-die disputes. Somewhat ironically, the development of a NuTech "Peaceful Pill" recipe that can be compounded by the user himself or herself would seem in some ways to resemble a return to the populist move that Humphry's publication of *Final Exit* involved—a populist move designed to put information, and thus control, into the hands of patients. But it goes a great deal further: *Final Exit* provided information about drugs that still required a physician's prescription to obtain; the new NuTech do-it-yourself suicide pill would eliminate this dependence on doctors, pharmacies, and state and federal prescription regulations altogether.

This might seem to produce the conditions for yet another compromise. NuTech would make an easier way of ending life available to dying patients who wanted it, and the proponents of assisted dying would see the central objective of their campaign achieved. At the same time, opponents would see one of their central objectives realized as well: to keep suicide and euthanasia—the deliberate, intentional causing of death—out of the hands of physicians. Thus both sides would win: an earlier, easier, self-controlled death would be possible, but the slippery slope that physician involvement seemed to risk, or at least most of it, could be avoided. For those whose opposition is based on slippery-slope warnings that fear legalization because it might lead to the abuse of patients by callous or over-worked physicians and greedy, cost-conscious health-care institutions that control the behavior of physicians, the development of a patient-compounded, patient-administered suicide pill would place decisionmaking about causing death squarely with the patient, not with the physician, the nurse, the hospital, the health-care organization, the government, or any external party, though of course alternative "deathing" providers might come into the market. It would thus decrease professional and institutional pressures on the patient and hence reduce the risk of abuse by other parties, though of course it would not protect the patient from his or her own irrationality. Of course, such a compromise would indeed be a compromise, with each side losing as well: proponents would give up the right to assistance in bringing about one's own death by a physician one trusts; and opponents would have to live with the fact that terminally ill patients were committing suicide with impunity.

A Change in the Model of Dying?

In contemplating the possibility of such a circumstance, it is important to note the similarities and differences of such an approach in the United States to those of other nations in the developed world. In the developed world, which is now in what is known as the fourth stage of the epidemiologic transition, the majority of the population dies at comparatively advanced ages of degenerative diseases with characteristically long downhill courses: it is this pattern that presents such dilemmas about the end of life. People in the developed world tend to die at late ages (average life expectancy in the developed world is in the late seventies, in some countries nearing eighty); they die of degenerative diseases (heart disease, cancer, stroke, liver, kidney, and other organ failure, rather than—with the exception of AIDS and pneumonia—parasitic and infectious diseases); and they inhabit worlds with sophisticated health care systems. There are three principal forms of response to this situation, three principal patterns or models of response to the dilemmas of dying in the contemporary developed world, represented respectively by three different countries—the United States, the Netherlands and Germany (see chapter 2, this volume). All three of these countries permit withholding and withdrawing care in order to "allow" a terminally ill patient to die rather than prolong treatment as long as possible, but the Netherlands also permits voluntary active euthanasia and physician-assisted suicide, which are now legal under a careful set of guidelines for due care, and Germany in effect allows non-physician-assisted suicide, since assisting a suicide is not illegal provided the person assisted is competent and in control of his or her own will.

Patterns of approach to end-of-life dilemmas in other developed nations resemble one of these three more or less closely. The approach taken by the United States in its primary reliance on withholding and withdrawing care but rejection of assisted dying is also taken by the United Kingdom and by Canada; the law of the Netherlands permitting voluntary active euthanasia and physician-assisted suicide has just been followed by a similar law permitting active euthanasia (though not assisted suicide) in Belgium; and Germany's distinctive legal situation, in which neither suicide nor assisted suicide are violations of the law and in which aid-in-dying may be provided by nonphysicians, is also the case in Switzerland.

Over the last several decades, proponents seeking legalization of physician-assisted suicide in the United States have been following more or less what might be described as the pattern or model set by the Netherlands. Here, physician involvement in the process of bringing about the patient's death is central and respected: provided the guidelines for due care are met, the Dutch physician may openly and legally perform active euthanasia or may assist directly in the patient's suicide. In Germany, physicians are not accorded a direct role in causing death and would have duties to rescue an unconscious patient who was in the process of suicide; however, in Germany and other German-speaking nations like Switzerland, assisting a suicide is not illegal (and has not been since the time of Frederick the

Great, 1742), provided, in Germany, that the person is competent and in control of his or her own will, or, in Switzerland, provided that the assister does not act out of self-interest. In Germany, suicide may be assisted, but not (according to the German physicians' code of ethics) by a physician; the primary role in assisting the suicide of a terminally ill person is instead likely to be taken by a family member, friend, or companion trained by the right-to-die society to provide such aid. The assister remains within the law in providing the means of suicide and perhaps in helping the person take it, but, because there is a generalized duty to rescue an unconscious person, cannot remain with the suiciding person after unconsciousness sets in. While the actual number of cases that take place does not appear to be high in either country, in the Netherlands the picture of response to end-of-life dilemmas—in addition, of course, to the far more frequent strategies of withholding and withdrawing care and the use of morphine that is foreseen but not intended to cause death—is one of professional, physician assistance; the picture in Germany is one of nonphysician assistance or self-performed suicide. Switzerland now has four or five organizations that provide direct assistance in suicide (but not euthanasia) to terminally ill patients, including "safe houses" where people can come to die; one of them has stirred considerable controversy by accepting patients from abroad.

So far, for the last several decades, all emphasis by proponents of assisted dying in the United States has been on making it legal for the physician to provide assistance to the patient. This is to follow in broad general outlines the approach of the Dutch. However, following the escalatory moves of the PRPA and the counterresponse of NuTech, the model the United States seems forced to follow in end-of-life dilemmas about assisted dying seems more nearly like the approach set by Germany, where physician involvement is strongly discouraged or prohibited, though a family member or friend can legally assist.

The difference between these two models, the Dutch and the German, is substantial. What is central in the Dutch picture is the interaction between physician and patient in the matter of assisted suicide: this model requires a long period of sustained consultation, so that the physician can be sure that the patient's decision is firm and well-considered; it expects the physician to be sure that the suffering (whether physical or psychological) is real and cannot be relieved by any treatment acceptable to the patient; it demands that the physician provide the patient with full information about his or her condition, about the prognosis, and about alternative forms of treatment; and it requires the physician to explore his or her own assessment of the situation by consulting with another physician. In Germany, in contrast, though apparently comparatively few patients choose this route, what is essential is independence from medical control: it may in part be a matter of the patient's search for a mode of dying—*Freitod,* or "free death"—that is free from the negative connotations of "suicide" and expressive of his or her own personal values, as well as a last resort when pain management fails. In general, suicide in terminal illness proceeds in Germany outside the medical establishment, though with other helpers, in contrast to the Netherlands, where it is a role willingly assumed by the medical community, even though it is often a difficult one for physicians to carry out.

The shift from roughly following the Dutch model to roughly following the German one is of substantial significance, not because it is the Netherlands that is left behind or Germany that is embraced but because the American populace does not have the several hundred years' worth of experience (since the time of Frederick the Great) in living in circumstances in which assistance in suicide under certain conditions is not illegal. To be sure, a turn toward the use of NuTech in the United States would not make *assistance* in suicide legal, but because NuTech is comparatively simple, needs no physician, and leaves no telltale evidence, it might make it easy: the issue is whether the American populace is prepared for a situation in which end-of-life suicide without physician assistance was a real and socially accepted possibility. Suicide itself is not illegal in virtually any of the states in the U.S.; it is assistance in suicide that violates the law in most. The provision of information about methods of suicide is also controversial; at the same time Philip Nitschke, the Australian NuTech researcher, was announcing the development of the "Peaceful Pill," the Australian government was announcing plans to ban websites that provide information about suicide, and Dr. Nitschke said that he would post the information on websites in the U.S. or Canada. But the very populism of the Peaceful Pill too brings challenges. Russel Ogden, an independent researcher who tracks NuTech, notes that if it can be compounded at home without technical expertise or prescription-only ingredients, one of the key safeguards—informed decision-making—may be lost, and it and any deathing services that might go along with it may further be prone to commodification, as well as misappropriation for killing of others.[14]

Yet whichever course is eventually chosen as a matter of public policy in the U.S. and other countries like Canada, the U.K, many countries in Europe, Australia, and other places where this issue is under debate—the medically-oriented one more similar to the Netherlands, or the amateur, self-reliant, do-it-yourself version more like that in Germany—it is not clear whether either would serve as a final, stable compromise. Neither opponents nor proponents in the U.S. or elsewhere are likely to be fully satisfied by any compromise situation, and if they are not, the question remains whether there will be a further escalatory move that ups the ante to a still higher level.

Long gone, it seems, is the possibility of what some early opponents and even some proponents said they wanted: a practice that would be available to those who really needed it but was out of sight, under the table, discreet and quiet, not the subject of legislation. To be sure, it would only have been the privilege of patients with a physician close enough to them to be willing to take this risk; but even this privilege may be disappearing. Now, it seems, with so many escalating, polarizing maneuvers already over the dam, the only possible route seems to be further escalation.

A Glimpse of the Future?

What might these further escalations be? Here, I think, we go beyond evidence from the current scene, but we can imagine various new moves: for example, opponents might try to have suicide—not just assisted suicide but suicide itself—recriminalized, as it was throughout Europe in medieval and early modern times, and in England until 1961. Of course, recriminalization would make psychiatric treatment for "ordinary" suicide attempts far more problematic if these patients were also labeled criminals; any attempt to avoid this result by legally distinguishing "ordinary" suicide from terminal-illness suicide, given the difficulties of prognostication and the even greater difficulties of assessing intent, would prove unworkable. To recriminalize suicide, even terminal-illness suicide, would invite such disruptive practices as greater surveillance of medical practices with high concentrations of terminally ill patients, like oncology or neurology, for example, where prescription patterns could be monitored and outlier physicians identified. Among other things, this would cause a profound change in the relationship between physicians and terminally ill patients, precluding the possibility of discreet understandings between physicians and patients about matters of dying, and inviting substantial invasions of privacy.

On the other hand, proponents might respond with, say, conceptual initiatives in the media, press, and literature that attempted to change the cultural understanding of the term "suicide," so that what had been opposed as physician-assisted *suicide* would no longer be seen—and opposed—as suicide at all. Many euphemisms have already been proposed—"self-deliverance," "aid-in-dying," "hastened death," to name but a few, but what we might expect is a more concerted effort at both linguistic and legal redefinition. Oregon's Death with Dignity Act, like all U.S. referenda so far, stipulates that actions taken in accord with the Act shall not constitute suicide.[15] This sort of redefinition would trade on altered cultural perceptions and would have something in common with changed perceptions of, say, pain as divine punishment for human sin or revenge killing as appropriate and justified: things we for the most part no longer assume. Playing an active role in bringing one's life to a close when one is terminally ill might no longer be seen as "suicide" at all, and thus not assumed to be wrong.

Such cultural redefinition is a long-term process, but by no means impossible, and indeed may already be partly underway. In the current stage of the dispute over physician-assisted suicide, voluntary active euthanasia, and other sorts of hastened death, neither sort of new move, made by opponents or made by proponents, would be an easy process, and it is difficult to predict what the long-term outcome might be. Yet given our history of escalatory moves by parties on both sides of the long and volatile debate, it is important to see what the next ante-upping moves might be—that is, how the dispute over physician-assisted suicide could get still worse, and what still further life might be fanned into this debate. Or perhaps some new move, for example, an effort at cultural redefinition in the circumstances of terminal illness, might be seen not as escalatory but as conciliatory after all, and put an end to this long and volatile debate with a resolution that would be more or less palatable to all, by allowing greater personal control in matters of bringing about one's own death without seeming to accept a physician's involvement in "suicide." This would be to some extent a smoke-and-mirrors solution, one of rhetorical rather than substantial change, but it might serve as a solution to our end-of-life dilemmas nevertheless.

Notes

From Albert Klijn, Margaret Otlowski, and Margo Trappenburg, eds., *Regulating Physician-Negotiated Death* (special issue of *Recht der Werkelijkheid,* Journal of the Dutch/Flemish Association for Socio-Legal Studies), 's-Gravenhage, Elsevier, 2001, pp. 49–63, revised and expanded by the author. © 2001 Reed Business Information. Reprinted by permission.

1. Not all observers see this pattern in quite the same way, and I'd like to thank Charles Baron—who sees it somewhat differently—for his response to this essay. I thank Russel Ogden for his comments as well.

2. See the historical account in Norman L. Cantor, "Twenty-Five Years after *Quinlan:* A Review of the Jurisprudence of Death and Dying," *Journal of Law, Medicine & Ethics* 29(2):182-196 (2001).

3. Humphry later left Hemlock to found Ergo! and still later Hemlock was renamed End-of-Life Choices.

4. By this time concern with active voluntary euthanasia had largely dropped out of the picture, and most of the referenda included no provision for it.

5. See Robert A. Kagan, *Adversarial Legalism: The American Way of Law.* (Cambridge, Mass., and Harvard University Press, 2000).

6. For an account of NuTech devices, see Russel D. Ogden, "Non-Physician Assisted Suicide: The Technological Imperative of the Deathing Counterculture," *Death Studies* 25: 387–401 (2001).

7. See Ogden, R. D. & Wooten, R. (2002). Asphyxial suicide using helium and a plastic bag. *American Journal of Forensic Medicine and Pathology,* 23(3), 234–237; Gallagher, K.E., Smith, D. M., & Mellen, P. F. (2003). Suicidal asphyxiation by using pure helium gas: Case report, review, and discussion of the influence of the Internet. *American Journal of Forensic Medicine and Pathology,* 24(4), 361–363; Gilson, T., Parks, B.O., & Porterfield, C.M. (2003). Suicide with inert gases: Addendum to Final Exit. *American Journal of Forensic Medicine and Pathology,* 24(3), 306–308.

8. Both in Philip Nitschke, report of the January 2004, Seattle, NuTech Conference.

9. Jonathan Imbody, "Euthanasia Supporters and their Strange Inventions," *Washington Times,* November 20, 1999, p. A12.

10. Russel Ogden, personal communication.

11. Justice Drion, a very well known and highly respected progressive legal scholar as well as member of the Supreme Court, asked whether persons over 75 years of age, under very limited conditions, should have the right to be supplied with a medicine with which they could choose their own moment of death and thus avoid being exposed to a situation of physical or mental deterioration; he did not, however, propose the development of such a pill and objected to having his name attached to it, though it is known that way nevertheless. See Griffiths, J., Bood, A., and Weyers, H., *Euthanasia and Law in the Netherlands,* Amsterdam: Amsterdam University Press (1998), p. 82.

12. Nijmegen, Netherlands: Stichting WOZZ, 2003.

13. Russel Ogden, personal communication.

14. Russel Ogden, personal communication.

15. The Oregon Death with Dignity Act, Section 3.14: "Actions taken in accordance with this Act shall not, for any purpose, constitute suicide, assisted suicide, mercy killing or homicide, under the law." As stipulated in the Act, such actions do not affect wills, contracts, insurance or annuity policies which might have conditions concerning suicide. The full text of the Act is available as Appendix D in Margaret P. Battin, Rosamond Rhodes, and Anita Silvers: *Physician-Assisted Suicide: Expanding the Debate* (New York: Routledge, 1998).

16

Empirical Research in Bioethics

The Method of "Oppositional Collaboration"

Chronicle of a Research Venture

Let me begin with personal experience in doing "empirical research" in bioethics. The year was 1988; the location, the Netherlands; the topic, the then newly emerging reality that, in a legal climate which tolerated these forms of hastening death, the Dutch were openly practicing physician-assisted suicide and euthanasia. As a bioethicist particularly interested in end-of-life issues, when this news about Holland began to spread abroad, I wanted to know what was happening. It didn't seem to me that one could sit in a philosopher's armchair and discuss the Dutch situation responsibly; one had to go there, talk to people, see for oneself first-hand, at close range, what was actually going on.

But I knew that if you went to see the situation for yourself, chances were you would succeed largely in reinforcing the antecedent view you'd taken with you. You'd meet the contacts your circle of informants supplied for you; you'd find the articles that supported the view you held; you'd hear what showed that what you already knew was true. So instead of going to the Netherlands solo or with a research associate of like mind, I went with someone of whom I could be sure that her antecedent view would be unlike mine, Corrine Bayley. She was a moderately conservative Catholic nun; I was a reasonably liberal secular philosopher. Together we traveled all over the Netherlands, interviewing doctors, lawyers, judges, family members, and a wide range of others, and the story was often the same. Corrine and I would be at the interview jointly; we would each be there the entire time; we would each take notes and engage in extended discussion with our interviewee—but riding the train on the way home from whatever town, Corrine would say, "Wasn't that interesting? That judge said *a, b, c*" and I would have to agree that it was interesting, but I had heard *d, e, f,* and sometimes not-*a* or not-*b;* in short, though we were both there all the time and equally attentive, we had heard quite different things. It was the same with the doctors, the lawyers, the family members: whatever they said, we heard sometimes strikingly different things. Of course we did not disagree about any of the so-called hard facts—specific dates or locations or technical names; but we had heard the softer parts—the intonations, the allusions, the subtle implications entirely differently, and from these absorbed different accounts of the overall picture of the facts. Corrine heard people's stories and accounts from her moderately conservative, Catholic, nun's perspective; I heard them from my fairly liberal, philosophical, secular perspective, and the stories and accounts just did not seem the same, even when compared in great detail. Nor were these differences easy to overcome; it took us at least three or four weeks of steady interviews—always conducted jointly, and always involving extensive comparison afterwards of whatever we each thought the interviewee had said—before we each got so we could hear what the other one had already heard.

As you may guess, this "research" trip proved enormously informative. It has seemed to me that the method we used—what one might call "oppositional collaboration"—has the potential to contribute to the resolution of many of the more difficult issues in bioethics, and it would be a good thing if it were more widely used. Indeed, I'm tempted to think that it should be the norm for the specific sorts of empirical research that go on in bioethics—not so much the physical-science, social-science, or medical-science research, but the distinctive kinds of empirical exploration that bioethicists often do. I'd like to explore here whether this is a realistic proposal or an idealistic fantasy.

A Method for Bioethics: Oppositional Collaboration

"Oppositional collaboration" is in a sense a method, a way of going about empirical research. It begins by noticing that "investigators" doing "empirical research" in a field like bioethics do not begin in a state of equipoise, in which they are genuinely neutral between competing alternatives; this is because empirical research in bioethics is about values, and individuals all come equipped with antecedent sets of values about the issues in question; they have all already developed characteristic ways of looking at things. (This is hardly news.) The method of *oppositional collaboration* involves pairing investigators on opposite sides of an issue—one for, one against, whatever the issue is, whether abortion, euthanasia, truthtelling in clinical encounters, whatever—or in more complex situations developing teams of investigators composed of approximately equal numbers of investigators on opposite (or all) sides of the fence. The researchers on the two sides collaborate in assembling their data: they visit the same locations at the same times; read the same articles and pore through the same books; interview the same people at the same time, so that they are always in the room together. If they need to conduct conventionally empirical studies or institute any sort of fact-finding research, they design the protocols together; if they formulate a reading list for themselves, both contribute to it. For the duration of the collaborative period, whether it is a day, a week, a number of months or years, they are like a pair of investigatorial Siamese twins, joined at the eyes and ears, so that they see and hear the same things wherever they go.

But they are not joined at the brain. What is crucial to this method is that the two (or more) researchers come from opposite sides of the issue, their antecedent values-commitments still intact, and while their collaboration consists in discussing, comparing, even quarreling over what they see and hear, they cannot be required to agree. They remain perfectly free in this collaboration to do their own thinking (and talking and writing) about it. They make ideal partners *because* they disagree. Nevertheless, if they enter the collaboration in good faith—that is, with a sincere interest in finding out what actually is the case in the matter they are exploring, what the people they contact actually think, and what values issues are at stake— they will seek agreement between themselves as providing the most nearly true account.

That's all there is to this "method." It is clearly not a social-science method, and while social-science researchers are trained in neutral, value-free, objective research, this is something different. It isn't anything like most social-science research, which may start with questionnaires or structured interviews or content analyses to try to discover what people are thinking; "oppositional collaboration" has little to do with attempts to identify and quantify attitudes or behaviors, or with efforts to find out how prevalent specific views are. Oppositional collaboration is adapted, rather, to the kind of very informal empirical research that characteristically goes on in bioethics: instead of working to find out what people think, empirical research in bioethics—at least one form of it, not borrowed from social science—explores what people think to try to get at the conceptual and moral roots of an issue. It goes to places to "see what's going on" in order to think about an issue, whether that issue is stem cell research or genetic engineering or contact-tracing in HIV/AIDS. This isn't the same as identifying the causes or political origins of an issue; what one looks for are the philosophical roots of an issue, what makes it a genuine issue and not just a bone of political contention.

Objections and Impossibilities

There are a great many reasons for thinking that oppositional collaboration as a *modus operandi* in empirical bioethics research couldn't really work. Here are some questions that might be raised:

1. Could you train researchers on opposite sides to work in collaborative ways? If so, what would you teach them? How would you check up on them?
2. Not all researchers have equally forceful and/or cooperative personalities. What would happen when one dominates the interaction, the other retreats or takes a largely subordinate role?

3. Some people with strong views in bioethics you can't seem to talk to at all, especially some highly visible people known for their stands concerning one values issue or another. Could this method be used to carry on a sustained interchange at all with such personality types?
4. Would there be any quantitative, qualitative, or other measures of success of such collaboration? How would you know when it worked?
5. What might count as abuses of this method? Excesses?

These concerns, all of them well taken, may suggest that "oppositional collaboration" just couldn't work. But I believe, on the contrary, that it can work, and further, that there are a great many areas in bioethics where it would be appropriate.

The Real Uses of Oppositional Collaboration

The key to the appropriateness of oppositional collaboration lies in using it in situations where the issue to be explored is primarily an issue of values, as indeed most issues in bioethics are. These issues are not subject to the kind of empirical confirmation and disconfirmation that issues in the natural sciences are, and they are not, as we've seen above, like the issues examined in the social sciences. In a sense, empirical issues in bioethics aren't exactly empirical in the usual sense at all, unless it is assumed that values are objective in some sense that permits direct observation. Of course bioethics discussion must always be supplemented with conventional empirical findings from the natural, social, and medical sciences, such as the mechanisms of gene transfer, the timing of the development of the primitive streak, the prevalence of reported pain and symptom distress (as measured by various methods) in patients who are dying. Yet bioethics' distinctive form of "empirical" observation still is relevant: the observation of what people think about when in moral dilemmas, how they respond to situations, when they are uncomfortable in what they are doing or uneasy about the consequences it will produce. These findings are all relevant in bioethical reflection, even if they do not have the status of ordinary fact and do not at all determine what conclusion will be reached. There are many, many issues to be explored in bioethics by going to see what the issues are: by looking closely at the environment of an issue, by talking to people affected by and involved in an issue, by reading what people write about an issue, and in general by rubbing one's nose in an issue until you get some sense of what it is, what the underlying tensions are, where the conceptual fracture lines fall, what issues of values are really at stake. What you see and hear is what prods you to think about the issue, not a collection of facts that decide the case. Empirical "research" in bioethics, as I see it, largely starts the process of worrying through issues, rather than ends it. But it does this for the parties on *both* sides of an issue, and it is this fact of which the method of oppositional collaboration wishes to take account. The call here is a way for making each partisan's approach to values issues more perceptive, with less likelihood of utter polarization and more likelihood of thoughtful mutual understanding.

I began with a personal note about the experiences Corrine Bayley and I had in 1988 in doing "empirical" research in bioethics on the newly exposed practice of physician-assisted suicide and euthanasia in the Netherlands. Neither Corrine nor I changed our minds about our original, antecedent positions, though we both stopped making unsupportable claims, both quit arguing only one side of the case, and both stopped insisting that the issues were "clear" or "obvious" or straightforward—all things we'd been doing beforehand, like many other bioethicists working on these issues. We both came to see what the other was seeing, and that was the real gain of this "method."

There are many other issues under discussion within bioethics that, I believe, could be moved away from fruitless polarization and towards more thoughtful resolution if the principal players on both sides were to come together for a period of oppositional collaboration. (Suggesting names of partisans—bioethicists ranged on opposites sides of values issues in bioethics—to pair with each other is best left as an exercise for the reader.) The issues include some of the most sensitive, difficult questions in bioethics, like convenience abortion or sex selection in intracytoplasmic sperm injection or the use of anencephalic infants as organ donors or genetically engineered foods or global surveillance in emerging and reemerging infectious diseases or any of the other myriad values issues bioethics addresses—even these highly volatile, starkly politicized issues would benefit from a period of collaborative effort by thinkers on opposing sides, in which they agreed to try to listen to what the other one was hearing, really see what the other one could see. I think this would change the face of much of bioethics.

Not only am I persuaded that despite many difficulties such a "method" is actually workable, but I think we should *expect* such commitment for some limited period from bioethicists working on issues such as these. This is only the commitment to be joined at the eyes and ears for a little while, not ever to be joined at the brain; but I believe it would make a real difference in the sensitivity, depth, and responsibleness of bioethics' reflections on issues of value—which is what, after all, bioethics actually has to offer.

Note

From *Notizie di Politeia* (Italy), 18:67 (2002): 15–19. © 2002 Notizie di Politeia. Reprinted by permission.

17

Safe, Legal, Rare?

Physician-Assisted Suicide and Cultural Change in the Future

Introduction

Cultural change is well recognized in the recent history of death and dying in the contemporary world. In the wake of Elizabeth Kübler-Ross's 1969 work *On Death and Dying,* not only has it become socially acceptable to talk about death and dying with someone who is terminally ill, but, as traditional religious and legal strictures loosen, it is becoming possible for a person facing death to consider what role he or she wants to play in the forthcoming death. The United States has seen rapid evolution in attitudes and practices about death and dying over the last several decades, beginning with the early legal recognition in the *California Natural Death Act* (1976) of a patient's right to refuse life-prolonging treatment in the face of terminal illness, to the increased public awareness of issues of personal autonomy in dying raised by Derek Humphry's how-to book of lethal drug dosages, *Final Exit,* to new sensitivity to physician roles in aiding dying, both in the maverick social activism of Dr. Jack Kevorkian and a New York grand jury's refusal to indict the respected physician Timothy Quill. This process of cultural evolution has reached legal recognition: in 1997, the U.S. Supreme Court jointly decided the cases *Washington v. Glucksberg* and *Vacco v. Quill,* and while it held that physician-assisted suicide is not a constitutional right, it by implication also decided that states are free to make their own laws in this matter. Indeed, Oregon has made it legal for a physician to provide a terminally ill patient who requests it with a prescription for a lethal drug, thus bringing above ground the practical manifestation of a long process of cultural change.

Cultural change like this draws on many factors, including changes in medical technology, in the epidemiology of death, and social and legislative recognition of civil and personal rights in many other areas. Or course, cultural change is not unidirectional; although Oregon legalized physician-assisted suicide, Maryland, among others, made it a felony. But it is possible to discern a pattern of increasing attention to end-of-life issues and, I believe, to the issue of individual self-determination in the matter of dying.

The story does not end here. This is the most important fact about cultural change—the fact that it is an ongoing process, one which we view only from some intermediate point. What I want to explore in this paper is the prospect of cultural change in the future, and the possibility that physician-assisted suicide may come to look very, very different from the desperation move that it is taken to be now.

Part One: The Way It Looks Now

Observe the current debate over physician-assisted suicide: on the one side, supporters of legalization appeal to the principle of autonomy, or self-determination, to insist that terminally ill patients have the right to extricate themselves from pain and suffering and to control as much as possible the ends of their lives. On the other, opponents resolutely insist on various religious, principled, or slippery-slope grounds that physician-assisted suicide cannot be allowed, whether because it is sacrilegious, immoral, or poses risks of abuse. As vociferous and politicized as these two sides of the debate have become, however, proponents and opponents (tacitly) agree on a core issue: that the patient may choose to avoid suffering and pain. They disagree, it seems, largely about the means the patient and his or her physician may use to do so.

They also disagree about the actualities of pain control. Proponents of legalization insist that currently available forms of pain and symptom control are grossly inadequate and unsatisfactory. Citing such data as the SUPPORT study,[1] they point to high rates of reported pain among terminally ill patients, inadequately developed pain-control therapies, physicians' lack of training in pain-control techniques, and obstacles and limitations to delivery of pain-control treatment, including restrictions on narcotic and other drugs. Pain and the suffering associated with other symptoms just aren't adequately controlled, proponents of legalization insist, so the patient is surely entitled to avoid them—if he or she so chooses—by turning to earlier, humanely assisted dying.

Opponents of legalization, on the other hand, insist that these claims are uninformed. Effective methods of pain control include timely withholding and withdrawal of treatment, sufficient use of morphine or other drugs for pain (even at the risk of foreseen, though unintended, shortening of life), and the discontinuation of artificial nutrition and hydration. When all other measures to control pain and suffering fail, there is always the possibility of terminal sedation: the induction of coma with concomitant withholding of nutrition and hydration, which, though it results in death, is not to be seen as killing. Proponents laugh at this claim. Terminal sedation, they retort, like the overuse of morphine, is functionally equivalent to causing death.

Despite these continuing disagreements about the effectiveness, availability, and significance of current pain control, both proponents and opponents in the debate appear to agree that *if* adequate pain control were available, there would be far less call for physician-assisted suicide. This claim is both predictive and normative. *If* adequate pain control were available, both sides argue, then physician-assisted suicide would be and should be quite infrequent—a "last resort," as Timothy Quill puts it, to be used only in exceptionally difficult cases when pain control really does fail. Borrowing use of an expression used by President Clinton to describe his view of abortion, proponents insist that physician-assisted suicide should be "safe, legal, and rare." Opponents do not believe that it should be legal, but they also think that if it cannot be suppressed altogether or if a few very difficult cases remain, it should be very, very rare. The only real disagreement between opponents and proponents seems to concern those cases in which adequate pain control cannot be achieved.

What accounts for the opposing sides' underlying agreement that physician-assisted suicide should be rare is, I think, an unexamined assumption they share. This assumption is the view that the call for physician-assisted suicide is what might be called a *phenomenon of discrepant development:* a symptom of the disparity in development between two distinct capacities of modern medicine, the capacity to extend or prolong life and the capacity to control pain. Research, development, and delivery of technologies for the prolongation of life have raced far ahead; those for control of pain lagged far behind. It is this situation of discrepant development that has triggered the current concern with physician-assisted suicide and the volatile public debate over whether to legalize it or not.

The opposing sides both also hold in common the view that what would lead to the resolution of the problem is whatever set of mechanisms would tend to equalize the degree of development of medicine's capacities to prolong life and to control pain. To achieve this equalization, two simultaneous strategies are recommended: cutting back on overzealous prolongation of life (as Dan Callahan, 1987, 1990, 1993, for example, has long recommended), and at the same time (as Hospice and others have been insisting[2]) accelerating the development of technologies, modes of delivery, and physician training for more effective methods of pain control. As life prolongation is held back a bit, pain control can catch up, and the current situation of discrepant development between the two can be alleviated. Thus calls for physician-assisted suicide can be expected to become rarer and rarer, and as medicine's capacities for pain control are finally equalized with its capacities for life prolongation, finally to virtually disappear. Almost no one imagines that there will not still be a few difficult situations in which life is prolonged beyond the point at which pain can be effectively controlled, but these will be increasingly infrequent, it is assumed, and in general, as the disparity between our capacities for life prolongation and for pain control shrinks, interest in and need for physician-assisted suicide will decrease and all but disappear.

Fortunately, this view continues, the public debate over physician-assisted suicide now so intense will not have been a waste, since it has both warned against the potential cruelty of overzealous prolongation of life and at the same time stimulated greater attention to imperatives of pain control. The current debate serves as social pressure for bringing equalization of the disparity about. Yet as useful as this debate is, this view holds, it will soon subside and disappear; we're just currently caught in a turbulent—but fleeting—little maelstrom.

Part Two: The Longer View

That's how things look now. But I think we can also see our current concern with physician-assisted suicide in a longer-term, historically informed view. Consider just three of the many profound changes that affect matters of how we die. First there has been a shift, beginning in the middle of the nineteenth century, in the ways in which human beings characteristically die. Termed the "epidemiological transition,"[3] this change involves a shift away from death due to parasitic and infectious disease (ubiquitous among humans in all parts of the globe prior to about 1850) to death in later life of degenerative disease—especially cancer and heart disease, which together account for almost two-thirds of deaths in the developed countries. This means dramatically extended lifespans and also deaths from diseases with characteristically extended downhill terminal courses. Second, there have been changes in religious attitudes about death: people are less likely to see death as divine punishment for sin, or to see suffering as a prerequisite for the afterlife, or to see suicide as a highly stigmatized and serious sin rather than the product of mental illness or depression. Third among the major shifts in cultural attitudes that affect the way we die is the increasing emphasis on the notion of individual rights of self-determination, reinforced in the latter part the twentieth century by the civil rights movement's attention to individuals in vulnerable groups: this shift has affected self-perceptions and attitudes toward the terminally ill, and patients, including dying patients, are now recognized to have a wide array of rights previously eclipsed by the paternalistic practices of medicine.

These three transitions, along with many other concomitant cultural changes, invite us to see our current concern with physician-assisted suicide in a quite different way—not just as a phenomenon resulting from the currently disparate development of life-prolonging and pain-controlling technologies, a temporary anomaly, but as a precursor, an early symptom of a much more substantial sea-change in attitudes about death. We might call this shift in attitudes a shift toward "directed dying," or "self-directed dying," in which the individual who is dying plays a far more prominent, directive role than in earlier eras in determining how and when his or her death shall occur. In this changed view, dying is no longer *something that happens to you* but *something you do*.

To be sure, this shift—if it is one—can be seen as already well underway. Taking its legally visible start with the California Natural Death Act, terminally ill patients have already gained dramatically enlarged rights of self-determination in matters of guiding and controlling their own deaths, including rights to refuse treatment, discontinue treatment, stipulate treatment to be withheld at a later date, designate decisionmakers, and to negotiate with their physicians, or have their surrogates do so, such matters as DNR orders, withholding and withdrawal of ventilators, surgical procedures, nutrition and hydration, the use of opioids, and even terminal sedation. Some patients also negotiate, or attempt to negotiate, physician-assisted suicide or physician-performed euthanasia with their physicians. In all of this, we already see the patient as playing a far more prominent role in determining the course of his or her dying process and in its character and timing, and far more willingness on the part of physicians, family members, the law, and other parties to respect the patient's preferences and choices in these matters.

But this may be just the tip of a looming iceberg. For we may ask whether, much as we human beings have made dramatic gains in control over our own reproduction, particularly rapidly in very recent times (the birth control pill was introduced just forty years ago), we human beings are beginning to make dramatic gains in control over our own dying, particularly rapidly in the last several decades. We cannot keep from dying altogether, of course. But by using directly caused death, as in physician-assisted suicide, it is possible to control many of dying's features: its timing in the downhill course of a terminal disease, its place, the exact agents which cause it, its observers, and so on. Indeed, as Robert Kastenbaum (1976) has argued, because it makes it possible to control the time, place, manner and people present at one's death, assisted suicide will become the *preferred* manner of dying.

But this conjecture doesn't yet show what could actually motivate such substantial social change, away from a culture which sees dying primarily as *something that happens to you* to a culture which sees it as *something you do*—a final, deliberate, planned activity, one's final and culminative activity. What might do this, I think, is a conceptual change, or, more exactly, a shift in decisional perspective in choicemaking about pain, suffering, and other elements of dying. It is the kind of shift in decisional perspective that evolves on a society-wide scale as a populace gains understanding of and control over a matter, a shift in choice-making perspective from a stance we might describe as immediately involved or "enmeshed" to one that is distanced and reflective (I'll use two Latin names for these stances later). This shift can occur for many features of human experience—it has already largely occurred in the developed world with respect to reproduction—but it has not yet occurred with respect to death and dying. It has not yet occurred—or rather, perhaps it has just begun.

Take a patient, an average man. This particular man is so average that he just happens to have contracted that disease which is the usual diagnosis (as we know from the Netherlands)[4] in cases of physician-assisted suicide—cancer—and he is also so average that this disease will kill him at just the average life expectancy for males in the United States, 72.8 years. Furthermore, he is also so average that if he does turn to physician-assisted suicide, he will choose to forgo just about the same amount of life that, on average, Dutch patients receiving euthanasia or physician-assisted suicide do, less than 3.3 weeks (Emanuel & Battin, 1998). He has been considering physician-assisted suicide since his illness was first diagnosed (since he is an average man, this was about 29.6 months ago), but now, as his condition deteriorates, he thinks more seriously about it. His motivation includes both preemptive elements, the desire to avoid some of the very worst things that terminal cancer might bring him, and reactive elements, the desire to relieve some of the symptoms and other suffering that he is already experiencing. *It's bad enough now,* he tells his doctor, *and it will probably get worse.* He asks his doctor for the pills. He is perfectly aware of what he may miss—a number of weeks of continued life, the possibility of an unexpected cure, the chance, even if it is a long shot, of spontaneous regression or remission, and—not to be overlooked—the possibility that the worst is over, so to speak, and that the remainder of his downhill course in terminal cancer won't be so bad. He is also well aware that even a bad agonal phase may nevertheless include moments of great intimacy and importance with his family or friends. But he makes what he sees as a rational choice, seeking to balance the risks and possible benefits of easy death now, versus a little more continuing life with a greater possibility of a hard death. He is making his choice *in medias res,* in the middle of things, as the physical, social, and emotional realities of terminal illness engulf him. He is enmeshed in his situation, caught in it, trapped between what seem like two bad alternatives—suffering, or suicide.

But, of course, he might have done his deciding about how his life shall end and whether to elect physician-assisted suicide in preference to the final stages of terminal illness from a quite different, more distanced perspective, a secular version of the view *sub specie aeternitatis.* This is not just an objective, depersonalized view—anybody's view—but his own, distinctively personal view not confined to a specific timepoint.[5] Rather than assessing his prospects from the point of view he has at the time at which he would continue or discontinue his life—that point late in the course of his illness when things have already become "bad enough" and are likely to get worse—he might have done his deciding, albeit rather more hypothetically, from the perspective of a more generalized view of his life. From this alternative perspective, what he would have seen is the overall shape of his life, and it is with respect to this that he would have made his choices about how it shall end. Of course, he could not know in advance whether he will contract cancer, or succumb to heart disease, or be hit by a bus—though he does know that he will die sometime or other. Consequently, his choices are necessarily conditional in form: "*if* I get cancer, I'll refuse aggressive treatment and use hospice care," "*if* I get AIDS, I'll ask for physician-assisted suicide," "*if* I get Alzheimer's, I'll commit suicide on my own, since no physician besides Jack Kevorkian would help me," and so on. Although conditional in form and predicated on circumstances that may not occur, these may be real choices nonetheless and, particularly because they are reiterated and repeated over the course of a lifetime, have real motive force.

The difference, then, between these two views is substantial. In the first, our average man with an average terminal cancer, doing his deciding *in medias res,* is deciding whether or not to take the pills his physician has given him now. It is his last possible couple of weeks or a month (on average, 3.3 weeks) that he is deciding about. Even if continuing life threatens pain and other suffering, it is still all he has left, and while it may be difficult to live this life—all he has left—it may also be very difficult to relinquish it.

In contrast, if our average man were doing his deciding *sub specie aeternitatis,* from a distanced though still personal viewpoint not tied to a specific moment in his life, he would have been deciding all along between two different conceptions of his own demise, between two possible lives for himself. One of his possible lives would, on average, be 72.8 years long, the average lifespan for a male in the United States, with the possibility of substantial suffering at the end—on average, as the SUPPORT study finds, a 50 percent chance of moderate to severe pain at least 50 percent of the time during the last three days before his death. The other of his possible lives would be about 72.7 years long, foreshortened on average 3.3 weeks by physician-assisted suicide, but with a markedly reduced possibility of substantial suffering at the end. (This shortening of the lifespan is not age-based but time-to-death–based, planned for, on average, 3.3 weeks before an unassisted death would have occurred; it occurs in this example at age 72.7 just because our man is so average.) This latter, shortened life also offers our man the opportunity to control the timing, the place, the manner, and so on of his death in the way he likes. Viewed *sub specie aeternitatis,* at any or many earlier points in one's life or from a vantage point standing outside life, so to speak, the difference between 72.8 and 72.7 seems negligible: these are both lives of average length not interrupted by grossly premature death. Why not choose the one in which the risk of agonal pain—as high as 50/50, according to the SUPPORT study—is far, far less great, and the possibility of conscious, culminative experience, surrounded by family members, trusted friends, and permitting final prayers and goodbyes, is far, far greater?

It may seem difficult to distinguish these two choices in practice. This is because we typically make our decisions about death and dying *in medias res,* not *sub specie aeternitatis,* and our medical practices, our bioethics discussions, and our background culture strongly encourage this. The call for assisted dying, like other patient pleas, is seen as a reaction to the circumstances of dying, not a settled, longer-term, preemptive preference (Prado, 1990). True, some independently minded individuals consider these issues in a kind of background, hypothetical way throughout their lives, but this is certainly not the practical norm. We can only really understand this view as involving a substantial cultural shift from our current perspective.

But if this shift occurs, a slightly abbreviated lifespan in which there is dramatically reduced risk of pain and suffering will not only seem to be preferable to one which is negligibly longer but carries substantial risk of pain and suffering in its agonal phase, it will also be seen as rational and normal to plan for this abbreviated lifespan and to plan the means of bringing it about. The way to ensure it, of course, is to plan for direct termination of life. After all, one cannot count on being able to discontinue some life-prolonging treatment or other—refusing antibiotics, disconnecting a respirator—to hasten death and thus avoid what might be the worst weeks at the end. This most likely means planning for physician-assisted suicide. From this distanced perspective, a 72.7-year life with a virtually assured good end looks much, much better than a 72.8-year life that has an even chance of coming to a bad end. Arguably, it would be rational for any individual, except those for whom religious commitments or other scruples rule out suicide altogether, to plan to ensure this. (This is a version of what can be called "advance personal policy making" about how you do and don't want your death to go.) But if it looks this way to one individual, it will look this way to many; and it is thus plausible to imagine that physician-assisted suicide would not be rare but rather a choice viewed as rational and preemptively prudent by many or most members of the culture. Thus it can come to be seen as a normal course of action, not a rarity or a "last resort." To be sure, there are other ways of abbreviating a lifespan to avoid terminal suffering—withdrawing or withholding treatment, overusing morphine or other pain-relieving drugs, discontinuing artificial nutrition and hydration, and terminal sedation—but these cannot be used unless the patient's condition has already worsened and thus is likely to involve that pain or suffering the person might choose to avoid. Thus these other modalities function primarily reactively; it is assisted suicide that can function preemptively.

But, as soon as planning for a normal, slight abbreviation in the lifespan by means of assisted suicide becomes conceptually possible not just for our average man but for actual persons in general, it also becomes possible to imagine a wide range of context-specific cultural practices which might emerge surrounding physician-assisted suicide. After all, that a person understands and expects his lifespan to be one which will end in an assisted death a few weeks before he might otherwise have died, while he is still conscious, alert, and capable of deciding what location he wants it to take place in, what family members, caregivers, clergy, or others he wants to have present, what ceremonies, religious or symbolic, he wants conducted, etc., suggests that more general social practices would grow up around these possibilities. After all, our average man sees his life this way; but it is possible for him to do this partly because the others in his society see their lives this way as well. Attitudes about death are heavily socially conditioned, and so are the perspectives from which choicemaking about death is seen.

This is the precondition for the development of a whole range of social practices supporting such choices. These might include various kinds of practical supports, such as legal, insurance, and other policies which treat assisted dying as acceptable and normal; various sorts of cultural and religious practices which similarly treat assisted dying as acceptable and normal (for instance, by developing rituals and rites concerning the forthcoming death); familial supports within the family, including family gatherings, preparing for the death, and sharing reminiscences and goodbyes; pre-death dispositions of wills and life insurance (we already recognize viaticums, pre-death payoffs of life insurance for terminally ill patients); and even such now-inconceivable practices as pre-death funerals, understood as ceremonies of leavetaking and farewell, expressions of both celebration of a life complete and grief at its loss. In turn, such social practices come to function as positive reasons for choosing a somewhat earlier, elective death—formerly and rudely called "physician-assisted suicide," even when pain control is no longer the issue at all, and the new social pattern—so different from our current one—reinforces itself. This has nothing to do with a *Soylent Green* sort of view, in which people are forced into choices they do not genuinely make (this film can be understood only from our current, *in medias res* view); but a world in which their normal choices have genuinely changed, and changed for reasons which seem to them good.

Furthermore, if the culture-wide view of choicemaking about death and dying were more fully held *sub specie aeternitatis* in this distanced, less enmeshed, and less merely reactive way, in which earlier, elective death becomes the norm, we could also expect the more frequent practice of "setting a date," as people who have contracted predictably terminal illnesses carry out the plans they had been developing all along for their own demises. Setting a date for one's own death— presumably, a couple of weeks or so before the date it might naturally have been, revisable of course in the light of any changes in the diagnosis or prognosis— would still be both preemptive and reactive in character, but far more preemptive than choices made *in medias res,* where choices will be highly reactive to the then-current circumstances the patient finds himself or herself in. The timing of such choices might always be revised in consultation with the physician; but what would be culturally reinforced would be the general commitment to advance planning for one's own death as well as a commitment to assuming a comparatively autonomist, directive role in it. Self-directed dying would be the norm, though of course different people would direct their deaths in quite different ways.

If the profound changes affecting matters of how we die that are already underway—the epidemiological transition, shifting from parasitic and infectious disease deaths to deaths of predictably degenerative disease; the changes in religious conceptions of suicide so that it is not understood primarily as sin; and the steadily increasing attention to patients' and terminally ill patients' rights of self-determination—continue, it is an open conjecture whether this is where we may be going. Are we in fact experiencing just a temporary aberration in our basic cultural patterns of death and dying, an aberration which is a function of the discrepant development of technologies for life prolongation and for pain control? Or are we seeing the first breaking waves of a sea-change from one perspective on death and dying to another, a far more autonomist and self-directive one?

Obviously, I can't say. But I can say that if this is what is happening, the assumption that physician-assisted suicide would or should be rare, an assumption still held by both sides in the current debate, will collapse. We would have no reason to assume that assisted dying should be rare, whatever the relationship between capacities for life prolongation and pain control. Of course, such a picture is very difficult to envision, since we do not think that way about death and dying now. But if we can at least see what is different about viewing personal choices about one's own death *sub specie aeternitatis* and in our current way, *in medias res,* enmeshed in particular circumstances, we can understand why it might occur.

Would it be a good thing, or a bad thing? I can hardly answer that question here, but let me close with a story I heard somewhere in the Netherlands several years ago. I do not remember the exact source of the story or the specific dates or names, and it is certainly not representative of current practice in Holland. But it was told to me as a true story, and it went something like this.

> Two friends, old sailing buddies, are planning a sailing trip in the North Sea in the summer. It is late February now, and they are discussing possible dates.
>
> "How about July 21?" says Willem. "The North Sea will be calm, the moon bright, and there's a music festival on the southern coast of Denmark we could visit."
>
> "Sounds great," answers Joost, "I'd love to get to the music festival. But I can't be gone then; the 21st is the date of my father's death."

"Oh, I'm so sorry, Joost," Willem replies. "I knew your father was ill. Very ill, with cancer. But I didn't realize he had died."

"He hasn't," Joost replies, "That's the day he will be dying. He's picked a date and made up his mind, and we all want to be there with him."

Such a story seems just that, a story, a fiction, somehow horrifying and also somehow liberating, but in any case virtually inconceivable to us. But it was not told to me as a fiction, but as a true story. I've tried to explore the conceptual assumptions that might lie behind such a story, and to consider whether in the future such stories might become more and more the norm, a form of advance personal policy making about one's own death reached long before one is enmeshed in what could become the desparate circumstances of dying. I have not tried to say whether this would be good or bad, but only that this might well be where we are going. In fact, I think it would be good—just as I think increasing personal control over reproduction is good—but I haven't argued for that view here.

Cultural change is an ongoing, long-term process of evolution, one which it is often hard to discern from a particular point in time. We see evolution in the past; but we have little way to think about the future. I've tried to suggest that our current point of view about personal autonomy in death and dying is unduly limited; while we recognize that substantial change has already occurred, we fail to realize that change as great or greater may be coming in the future. Indeed, it could involve a full reversal of earlier cultural attitudes about one's own role in one's own death. Of course cultural change is not unidirectional, and there may be backward as well as forward motion; nor do the attitudes of all members of a culture evolve at the same rate at the same time. Factors like wars, plagues, famines, scientific discoveries, and technological advances have reversed or hastened cultural change in the past, and could of course do so in the future. Just the same, I think it is possible to discern motion beyond the current view that physician-assisted suicide should be rare, a desperation move when nothing else works, toward the view that one's own death at the conclusion of terminal illness may be self-directed, that individuals can and should have the psychological and social freedom to reflect in a longer-term way about their own future choices when they embark on the dying process, perhaps making physician-assisted suicide an eventual part of their plans, as well as the practical and legal freedom to plan whatever family gatherings, ceremonies, and religious observances they might wish—not as a desperate last resort or reactive escape from bad circumstances, but as a preemptively prudent, significant, culminative experience. How long this process of cultural change might take, and what might interrupt it or hasten it, only time will tell.

Notes

From Margaret P. Battin, Rosamond Rhodes, and Anita Silvers, eds., *Physician-Assisted Suicide: Expanding the Debate,* Routledge, 1998) pp. 63–74; revised and expanded version in Loretta Kopelman and Kenneth DeVille, ed., *Physician-Assisted Suicide* (Kluwer, 2001), pp. 187–201, and in Diego DeLeo, ed., *Suicide and Euthanasia in Older Adults: A Transcultural Journey.* (Hogrefe & Huber, 2001). © Kluwer Academic Publishers. Reprinted by permission.

1. According to the SUPPORT study, about 50 percent of dying hospitalized patients were reported to have experienced moderate to severe pain at least 50 percent of the time in their last three days of life.

2. See especially the work of Foley, K. (1995), "Pain, physician-assisted suicide, and euthanasia." *Pain Forum,* 4(3): 163–178, and other works.

3. The term originates with Omran (1971), and the theory is augmented in Olshansky & Ault (1987).

4. Data on physician-assisted suicide and euthanasia in the Netherlands are provided by what is called the Remmelink Commission Report (van der Maas, van Delden, & Pijnenborg, 1992). A five-year update is available in van der Maas, van der Wal, et al., 1996.

5. The distinction I am drawing here between personal views *in medias res* and *sub specie aeternitatis* is thus not quite the same as that drawn by Thomas Nagel between subjective and objective views, though it has much in common with Nagel's distinction in contexts concerning death. See Nagel (1986), especially chap. 11, sec. 3, on death.

References

Callahan, D. (1987). *Setting Limits: Medical Goals in an Aging Society.* New York: Simon and Schuster.

Callahan, D. (1990). *What Kind of Life? The Limits of Medical Progress.* New York: Simon and Schuster.

Callahan, D. (1993). *The Troubled Dream of Life: Living with Mortality.* New York: Simon and Schuster.

Connors, A. F., Jr., Dawson, N. V., Desbiens, N. A., Fulkerson, W. J., Jr., Goldman, L., Knaus, W. A., Lynn, J., & Oye, R. K. [SUPPORT principal investigators] (1995). A Controlled Trial to Improve Care for Seriously Ill Hospitalized Patients. *Journal of the American Medical Association, 274,* 1951–98.

Emanuel, E. J., & Battin, M. P. (1998). The Economics of Euthanasia: What are the Potential Cost Savings from Legalizing Physician-Assisted Suicide? *New England Journal of Medicine,* 339, 167–72.

K. Foley. (1995). Pain, Physician-Assisted Suicide, and Euthanasia. *Pain Forum, 4,* 163–178.

Kastenbaum, R. (1976). Suicide as the Preferred Way of Death. In E. S. Shneidman (Ed.), *Suicidology: Contemporary Developments* (pp. 425–41). New York: Grune & Stratton.

Nagel, T. (1986). *The View from Nowhere.* New York: Oxford University Press.

Olshansky, A. J., & Ault, A. B. (1987). The Fourth Stage of the Epidemiologic Transition: The Age of Delayed Degenerative Disease. In T. M. Smeeding (Ed.), *Should Medical Care Be Rationed by Age?* (pp. 11–43). Totowa, N.J.: Rowman & Littlefield.

Omran, A. R. (1971). The Epidemiologic Transition: A Theory of the Epidemiology of Population Change. *Milbank Memorial Fund Quarterly, 49,* 509–38.

Onwuteaka-Philipsen, Bregje D., et al. (2003). Euthanasia and other end-of-life decisions in the Netherlands in 1990, 1995, and 2001. *Lancet,* 263, 395–399.

Prado, C. G., (1990). *The Last Choice: Preemptive Suicide in Advanced Age.* Westport, Conn.: Greenwood Press.

Van der Maas, P. J. van Delden, J. M. M., & Pijnenborg, L. (1992). Euthanasia and Other Medical Decisions Concerning the End of Life. *Health Policy,* 22 (1,2).

Van der Mass, P. J., van der Wal, G., Haverkate, I., de Graaff, C. C., Kester, J. G., Onwuteaka-Philipsen, B. D., van der Heide, A., Bosma, J. M., & Willems, D. L. (1996). Euthanasia, Physician-Assisted Suicide, and Other Medical Practices Involving the End of Life in the Netherlands, 1990–1995. *New England Journal of Medicine, 335,* 1699–05.

INDEX

Jehovah's Witnesses, 190–191, 194, 195–196,
205, 207, 208, 212, 213–214, 217, 220–221
Jesus Christ, 171, 192, 193, 204, 209, 217
jihad, 5, 173, 244, 246
Job, 172
Josephus, 166, 170
Journal of the American Medical Association,
196
Judaism
deaths during Passover, 177
ethics of suicide and, 165, 166, 167, 169
rejection of suicide in, 5, 245
Tays-Sachs disease among Ashkenazi Jews,
253–254, 259, 270
and wrongness of killing, 21
Judeo-Christian tradition, suicide in, 241, 245,
247
Justice Department, U.S., 306

Kagan, Robert, 304
kamikaze, 164, 166, 169
Kamisar, Yale, 27
Kant, Immanuel, 5, 21, 214, 243, 291
Kass, Leon, 24, 33
Kastenbaum, Robert, 325
Keown, John, 27
Kevorkian, Jack, 30, 85, 301, 303, 321
killing, wrongness of, in assisted-dying
argument, 8, 18, 21–24, 39, 57–58, 93, 94,
95–96, 97
Kübler-Ross, Elizabeth, 19, 321
Kuhse, Helga, 20

Lactantius, 167, 170
Lamm, Richard, 280
Landsberg, Paul-Louis, 170
last resort
physician's assistance in suicide as a, 30, 31,
323, 328
suicide in Germany as a, 55
Last Rights Publications, 38, 307
Last Will Pill, 309
late-onset genetic diseases, 257–259, 268n. 3
legislation, physician-assisted suicide, 88–89, 93,
96, 99, 105n. 2, 302, 304–307
Lesotho, 292
Lethal Drug Abuse Prevention Act of 1998, 306
"letting die", not "killing" practices, 6, 23–24,
25, 58, 169
life choices, size of one's life and basic, 265–
266
life-ending on request (voluntary active
euthanasia), 50
life expectancy, 47, 164
average, 262, 281
in the developed world, 311

in duty-to-die argument, 281, 282, 284–285,
291, 292, 293
in early human history, 18, 255
for Huntington's disease, 258
for males in the United States, 325, 327
life insurance, 288, 299n. 24, 328
life-prolonging care
duty-to-die argument and, 284, 286, 290, 291,
297
pain controlling technologies and, 323, 324
patient's right to refuse, 321
life span. *See* ethical aspects of increased life
span
"like-family" relationship, duty-to-die argument
and, 287–289
living-will legislation, 19, 302
living wills, 48, 55, 273
longer-decline scenario, 270, 276
longer-dying scenario, 269–270, 272, 275, 276
longer-health scenario, 269, 272, 276
Lotus Sutra, 167
Lou Gehrig's disease patients. *See* amyotrophic
lateral sclerosis (ALS) patients
Lucretia, 170
Lucretius, 21
Luria, 166
Lynn, Joanne, 31

Maine, 9, 304
malaria, 254, 285, 295
Malawi, 281
malpractice actions, in the U.S., 62–63
malpractice insurance, clergy, 220
Maltsberger, John T., 108–110
Mao Zedong, 170, 173
Margoliouth, 166
Martens, Evelyn, 309
martyrdom, suicide and, 5, 169, 170, 172, 240,
241, 243, 245, 247
Masada, 170
maternal mortality, 292–293
maximax and maximin decision makers, AIDS
and, 77–78, 81, 86
Mayo, David, 19
Measure 16 (Oregon), 88, 304, 305, 306
Médecins Sans Frontières, 294
medical profession integrity, in assisted-dying
argument, 24–25
medical treatment, refusal of
Christian Science beliefs and, 189–190, 195,
200, 204, 205, 213
Faith Assembly group and, 189, 191–192,
195, 199, 213, 217
Jehovah's Witnesses and, 189, 190–191, 195–
196, 205, 208, 213–214, 217, 220–221
Meier, Diane, 25